Epidemiology, Evidence-based Medicine and Public Health
Lecture Notes

Yoav Ben-Shlomo

Professor of Clinical Epidemiology
School of Social and Community Medicine
University of Bristol

Sara T. Brookes

Senior Lecturer in Health Services Research & Medical Statistics
School of Social and Community Medicine
University of Bristol

Matthew Hickman

Professor in Public Health and Epidemiology
School of Social and Community Medicine
University of Bristol

Sixth Edition

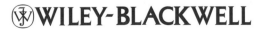
WILEY-BLACKWELL

A John Wiley & Sons, Ltd., Publication

Blackwell Publishing was acquired by John Wiley & Sons in February 2007. Blackwell's
publishing program has been merged with Wiley's global Scientific, Technical and Medical
business to form Wiley-Blackwell.

Registered office: John Wiley & Sons, Ltd, The Atrium, Southern Gate, Chichester,
West Sussex, PO19 8SQ, UK

Editorial offices: 9600 Garsington Road, Oxford, OX4 2DQ, UK
                       The Atrium, Southern Gate, Chichester, West Sussex, PO19 8SQ, UK
                       111 River Street, Hoboken, NJ 07030-5774, USA

For details of our global editorial offices, for customer services and for information about
how to apply for permission to reuse the copyright material in this book please see our
website at www.wiley.com/wiley-blackwell.

Library of Congress Cataloging-in-Publication Data

Ben-Shlomo, Yoav.
   Lecture notes. Epidemiology, evidence-based medicine, and public health / Yoav
Ben-Shlomo, Sara T. Brookes, Matthew Hickman. – 6th ed.
      p. ; cm.
   Epidemiology, evidence-based medicine, and public health
   Rev. ed. of: Lecture notes. Epidemiology and public health medicine / Richard Farmer,
Ross Lawrenson. 5th. 2004.
   Includes bibliographical references and index.
   ISBN 978-1-4443-3478-4 (pbk. : alk. paper)
   I. Brookes, Sara.   II. Hickman, Matthew.   III. Farmer, R. D. T. Lecture notes.
Epidemiology and public health medicine.   IV. Title.   V. Title: Epidemiology,
evidence-based medicine, and public health.
   [DNLM: 1. Epidemiologic Methods.   2. Evidence-Based Medicine.   3. Public
Health.   WA 950]
   614.4–dc23

                                                             2012025764

A catalogue record for this book is available from the British Library.

Cover design by Grounded Design

Set in 8.5/11pt Utopia by Aptara® Inc., New Delhi, India
Printed and bound in Malaysia by Vivar Printing Sdn Bhd

1   2013

Contents

Preface

It was both an honour and a challenge to take on the revision of a 'classic' textbook such as *Lecture Notes in Epidemiology and Public Health Medicine* already in its fifth edition (originally written by Richard Farmer and David Miller, the latter author being subsequently replaced by Ross Lawrenson). Much has changed in the field of epidemiology, public health and the scientific world in general since the first edition was published almost 35 years ago. When the current editors sat down to plan this new sixth edition, we felt there was now a need to restructure the book overall rather than updating the existing chapters. In the intervening period, we have seen the rise of new paradigms (conceptual ideas) such as life course and genetic epidemiology and the advance of evidence-based medicine. The latter was first covered in the fifth edition by a single chapter. We felt the need to rebalance the various topics so this new edition has now got three main subsections: Epidemiology, Evidence Based Medicine (EBM) and Public Health. Whilst much of the epidemiology section will appear familiar from the previous edition, we have added a new chapter on genetic epidemiology and there is a whole chapter on causality as this is so fundamental to epidemiological research and remains an issue with conventional observational epidemiology. The new section on EBM is very different with separate chapters on diagnosis, prognosis, effectiveness, systematic reviews and health economics. The Public Health section is less focussed on the National Health Service and we now have a new chapter on global health; a major topic given the challenges of 'climate change' and the interrelated globalised world that we all now live in. We have also included a new chapter specifically on the difficult task of evaluating public health interventions, which presents unique challenges not found with more straightforward clinical trials. Inevitably, we have had to drop some topics but we believe that overall the new chapters better reflect the learning needs of contemporary students in the twenty-first century. We hope we have remained faithful to the original aims of this book and the previous authors would be proud of this latest edition.

In redesigning the structure of the book we have been guided by three underlying principles:

(1) To fully utilise our collective experience based on decades of teaching undergraduate medical students (Ben-Shlomo, 2010). We have therefore used, where appropriate relevant materials from the courses we run at the University of Bristol that have been refined over many years. We wish to thank the many students we have encountered who have both challenged, provoked and rewarded us with their scepticism as well as enthusiasm. We fully appreciate that some students are put off by the more statistical aspects of epidemiology (a condition we termed 'numerophobia (Ben-Shlomo *et al.*, 2004)). Other students feel passionately about issues such as global health and/or the marked inequalities in health outcomes seen in both developing and developed countries (see http://www.medsin.org/ for more information around student activities).

(2) The need to have a wide range of expertise to stimulate and inspire students. We therefore decided to make this new edition a multiauthor book rather than relying on our own expertise.

(3) The desire to make our textbook less anglocentric and of interest and relevance to health professionals and students other than those studying medicine. We appreciate that the examples we have taken are predominantly from a developed world perspective but the fundamental principles and concepts are generic and should form a sound scientific basis for someone wishing to learn about epidemiology, evidence based medicine and public health regardless of their country of origin. It would be wonderful to produce a companion book that specifically uses examples and case studies that are more relevant to developing countries. But that is for the future.

As we work in the United Kingdom, our curriculum is heavily influenced by the recommendations of the UK General Medical Council and the latest version of *Tomorrow's Doctors* (GMC, 2009). We have tried to cover most of the topics raised in sections 10–12 of *Tomorrow's Doctors* though this book will be inadequate on its own for areas such as medical sociology and health psychology, covered in more specialist texts. We appreciate that students are usually driven by the need to pass exams, and the medical curriculum is particularly dense, if you forgive the pun, when it comes to factual material. We have, however, tried to go beyond the simple basics and some of the material we present is somewhat more advanced than that usually presented to undergraduates. This was a deliberate choice as we believe that the inevitable over-simplification or 'dumbing down' can turn some students off this topic. We feel this makes the book not merely an 'exam-passing tool' but rather a useful companion that can be used at a postgraduate level. We believe that students and health-care professionals will rise to intellectual challenges as long as they can see the relevance of the topic and it is presented in an interesting way. We have therefore also included further readings at the end of some chapters for those students who want to learn more about each topic.

We have provided a glossary of terms at the end of the book to help students find the meaning of terms quickly and also highlighted **key terms** in **bold** that may help students revise for exams. Finally we have included some self-assessment questions and answers at the end of each section that will help the student test themselves and provide some feedback on their comprehension of the knowledge and concepts that are covered in the book. We appreciate that very few medical students will become public health practitioners, though somewhat more will become clinical epidemiologists and/or health service researchers. However the knowledge, skills and '*scepticaemia*' that we hope students gain from this book, will serve them well as future doctors or other health care professionals regardless of their career choice. Improving the health of the population and not just treating disease is the remit of all doctors. As it states in *Tomorrow's Doctors:*

Today's undergraduates – tomorrow's doctors – will see huge changes in medical practice. There will be continuing developments in biomedical sciences and clinical practice, new health priorities, rising expectations among patients and the public, and changing societal attitudes. Basic knowledge and skills, while fundamentally important, will not be enough on their own. Medical students must be inspired to learn about medicine in all its aspects so as to serve patients and become the doctors of the future.

Yoav Ben-Shlomo
Sara T. Brookes
Matthew Hickman

 ## REFERENCES

Ben-Shlomo Y. Public health education for medical students: reflections over the last two decades. *J Public Health* 2010; **32**: 132–133.

Ben-Shlomo Y, Fallon U, Sterne J, Brookes S. Do medical students without A-level mathematics have a worse understanding of the principles behind Evidence Based Medicine? *Medical Teacher* 2004; **26**:731–733.

GMC (2009) *Tomorrow's Doctors: Outcomes and standards for undergraduate medical education.* London: General Medical Council.

Contributors

Yoav Ben-Shlomo Professor of Clinical
Epidemiology
School of Social and Community Medicine
University of Bristol

Bruce Bolam Executive Manager
Knowledge & Environments for Health
VicHealth Victorian Health Promotion
Foundation

Sara T. Brookes Senior Lecturer in Health
Services Research & Medical Statistics
School of Social and Community Medicine
University of Bristol

Rona Campbell Professor of Health Services
Research and Co Director of the UKCRC Public
Health Research Centre of Excellence
School of Social and Community Medicine
University of Bristol

George Davey Smith Professor of Clinical
Epidemiology, Scientific Director of ALSPAC &
MRC CAiTE Centre
Oakfield House
University of Bristol

Ian N. M. Day Professor of Genetic and Molecular
Epidemiology and Deputy Director of MRC
CAiTE Centre
Oakfield House
University of Bristol

Jenny Donovan Head of School & Professor of
Social Medicine
School of Social and Community Medicine
University of Bristol

Shah Ebrahim Professor of Public Health
London School of Hygiene and Tropical
Medicine and Director, South Asia Network for
Chronic Disease
PHFI, New Delhi, India

David M. Evans Senior Lecturer in Biostatistical
Genetics
Oakfield House
University of Bristol

Bruna Galobardes Senior Research Fellow
Oakfield House
University of Bristol

Maya Gobin Consultant Regional Epidemiologist,
Health Protection Services
South West

David Gunnell Head of Research
Professor of Epidemiology
School of Social and Community Medicine
University of Bristol

David Heymann Professor of Infectious Disease
Epidemiology
London School of Hygiene and Tropical
Medicine

Matthew Hickman Professor in Public Health
and Epidemiology
School of Social and Community Medicine
University of Bristol

William Hollingworth Reader in Health
Economics
School of Social and Community Medicine
University of Bristol

Mona Jeffreys Senior Lecturer in Epidemiology
School of Social and Community Medicine
University of Bristol

Sanjay Kinra Senior Lecturer in
Non-communicable Disease Epidemiology
London School of Hygiene and Tropical
Medicine

Ruth Kipping Consultant and Research Fellow in
Public Health
School of Social and Community Medicine
University of Bristol

Debbie A. Lawlor Professor of Epidemiology;
Head of Division of Epidemiology,
University of Bristol; Deputy Director of MRC
CAiTE Centre
Oakfield House
University of Bristol

John MacLeod Professor in Clinical
Epidemiology and Primary Care
School of Social and Community Medicine
University of Bristol

Richard Martin Professor of Clinical
  Epidemiology
  School of Social and Community Medicine
  University of Bristol

Sian Noble Senior Lecturer in Health Economics
  School of Social and Community Medicine
  University of Bristol

Isabel Oliver Regional Director
  South West Health Protection Agency

Angela Raffle Consultant in Public Health,
  NHS Bristol
  Honorary Senior Lecturer, School of Social and
  Community Medicine
  University of Bristol

Gabriel Scally Professor of Public Health
  WHO Centre for Healthy Urban Environments
  University of West of England

Joanne Simon Research Manager
  School of Social and Community Medicine
  University of Bristol

Jonathan Sterne Head of HSR Division &
  Professor of Medical Statistics and
  Epidemiology
  School of Social and Community Medicine
  University of Bristol

Kate Tilling Professor of Medical Statistics
  School of Social and Community Medicine
  University of Bristol

Caroline Trotter Senior Research Fellow
  School of Social and Community Medicine
  University of Bristol

Penny Whiting Senior Research Fellow
  School of Social and Community Medicine
  University of Bristol

Part 1

Epidemiology

Epidemiology: defining disease and normality

Sara T. Brookes and Yoav Ben-Shlomo
University of Bristol

Learning objectives

In this chapter you will learn:

✓ what is meant by the term epidemiology;
✓ the concepts underlying the terms 'normal, abnormal and disease' from a (i) sociocultural, (ii) statistical, (iii) prognostic, (iv) clinical perspective;
✓ how one may define a case in epidemiological studies.

What is epidemiology?

Trying to explain what an epidemiologist does for a living can be complicated. Most people think it has something to do with skin (so you're a dermatologist?) wrongly ascribing the origin of the word to epidermis. In fact the Greek origin is *epidēmia* – 'prevalence of disease' (taken from the Oxford online dictionary) – and the more appropriate related term is epidemic. The formal definition is

'The study of the occurrence and distribution of health-related states or events in specified populations, including the study of the determinants influencing such states and the application of this knowledge to control the health problems' (taken from the 5th edition of the Dictionary of Epidemiology)

An alternative way to explain this and easier to comprehend is that epidemiology has three aims (3 Ws).

Whether	To describe *whether* the burden of diseases or health-related states (such as smoking rates) are similar across different populations (descriptive epidemiology)
Why	To identify *why* some populations or individuals are at greater risk of disease (risk-factor epidemiology) and hence identify causal factors
What	To measure the need for health services, their use and effects (evidence-based medicine) and public policies (Public Health) that may prevent disease – *what* we can do to improve the health of the population

---

Epidemiology, Evidence-based Medicine and Public Health Lecture Notes, Sixth Edition. Yoav Ben-Shlomo, Sara T. Brookes and Matthew Hickman.
© 2013 Y. Ben-Shlomo, S. T. Brookes and M. Hickman. Published 2013 by John Wiley & Sons, Ltd.

Population versus clinical epidemiology – what's in a name?

The concept of a population is fundamental to epidemiology and statistical methods (see Chapter 3) and has a special meaning. It may reflect the inhabitants of a geographical area (lay sense of the term) but it usually has a much broader meaning to a collection or unit of individuals who share some characteristic. For example, individuals who work in a specific industry (e.g. nuclear power workers), born in a specific week and year (birth cohort), students studying medicine etc. In fact, the term population can be extended to institutions as well as people; so, for example, we can refer to a population of hospitals, general practices, schools etc.

Populations can either consist of individuals who have been selected irrespective of whether they have the condition which is being studied or specifically because they have the condition of interest. Studies that are designed to try and understand the causes of disease (**aetiology**) are usually population-based as they start off with healthy individuals who are then followed up to see which risk factors predict disease (**population-based epidemiology**). Sometimes they can select patients with disease and compare them to a control group of individuals without disease (see Chapter 5 for observational study designs). The results of these studies help doctors, health-policy-makers and governments decide about the best way to prevent disease. In contrast, studies that are designed to help us understand how best to diagnose disease, predict its natural history or what is the best treatment will use a population of individuals with symptoms or clinically diagnosed disease (**clinical epidemiology**). These studies are used by clinicians or organisations that advise about the management of disease. The term clinical epidemiology is now more often referred to as evidence-based medicine or health-services research. The same methodological approaches apply to both sets of research questions but the underlying questions are rather different.

One of the classical studies in epidemiology is known as the Framingham Heart Study (see http://www.framinghamheartstudy.org/about/history.html). This study was initially set up in 1948 and has been following up around 5200 men and women ever since (prospective cohort study). Its contribution to medicine has been immense, being one of the first studies to identify the importance of elevated cholesterol and high blood pressure in increasing the risk of heart disease and stroke. Subsequent randomised trials then went on to show that lowering of these risk factors could importantly reduce risk of these diseases. Furthermore the Framingham risk equation, a prognostic tool, is commonly used in primary care to identify individuals who are at greater risk of future coronary heart disease and to target interventions (see http://hp2010.nhlbihin.net/atpiii/calculator.asp).

Regardless of the purpose of epidemiological research, it is always essential to define the disease or health state that is of interest. To understand disease or pathology, we must first be able to define what is normal or abnormal. In clinical medicine this is often obvious but as the rest of this chapter will illustrate, epidemiology has a broader and often pragmatic basis for defining disease and other health-related states.

What is dis-ease?

Doctors generally see a central part of their job as treating people who are not 'at ease' – or who in other words suffer 'dis-ease' – and tend not to concern themselves with people who are 'at ease'. But what is a disease? We may have no difficulty justifying why someone who has had a cerebrovascular accident (stroke), or someone who has severe shortness of breath due to asthma, has a disease. But other instances fit in less easily with this notion of disease. Is hypertension (high blood pressure) a disease state, given that most people with raised blood pressure are totally unaware of the fact and have no symptoms? Is a large but stable port wine stain of the skin a disease? Does someone with very protruding ears have a disease? Does someone who experiences false beliefs or delusions and imagines her/him-self to be Napoleon Bonaparte suffer from a disease?

The discomfort or 'dis-ease' felt by some of these individuals – notably those with skin impairments – is as much due to the likely reaction of others around the sufferer as it is due to the intrinsic features of the problem. Diseases may thus in some cases be dependent on subjects' sociocultural environment. In other cases this is not so – the sufferer would still suffer even if marooned alone on a desert island. The purpose of this next section is to offer a structure to the way we define disease.

A sociocultural perspective

Perceptions of disease have varied greatly over the last 400 years. Particular sets of symptoms and signs have been viewed as 'abnormal' at one point in history and 'normal' at another. In addition, some sets of symptoms have been viewed simultaneously as 'abnormal' in one social group and 'normal' in another.

Examples abound of historical diseases that we now consider normal. The ancient Greek thinker Aristotle believed that women in general were inherently abnormal and that female gender was in itself a disease state. In the late eighteenth century a leading American physician (Benjamin Rush) believed that blackness of the skin (or as he termed it 'negritude') was a disease, akin to leprosy. Victorian doctors believed that women with healthy sexual appetites were suffering from the disease of nymphomania and recommended surgical cures.

There are other examples of states that we now consider to be diseases, which were viewed in a different light historically. Many nineteenth-century writers and artists believed that tuberculosis actually enhanced female beauty and the wasting that the disease produces was viewed as an expression of angelic spirituality. In the sixteenth and seventeenth centuries gout (joint inflammation due to deposition of uric acid) was widely seen as a great asset, because it was believed to protect against other, worse diseases. Ironically, recent research interest has suggested a potential protective role of elevated uric acid, which may cause gout, for both heart and Parkinson's disease.

In Shakespeare's time melancholy (what we would now call depression) was regarded as a fashionable state for the upper classes, but was by contrast stigmatised and considered unattractive among the poor. The modern French sociologist Foucault points out that from the eigtheenth century onwards those who showed signs of what we would now call mental illness were increasingly confined in institutions, as tolerance of 'unreason' declined. Whereas previously 'mad' people had often been viewed as having fascinating and desirable powers (and were legitimised as holy fools and jesters), increasingly they were seen as both disruptive and in need of treatment. Other examples exist of the redefinition of socially unacceptable behaviour as a disease. Well into the second half of the last century single mothers were viewed as being ill and were frequently confined for many years in psychiatric institutions.

As some diseases have been accepted as part of the normal spectrum of human behaviours so new ones have been labelled. Newly recognised diseases include alcoholism (previously thought of simply as heavy drinking), suicide (previously thought of as a criminal offence, it was illegal in the UK until the 1960s so that failed suicides were prosecuted and successful suicides forfeited all their property to the State), and psychosomatic illness (previously dismissed as mere malingering).

Some new disease categories have arisen simply because new tests and investigations allow important differences to be recognised among what were previously thought of as single diseases. For example people died in past times of what was believed to be the single disease of dropsy (peripheral oedema), which we now know to be a feature of a wide range of diseases ranging across primary heart disease, lung disease, kidney disease and venous disease of the legs. There are still disagreements in modern medicine about the classification of disease states. For example, controversy remains around the underlying pathophysiology of chronic fatigue syndrome (myalgic encephalomyelitis) and Gulf War syndrome.

The sociocultural context of health, illness and the determinants of health-care-seeking behaviour as well as the potential adverse effects of labelling and stigma are main topics of interest for medical sociologists and health psychologists and the interested reader may wish to read further in other texts (see Further reading at the end of this chapter).

Abnormal as unusual (statistical)

In clinical medicine – especially in laboratory testing – it is common to label values that are unusual as being abnormal. If, for example, a blood sample is sent to a hospital haematology laboratory for measurement of haemoglobin concentration the result form that is returned may contain the following guidance (the absolute values will differ for different laboratories and units will differ by country):

Male reference range	Female reference range
130–170 g/L	115–155 g/L

This **reference range** is derived as follows: a large number (several hundred) of **samples** from people believed to be free of disease (usually blood donors) are measured and the reference range is defined as that central part of the range which contains 95% of the values. By definition, this approach will result in 5% of individuals who may be completely well, being classified as having an **abnormal** test result.

Normal (Gaussian) distributions

In practice, as with haemoglobin concentration above, many distributions in medical statistics may be described by the **Normal**, also known as **Gaussian distribution**. It is worth noting that the statistical term for 'Normal' bears no relation to the general use of the term 'normal' by clinicians. In statistics, the term simply relates to the name of a particular form of frequency distribution. The curve of the Normal distribution is symmetrical about the **mean** (see Chapter 2) and bell-shaped.

The theoretical Normal distribution is continuous. Even when the variable is not measured precisely, its distribution may be a good approximation to the Normal distribution. For example in Figure 1.1, heights of men in South Wales were measured to the nearest cm, but are approximately Normal.

Abnormal as increased risk of future disease (prognostic)

An alternative definition of abnormality is one based on an increased risk of future disease. A biochemical measure in an asymptomatic (undiagnosed) individual may or may not be associated with future disease in a **causal** way (see Chapter 7). For example, a raised C-reactive protein level in the blood indicates infection or inflammation. Whilst noncausally related, epidemiological studies demonstrate that C-reactive protein can also predict those at an increased future risk of coronary heart disease (CHD). Treatments focused on lowering C-reactive protein will not necessarily reduce the risk of CHD.

In a man of 50 years a systolic blood pressure of 150 mm Hg is well within the usual range and may not produce any clinical symptoms. However, his risk of a fatal myocardial infarction (heart attack) is about twice that of someone with a low blood pressure.

• Does he have a disease, and should he be treated?
• What factors might influence this decision?

These are important questions to consider when we come to think of disease in terms of increased risk of future adverse health outcomes.

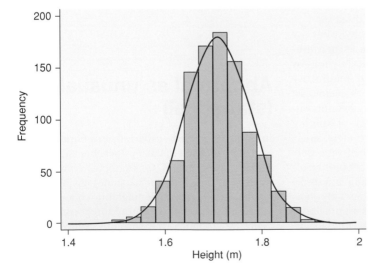

Figure 1.1 Heights of 1,000 men in South Wales.
Note: This figure is known as a **histogram** and is used for displaying grouped numerical data (see Chapter 2) in which the relative frequencies are represented by the areas of the bars (as opposed to a **bar chart** used to display categorical data, where frequencies are represented by the heights of the bars).
The superimposed continuous curve denotes the theoretical Normal distribution.

Thresholds for introducing treatment for blood pressure have changed over the years, generally drifting downwards. This is due to two main factors:

(1) researchers have gradually extended their limits of interest as they have become more confident that blood pressure well within usual limits may have adverse effects in the future.
(2) newer drugs have tended to have fewer and less dangerous side effects, making it reasonable to consider extending treatment to lower levels of blood pressure, where the benefits – though present – are less striking.

Blood glucose levels provide similar problems to blood pressure levels – specifically, for type II diabetes which is treated with diet control, tablets and occasionally insulin (rather than type I which requires insulin as a life-saving measure). At what blood glucose level should one attach the label 'diabetic' and consider starting treatment? To address these questions large prospective studies (called **cohort studies**) are required. In such studies, subjects have a potential risk factor such as blood glucose levels measured at the beginning of the study. They are then followed up, sometimes for many years, to examine whether rates of disease differ according to levels of blood glucose at the start of the study.

Does a fasting glucose in a healthy individual have any implication for their future health?

The glucose tolerance test is commonly used as a diagnostic aid for diabetes. In one of the very early epidemiological studies, conducted in Bedford UK (Keen *et al.*, 1979), 552 subjects had their blood glucose measured when fasting and again two hours after a 50 g glucose drink. On the basis of this they were classified as having high, medium or low glucose levels. The cohort was then followed for ten years, at which point the pattern of deaths that had occurred was as illustrated in Table 1.1.

Amongst both men and women, those with high levels of glucose following the glucose tolerance test had an increased risk of all causes and cardiovascular death. In addition, the female medium glucose group had an increased risk compared to the low glucose group. This additional risk is far less dramatic amongst the men in this study. Basing a definition of abnormality on future 10-year risk of death, treatment might be considered for women with a medium glucose level in addition to those with a high glucose level.

Based on studies such as this, the World Health Organisation (WHO) recommends levels of blood glucose, which should be regarded as indicating diabetes and therefore considered for treatment (fasting glucose ≥ 7.0 mmol/L (126 mg/dl) and/or 2 hour post-load glucose ≥ 11.1 mmol/L (200 md/dl). It also identifies an intermediate risk group who are said to have Impaired Glucose Tolerance or borderline diabetes (fasting glucose <7.0 mmol/L and 2 hour post-load glucose ≥ 7.8 mmol/L but <11.1 mmol/L). Such individuals are not generally treated but may legitimately be kept under increased surveillance. However, the increased risk of cardiovascular disease appears to show a linear relationship with fasting glucose with no obvious threshold. A recent WHO report concluded 'there are insufficient data to accurately define normal glucose levels, the term normoglycaemia should be used for glucose levels associated with low risk of developing diabetes or cardiovascular disease' (WHO/IDF, 2006).

Abnormal as clinical disease

It is better to define values of a particular test as abnormal if they are clearly associated with the presence of a disease state – rather than simply being unusual. However this is often less than straightforward.

The range of values describing diseased individuals is rarely clearly and completely separated from that for healthy individuals. The nice bell shaped curve described above may actually be bimodal with a second superimposed distribution either at the top (see Figure 1.2) or bottom end or both. This overlap means that there will be healthy people with 'abnormal' results and people with disease with apparently 'normal' results (see Chapter 9 on diagnostic tests for more details).

For example, it is widely believed by many doctors that chronic (i.e. of long duration) mildly reduced haemoglobin (Hb) levels (of 100–110 g/L) or anaemia, such as might be seen in menstruating females, may account for fatigue and tiredness. In a study of 295 subjects in South Wales no association was found between Hb level and fatigue until the Hb level fell to well below 100 g/L (Wood

Table 1.1 Glucose tolerance[a] and mortality in the Bedfordshire cohort.

Glucose group	Men			Women		
	Number	All deaths	Cardiovascular deaths	Number	All deaths	Cardiovascular deaths
High glucose	51	19 (37.2%)	15 (29.4%)	63	25 (39.7%)	18 (28.5%)
Medium glucose	130	29 (22.3%)	19 (14.6%)	119	35 (29.4%)	25 (21.0%)
Low glucose	104	20 (19.2%)	12 (11.5%)	85	9 (10.6%)	4 (4.7%)

[a] Oral glucose tolerance test: After an overnight fast the participant is asked to drink a solution containing 1.75 g/kg body weight (maximum 75 g) of glucose dissolved in 250 ml of water within 2–3 minutes. Blood samples are taken just before and two hours after ingestion of the glucose solution.

and Elwood, 1966). Fatigue is common in the population generally for a wide range of reasons and is only strongly associated with Hb level among severely anaemic individuals. A longstanding Hb of between 100 and 115 g/L (which it should be noted is outside the laboratory reference range, whose lower limit is 115 in women and 130 in men) in an otherwise healthy person who is complaining only of fatigue shouldn't therefore generally be considered as responsible for this symptom.

In general, the definition of abnormality as clinical abnormality is both logical and clear. It is nevertheless an approach that usually involves thinking in terms of the probability of disease being present, rather than the certainty.

Defining a case in epidemiological studies

Before an epidemiologist is able to study any disease s/he needs to develop and agree upon a case definition: a definition of disease that is as free as possible of ambiguity. This should enable researchers to apply this definition reliably on a large number of subjects, without access to sophisticated investigations. Because epidemiological case definitions are not used as a guide to the treatment of individuals they may differ from the sorts of definitions used in routine clinical practice.

Chronic Fatigue Syndrome provides a good example of the problems of agreeing on a case definition for a rather ill-defined condition. At a meeting in Oxford in 1990, 28 UK experts met to agree a case definition for Chronic Fatigue Syndrome (Sharpe *et al.*, 1991). They came up with the following:

- Fatigue must be the principal symptom.
- There must be a definite point of onset (fatigue must not have been lifelong).
- Fatigue must have been present for at least 6 months and present for at least 50% of that time.
- Other symptoms may be present – e.g. myalgia (muscle pain), mood and sleep disturbance.
- Certain patients should be excluded: those with medical conditions known to produce chronic fatigue (such as severe anaemia); patients with a current diagnosis of schizophrenia, manic-depressive illness, substance abuse, eating disorder.

What is being attempted here is to produce a reasonably reliable definition (one that will classify the same person in the same way when used repeatedly by different observers) that can be applied without recourse to sophisticated tests, that excludes already well recognised causes of fatigue such as anaemia but which encompasses relevant patients.

This has now been updated in the UK by NICE guidelines (2007) that state a diagnosis should be

Unimodal curve

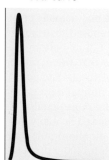

Bimodal curve

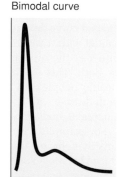

Figure 1.2 Potential distributions (taken from WHO report (2006) Definition and diagnosis of diabetes mellitus and intermediate hyperglycaemia).

made after other possible diagnoses have been excluded and the symptoms have persisted for 4 months in an adult and 3 months in a child or young person (a shorter duration than previously stated). They suggest guidelines based on expert consensus opinion (see Box 1.1).

The use by both UK and American epidemiologists of the descriptive term 'Chronic Fatigue Syndrome' rather than 'Post-viral Fatigue Syndrome' is deliberate. The term implies no particular aetiology (cause) unlike 'Post-viral Fatigue Syndrome', which presupposes that a viral cause is established and which may therefore inhibit exploration of other possible causes.

The NICE definition is intended to be used by clinicians and often 'research case definitions' are stricter so that some true cases are missed but you are less likely to include any false positive cases. So for example the USA Centre for Disease Control and Prevention case definition still has a requirement for a 6-month minimum period of symptoms.

Box 1.1 Symptoms that may indicate CFS/ME.

Consider the possibility of CFS/ME if a person has:

- fatigue with all of the following features:
  - new or a specific onset (i.e. not lifelong)
  - persistent and/or recurrent
  - unexplained by other conditions
  - has resulted in a substantial reduction in *activity* level characterised by post-exertional malaise and/or fatigue (typically delayed, e.g. by at least 24 hours, with slow recovery over several days)

and

- one or more of the following symptoms:
  - difficulty with sleeping, such as insomnia, hypersomnia, unrefreshing sleep, a disturbed sleep–wake cycle
  - muscle and/or joint pain that is multi-site and without evidence of inflammation
  - headaches
  - painful lymph nodes without pathological enlargement
  - sore throat
  - cognitive dysfunction, such as difficulty thinking, inability to concentrate, impairment of short-term memory, and difficulties with word-finding, planning/organising thoughts and information processing
  - physical or mental exertion makes symptoms worse
  - general malaise or 'flu-like' symptoms
  - dizziness and/or nausea
  - palpitations in the absence of identified cardiac pathology

The symptoms of CFS/ME fluctuate in severity and may change in nature over time.
Source: NICE (2007) *NICE Quick Reference Guide – Chronic Fatigue Syndrome/myalgic Encephalomyelitis (or Encephalopathy*. NICE, UK).

 KEY LEARNING POINTS

- Epidemiology is the study of the population determinants and distribution of disease in order to understand its causes and prevention
- Epidemiology studies populations of either healthy individuals (before disease onset) or patients with symptoms or established disease
- The acceptance of what is a disease changes over time with some disease disappearing e.g. homosexuality, and others appearing, e.g. Attention Deficit Hyperactivity Disorder
- Sociocultural factors can influence whether some societies label different phenomena as disease
- Doctors often define abnormality as lying outside the normal range which reflects a statistical definition but may not be due to disease
- Screening can identify risk factors, not associated with symptoms, which predict future disease (prognostic) and may be amenable to intervention thereby preventing disease
- Doctors usually have to diagnose disease from patients, symptomatic complaints and/or physical abnormalities
- Epidemiological studies have to specify clear objective criteria, usually more rigorous than that used by doctors in everyday practice, that they use to identify cases in research

 REFERENCES

Keen H, Jarrett RJ, Alberti KGMM (1979) Diabetes mellitus: a new look at diagnostic criteria. *Diabetologia* **6**: 283–5.

Sharpe MC, Archard LC, Banatvala JE, *et al.* (1991) A report – chronic fatigue syndrome: guidelines for research. *J Roy Soc Med* **84**: 118–21.

WHO/IDF (2006) Definition and diagnosis of diabetes mellitus and intermediate hyperglycaemia. Report of a WHO/IDF Consultation. Geneva: World Health Organisation.

Wood MM, Elwood PC (1966) Symptoms of iron deficiency anaemia: A community survey, *Brit J Prev Soc Med* **20**: 117–21.

 ## FURTHER READING

Dowrick C (ed.) (2001) *Medicine in Society: Behavioural Sciences for Medical Students.* London: Arnold Publishers.

Scambler G (2003) *Sociology as Applied to Medicine.* 5th edn. London: Saunders.

2

Measuring and summarising data

Sara T. Brookes and Yoav Ben-Shlomo
University of Bristol

Learning objectives

In this chapter you will learn:

✓ how we classify different types of variables;

✓ to recognise and define measures of central tendency, variability and range;

✓ four measures of disease frequency: prevalence, risk, incidence rate and odds;

✓ to identify exposure and outcome variables;

✓ to define and calculate absolute and relative measures of association between an exposure and outcome.

Epidemiology is a **quantitative** discipline. It involves the collection of data within a **study sample** and analyses using statistical methods to summarise, examine associations and test specific hypotheses from which it infers generalisable conclusions about **aetiology** (causes of disease) and **health care evaluation** in the **target population**. In order to be able to understand epidemiological research, one must have a basic understanding of the statistical tools that are used for data analysis both in epidemiological and basic science research.

Types of variables

A **variable** is a quantity that varies; for example, between people, occasions or different parts of the

body. A variable can take any one of a specified set of values. Medical data may include the following types of variables.

Numerical variables

There are two types of **numerical variables**. **Continuous variables** are measurements made on a continuous scale; for example, height, haemoglobin or systolic blood pressure. **Discrete variables** are counts, such as the number of children in a family, or the number of asthma attacks in a week.

Categorical variables

There are two basic types of **categorical variable**, which are variables that take nonnumeric values

---

Epidemiology, Evidence-based Medicine and Public Health Lecture Notes, Sixth Edition. Yoav Ben-Shlomo, Sara T. Brookes and Matthew Hickman.

and refer to categories of data. Firstly, **unordered categorical variables** are used to class observations into a number of named groups; for example, ethnic group, marital status (single, married, widowed, other), or disease categories. A special case of the unordered categorical variable is one which classes observations into two groups. Such variables are known as **dichotomous** or **binary** and generally indicate the presence or absence of a particular characteristic. Presence versus absence of chest pain, smoker versus nonsmoker, and vaccinated versus unvaccinated are examples of dichotomous or binary variables.

Secondly, **ordered categorical variables** are used to rank observations according to an ordered classification, such as social class, severity of disease (mild, moderate, severe), or stages in the development of a cancer. Often in epidemiological studies a variable may be measured as numerical and then subsequently categorised. For example height may be measured in feet and inches and then categorised as: <5ft, 5ft–5ft 5in, 5ft 5in–6ft, >6ft.

The type of variable will determine how that variable is displayed and what subsequent analyses are carried out. In general, continuous and discrete variables are treated in the same way.

Descriptive statistics for numerical variables

Most medical, biological, social, physical and natural phenomena display variability. Frequency distributions express this variability and are summarised by measures of **central tendency** ('location') and of **variability** ('spread'). We will explore these measures using the following hypothetical data on the number of days spent in hospital by 19 patients following admission with a diagnosis of an acute exacerbation of chronic obstructive airways disease.

3 4 4 6 7 8 8 8 10 10 12 14 14 17 20 25 27 37 42

Measures of central tendency

There are three important measures of central tendency or location.

(1) **Mean**

The mean is the most commonly used 'average'. It is the sum of all the values in a set of observations divided by the number of observations in that set.

So the mean number of days spent in hospital by the 19 patients is

$$(3 + 4 + 4 + 6 + 7 + 8 + 8 + 8 + 10 + 10$$
$$+ 12 + 14 + 14 + 17 + 20 + 25 + 27$$
$$+ 37 + 42)/19 = 276/19 = 14.53 \text{ days.}$$

The algebraic formula for this calculation is given in Table 2.1.

(2) **Median**

The median is the middle value when the values in a set are arranged in order. If there is an even number of values the median is defined as the mean of the two middle values.

Thus, the median number of days spent in hospital is 10 days (see Figure 2.1).

(3) **Mode**

The mode is the most frequently occurring value in a set. It is rarely used in epidemiological practice.

The modal number of days spent in hospital is 8 days.

For data presented in grouped form, e.g. if hospital stay were grouped as 0–10, 11–20, 21–30 and 30+ days, we can identify the modal class in this instance as 0–10 days. Thought of in this way, it is a peak on a frequency distribution or histogram. When there is a single mode, the distribution is known as **unimodal**. If there is more than one peak the distribution is said to be **bimodal** (two peaks) or **multimodal**.

Let us assume in the above example that the patient with the longest length of stay actually spent 120 days rather than 42 days in hospital because they could not be sent back home but required placement in a nursing home. This 'unusual' observation (outlier) would have a large effect on the mean value (now 18.6 days) whilst having no effect on the median and could make the performance of one hospital look worse than another depending on which summary statistic was being used for the comparison.

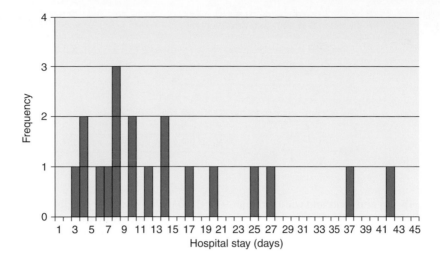

Figure 2.1 Distribution of hospital stay in sample of 19 patients.

Measures of variability

The extent to which the values of a variable in a distribution are spread out a long way or a short way from the centre indicates their variability or spread. There are several useful measures of variability.

(1) Range

The range is simply the difference between the largest and the smallest values.

The range of the number of days spent in hospital following operation for the 19 patients is:

$$42 - 3 = 39 \text{ days.}$$

As a measure of variability, the range suffers from the fact that it depends solely on the two extreme values which may give a quite unrepresentative view of the spread of the whole set of values.

(2) Interquartile range

Quantiles are divisions of a set of values into equal, ordered subgroups. The median, as defined above, delimits the lower and upper halves of the data. Tertiles divide the data into three equal groups, quartiles into four, quintiles into five, deciles into ten, and centiles into 100 subgroups. Measures of variability may thus be the interquartile range (from the first to the third quartile), the 2.5th to 97.5th centile range (containing the 'central' 95% of observations, and so on).

For example, the quartiles for the data on days spent in hospital are 7, 10 and 20 days, so the interquartile range is: 7 days to 20 days

(3) Standard deviation

The standard deviation (SD) is a measure of spread of the observations about the mean. It is based on the deviations (differences) of each observation from the mean value: these deviations are squared to remove the effect of their sign. The SD is then calculated as the square root of the sum of these squared deviations divided by the number of observations minus 1.

The SD of the data on days spent in hospital is calculated as:

$$\sqrt{\frac{(3 - 14.53)^2 + (4 - 14.53)^2 + \ldots + (42 - 14.53)^2}{19 - 1}}$$
$$= \sqrt{\frac{2220.7}{18}} = 11.11 \text{ days.}$$

The algebraic formula for this calculation is given in Table 2.1. The square of the SD (that is, SD $\times$ SD) is known as the **variance**.

The **Normal** (or **Gaussian**) **distribution** (introduced in Chapter 1) is described entirely by its mean and standard deviation (SD). The mean, median and mode of the distribution are identical and define the location of the curve. The SD determines the shape of the curve, which is tall and

Table 2.1 Formulae for the mean and standard deviation.

Mean	In algebraic notation, the mean of a set of n values $\{X_1, X_2, \ldots, X_n\}$ is:
	$$\bar{X} = \frac{\sum\limits_{i=1}^{n} X_i}{n} = \frac{X_1 + X_2 + X_3 + \ldots + X_n}{n}$$
Standard deviation	The algebraic notation for the SD of a set of n values $\{X_1, X_2, \ldots, X_n\}$ is:
	$$SD = \sqrt{\frac{\sum\limits_{i=1}^{n} (X_i - \bar{X})^2}{n-1}} = \sqrt{\frac{(X_1 - \bar{X})^2 + (X_2 - \bar{X})^2 + (X_3 - \bar{X})^2 + \ldots + (X_n - \bar{X})^2}{n-1}}$$

narrow for small SDs and short and wide for large ones (see Figure 2.2).

We can use the mean and SD of the Normal distribution to determine what proportion of the data lies between any two particular values. Regardless of the values of the mean and SD, the following rules apply:

(1) 68.3% of the observations lie within 1 SD of the mean: (mean – 1 × SD to mean + 1 × SD); 95.4% lie between mean ± 2 × SD: (mean – 2 × SD to mean + 2 × SD); 99.7% lie between mean ± 3 × SD: (mean – 3 × SD to mean + 3 × SD).
(2) Because of symmetry the following properties also hold:
15.85% of the observations lie above mean + 1 × SD, and 15.85% lie below mean – 1 × SD; 2.3% lie above mean + 2 × SD, and 2.3% lie below mean – 2 × SD.
(3) 95.0% of the observations are enclosed between mean – 1.96 × SD to mean + 1.96 × SD.

Reference range

These properties lead to an additional measure of spread in a set of observations or measurements.

If the data are normally distributed the 95% reference range is given by the mean – 1.96 × SD to mean + 1.96 × SD. From property (3) above, we know that 95% of our data lie in the 95% reference range. We can also define a 90% reference range, a 99% reference range, and so on in much the same way. The assumption of normality is an important one and it is important to ensure that the data are normally distributed before calculating a 95% reference range.

Descriptive statistics for binary/dichotomous variables

Clinicians see patients who present with some problem. If they are specialists they will often collect a large group of patients with the same condition, for example diabetes. They may notice certain characteristics about their patients, which can give clues as to the possible origin or aetiology of their disease, e.g. a disease being more common for a specific occupation. Sometimes they describe the frequency of these characteristics in their patient sample. This is known as a **case series**. However to make sense of these data, it is essential to

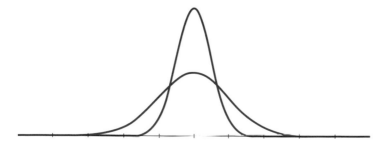

Figure 2.2 Normal distribution curves. The flatter, wider curve has a greater standard deviation.

know something about the population from which these cases arose. For example if a GP had seen three male cases of Parkinson's disease over the last year and all had worked in the local pesticide factory, he may suspect a neurotoxic aetiology. But if 95% of his male catchment population worked at the factory, this would be less suspicious. It is therefore essential that clinical data are related to a population at risk.

Often, we can classify each individual in our study as having or not having the disease of interest (disease is then a binary variable). We can then measure the proportion of individuals with disease. The numerator in the proportion is the number of individuals with disease, and the denominator is the total number of individuals.

$$\text{Proportion} = \frac{\text{number with disease (numerator)}}{\text{total number (denominator)}}.$$

Proportions are often multiplied by 100 and expressed as a percentage. The two most important types of proportion are the **prevalence** and the **cumulative incidence (risk)**.

Prevalence and incidence

Prevalence is defined as the proportion (or %) with the disease at a particular point in time:

$$\text{Prevalence} = \frac{\begin{array}{c}\text{number with disease at}\\ \text{particular time}\end{array}}{\begin{array}{c}\text{total number in population}\\ \text{at that time}\end{array}}.$$

Example: among 878 children aged 5 to 15 registered with a general practitioner 173 are being treated for asthma. The prevalence of asthma is $173/878 = 0.197$ (19.7%).

Risk is defined as the proportion (or %) of new cases of disease occurring in a specified time period (for example 1 year or 5 years):

$$\text{Risk} = \frac{\text{number of new cases of disease in period}}{\text{number initially free of disease}}.$$

The risk is also known as the **cumulative incidence**.

Example: A total of 5,632 women aged 55–64 attended their local breast cancer screening service during 1990 and were found to be free of breast cancer. Over the next five years, 58 were diagnosed with breast cancer. The risk of breast cancer over the

five-year period was therefore $58/5,632 = 0.0103$ (1.0%).

When we wish to calculate how fast new cases of disease are occurring, we may calculate the **incidence rate**.

$$\text{Incidence rate} = \frac{\text{number of new cases of disease}}{\text{total number} \times \text{time interval}}.$$

Example: The incidence of breast cancer among the 5,632 women described earlier was $58/(5 \times 5,632) = 0.0020$ per year, or 2.0 per 1,000 person-years. We have used the term person-year to indicate a denominator that includes both people and time. Note, however, that a 1,000 person years could be generated by observing 1,000 people for 1 year or 500 people for 2 years.

Under certain conditions, it is possible to relate prevalence to incidence by the following formula:

$$\text{prevalence} = \text{incidence} \times \text{average duration of disease}.$$

This can be illustrated simply by a figure of a funnel with water coming in at the top (incidence) and leaving at the bottom (death, emigration, recovery) so that at any one moment we have a pool of water in the funnel (prevalence) (see Figure 2.3).

Thus the prevalence of a disease in a population can increase either because the incidence has increased and/or the average duration of people with that disease has increased. For example, repeat surveys of multiple sclerosis in North East

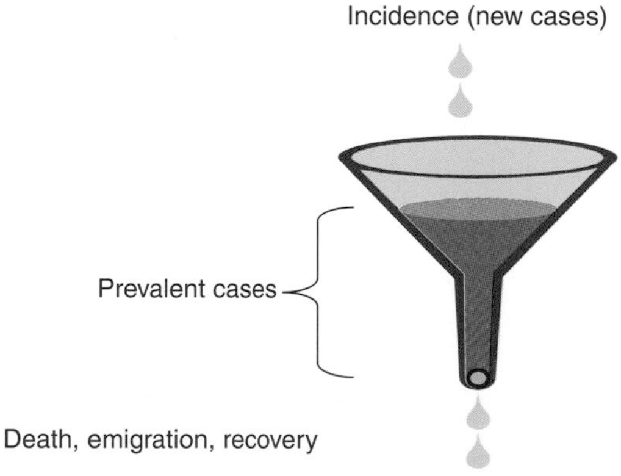

Figure 2.3 The relationship between prevalence, incidence and disease duration.

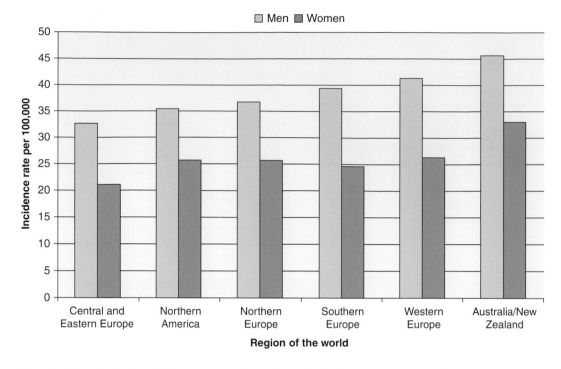

Figure 2.4 Age standardised incidence rates for colorectal cancer (2008) for men and women in different regions of the developed world.
Source: Data taken from Cancer Research UK website
http://info.cancerresearchuk.org/cancerstats/world/colorectal-cancer-world

Scotland have shown an increase in disease prevalence over a 15-year period. Assuming that the incidence rate has not changed over this short period and the methods of case ascertainment were the same, then the increased prevalence probably reflects an increase in survival for patients with MS today so there is an increase in the pool of prevalent cases.

Descriptive epidemiology

It is common for epidemiologists to often describe disease patterns in **T**ime, **P**lace and **P**erson (TPP). For example in Figure 2.4 we have plotted the annual incidence rate for colorectal cancer from several developed regions in the world for men and women. There is marked geographical variability so that there is a 50% increase across the lowest and highest risk areas. In each area, men have a greater risk than women. These figures are both helpful in planning health care services, e.g. number of specialists required, as well as generating hypotheses as to what may cause colorectal

cancer. Many Australians are European migrants and hence the higher risk seen in this population may reflect differences in environmental exposures (e.g. diet, sunlight exposure etc.) rather than genetic differences or better health care ascertainment. (See Chapter 15 for an example as to how suicide mortality rates have changed over time and possible explanations.)

When examining disease trends over time, it is important to consider the following potential explanations for any increase or decreased risk:

(1) Chance: variations may be due to *random* fluctuations. Statistical methods will address this.

(2) Ascertainment: change in *diagnostic* techniques so that disease is more likely to be diagnosed e.g. increase in diagnosis of brain tumours with introduction of CT brain scanning.

(3) Demography: change in *age distribution* of population. An ageing population will result in an apparent increase in crude disease rates but will not alter age-specific rates.

(4) **Coding**: changes in the rules by which mortality is coded (International Classification of Diseases, ICD) can produce spurious effects. This can be demonstrated by use of bridge coding i.e. compare new rates using the old coding rules.

(5) **Treatment effects**: new medical therapies may have a beneficial effect on disease frequency or rarely actually result in an increase in mortality due to iatrogenic causes e.g. isoprenaline inhalers and increased asthma mortality.

(6) **True changes in incidence**: changes in risk factors may have resulted in a true increase or decrease in the *incidence* of the disease. This suggests the potential role of prevention by altering these risk factors.

Examining the associations between two variables

One of the main aims of epidemiology is to understand the causes of disease or health-related risk factors (that is an individual characteristic, such as smoking status, that can influence one's future risk of developing a disease). Occasionally, as with cross-sectional studies (see Chapter 5), a study simply measures the frequency (prevalence) of a disease. However, the aim is usually to examine the association between an **exposure** and an **outcome** and to test a specific **hypothesis** about the association. For example, we may test the hypothesis that there is no association between the exposure and outcome – known as the **null hypothesis**. The exposure may be a lifestyle characteristic (e.g. physical activity) or a physiological (e.g. height) or even genetic (e.g. presence of specific genetic polymorphism) measure. The outcome is usually a disease state (e.g. heart attack) but may also be a behaviour related to subsequent disease (e.g. smoking status). The notion behind the research is that the presence or absence of exposure may change the likelihood of an individual developing the outcome.

For example if we want to test whether moderate physical activity protects against heart disease then physical activity is our exposure whilst heart disease is our outcome. Similarly, if we want to see if men are more physically active than women,

then gender is our exposure whilst physical activity is our outcome. As you can see a variable can be both an exposure and an outcome depending on the specific question that is being asked.

Absolute and relative measures of association

Different measures are available to measure the association between an exposure and outcome. When the outcome is numerical (and the exposure dichotomous/binary) we generally calculate the **difference in means** between exposure groups as follows:

$$\text{difference in means} = \text{mean in exposed} - \text{mean in unexposed}.$$

For example, does cognitive function score differ between those less than and greater than 65?

When the outcome and exposure are dichotomous/binary we can calculate the difference in proportions or the **risk difference** (or **attributable risk**) as follows:

$$\text{risk difference} = \text{risk among exposed} - \text{risk among unexposed}.$$

For example, we could calculate the risk difference of lung cancer amongst smokers compared to nonsmokers. If there is no difference in risk between exposure groups then the risk difference will be zero. A positive value indicates that exposure increases risk whilst a negative value indicates a reduced risk.

The risk difference and difference in means are absolute measures, that is, they provide an indication of the magnitude of excess risk or excess disease relating to exposure. Another absolute measure is the **population attributable risk** which is calculated as follows:

$$\text{population AR} = \text{overall risk} - \text{risk among unexposed}.$$

For example, how much of the overall population risk of lung cancer is due to smoking? If we compared two countries where smoking was common (A) or rare (B), if we assume that the risk associated with lung cancer is identical in countries A and B for both smokers and nonsmokers, then the risk difference for each country would be the same but the population attributable risk would be far greater for country A. To put this another way, if we could abolish smoking we would have a far greater impact in reducing lung cancer risk in country A.

When the outcome and exposure are both dichotomous/binary a relative measure of association can alternatively be calculated such as the **risk ratio** (also known as a **relative risk**). Such a measure tells us how much more likely the outcome is among those exposed compared to those unexposed and is calculated as follows:

$$\text{Risk ratio} = \frac{\text{risk in exposed individuals}}{\text{risk in unexposed individuals}}.$$

If there is no difference in risk between exposure groups then the ratio measure will be one (unity). A value larger than one indicates a relative increased risk whilst a value less than one indicates a reduced risk. For example if the risk of developing lung cancer amongst smokers is 9 per 1,000 person-years whilst for nonsmokers it was 3 per 1,000 person-years then the ratio for smoking and lung cancer will be 3 (9 per 1,000/3 per 1,000). This indicates that smokers have a threefold relative risk of developing lung cancer. Alternatively, nonsmokers have a risk ratio of 0.33 (inverse of previous result) or a 67% relative reduction in risk.

An alternative to calculating the risk of disease is to calculate the **odds of disease**. You may have come across odds in the context of gambling, for example horse racing. In a race with 5 horses the probability of each horse winning might be 0.4, 0.3, 0.2 and 0.1 or 40%, 30%, 20% and 10%. In other words, horse 1 has a probability of 60% of losing compared to 40% of winning; horse 2 has a 70% chance of losing compared to a 30% chance of winning and so on. These horses would then have odds against winning (or odds of losing) of 3 to 2, 7 to 3, 4 to 1 and 9 to 1 respectively. These true odds against winning are then reduced by bookmakers to ensure that they make a profit. Odds of 9 to 1 for horse 5 for example might be reduced to 4 to 1 meaning that for each pound bet four pounds will be received if the horse wins the race.

In epidemiology, if 100 heavy smokers are followed up for 10 years and 70 get lung cancer, then the probability or risk of lung cancer is $70/100 = 0.7$ or 70%. The probability of not getting lung cancer within this sample is therefore 30%, so the odds of lung cancer are 70 to 30 or 7 to 3, which can be written as $7/3 = 2.33$. The odds of disease is the number of people with disease divided by the number of people without disease:

$$\text{Odds of disease} = \frac{\text{number of individuals with disease}}{\text{number of individuals without disease}}.$$

If the disease is rare, so that the number of individuals without disease is approximately the same as the total number of individuals then the odds of disease is approximately the same as the risk of disease. For example, if 1,000 light smokers are followed up for 10 years and 7 develop lung cancer then the risk of lung cancer is $7/1,000 = 0.007$ or 0.7%. There are 993 light smokers without lung cancer so the odds of lung cancer is $7/993 = 0.007$ – the same as the risk to three decimal points.

An odds ratio is calculated as follows:

$$\text{Odds ratio} = \frac{\text{odds of disease in exposed individuals}}{\text{odds of disease in unexposed individuals}}.$$

Note that the odds ratio also equals the ratio of the odds of exposure in individuals with disease to the odds of exposure amongst individuals without the disease:

$$\text{Odds ratio} = \frac{\text{odds of exposure in individuals with disease}}{\text{odds of exposure in individuals without disease}}$$

$$= \frac{d_1/d_0}{h_1/h_0} = \frac{d_1 \times h_0}{d_0 \times h_1},$$

where d_1 is the number of exposed in the disease group, d_0 is the number of unexposed in the disease group, h_1 is the number of exposed in the healthy group, h_0 is the number of unexposed in the healthy group. This form of the odds ratio is used within case-control studies (see Chapter 5). (Another relative measure of risk which is used for time to event data as in survival analysis is called the hazard ratio – see Chapter 10.)

Note that absolute measures of association, such as a risk difference must have units e.g. per 1,000, per 10,000 etc. whilst ratio measures such as the risk or odds ratio are unitless. Similarly, if you reverse the exposure groups then a risk difference or difference in means measure will be the same but the sign or direction will have changed, but a ratio measure will be either above or below one and this will not be symmetrical as an increased risk can go from 1 to infinity whilst a reduction in risk can only go down from 1 to zero.

KEY LEARNING POINTS

- Medical data includes both numerical and categorical variables – the type of variable will determine how the data is summarised and analysed

- Numerical variables are summarised by measures of central tendency (such as mean and median) and variability (such as standard deviation (SD) and range)

- The Normal distribution is explained entirely by its mean and SD. These two measures can be used to determine the proportion of data that lies between any two values – for example 95% will lie between the mean and $+/-$ 1.96 SDs. This is known as the 95% reference range

- It is essential that binary variables such as the presence (or absence) of disease are related to the population at risk

- The prevalence of a disease tells us something about the burden of disease

- Incidence tells us how fast new cases of disease are occurring

- The aim of epidemiological studies is generally to examine an association between an exposure (risk factor) and an outcome (disease) and to test a specific hypothesis

- Absolute measures of the association between an exposure and outcome include the difference in means, risk difference and population attributable risk

- Relative measures include risk and odds ratios which tell us how much more likely the outcome is among those exposed compared to those unexposed

3

Epidemiological concepts

Sara T. Brookes and Yoav Ben-Shlomo
University of Bristol

Learning objectives

In this chapter you will learn:

- ✓ how to distinguish between validity and reliability;
- ✓ how results may be misleading due to bias and the difference between selection, measurement, differential and nondifferential biases;
- ✓ what is meant by the term confounding and the different approaches to try and control confounding.

This chapter will introduce you to some key concepts in epidemiology that are essential to understand when trying to interpret the results of epidemiological studies. These are validity, reliability, bias and confounding. We often use these terms in everyday conversation but as you will see the epidemiological definitions may sometimes not exactly match our lay definitions.

Validity (accuracy) and reliability (precision)

It is important to distinguish between the **validity** (**accuracy**) and **reliability** (**precision**) of a sample statistic. Consider shooting a target where the bullseye in the centre represents the population parameter we are trying to estimate. We take seven shots at this target, representing seven statistics calculated from seven samples. Then we might see one of the patterns of shots illustrated in Figure 3.1.

The validity relates to how representative the sample is of the population. If systematic bias is introduced into the study then on average any sample estimate will differ from the population parameter and the statistic will be inaccurate. If there is no systematic bias then on average sample statistics will be the same as the population parameter. We discuss different reasons for bias later in this chapter. Similarly, if the study sample is not representative of the target population, then the study sample result may be different to the true result in the population. In this case the results from the study sample cannot be generalised to the population and are thus an inaccurate reflection of the true population value.

The reliability concerns the amount of variation between sample statistics. The more precise the statistics, the smaller the variability between the sample statistics and the more we can narrow down the likely values of the population

---

Epidemiology, Evidence-based Medicine and Public Health Lecture Notes, Sixth Edition. Yoav Ben-Shlomo, Sara T. Brookes and Matthew Hickman.

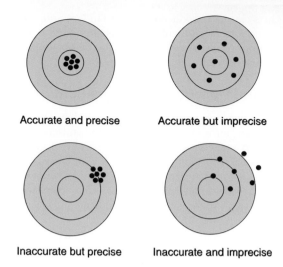

Accurate and precise Accurate but imprecise

Inaccurate but precise Inaccurate and imprecise

Figure 3.1 Illustration of the concepts of validity and reliability.

parameter. The precision of a single sample statistic can be considered by calculation of a confidence interval, which is introduced in Chapter 4.

We would ideally like to achieve accurate and precise results but research occurs cumulatively so even if our results are accurate but imprecise, this is better than inaccurate but precise as in the longer term it is likely the data of one study will be pooled with other studies (see Chapter 12) which will increase precision.

Bias in epidemiological studies

In an epidemiological study we aim to estimate a population parameter with as much accuracy (and precision) as possible. In a **cross-sectional** study this is generally the prevalence of a particular exposure or disease, and in an analytical study (such as a **randomised controlled trial**, **cohort** or **case control**) we measure the association between an exposure and an outcome (analytical studies). All of these studies will be dealt with in later chapters. Bias in such studies relates to a departure from the true value that we are trying to estimate.

There are many different names that have been given to the various types of bias that can affect different epidemiological studies and we will introduce many of these throughout the book.

However, in practice bias can be classified as relating either to the selection of participants into (or out of) a study or to the measurement of exposure and/or outcome.

Selection bias

As stated above, in a cross-sectional study interest lies in the estimate of the prevalence of a particular exposure or outcome. If there is systematic bias in the selection of participants we may end up answering a different question to that intended. If the way in which people are selected for the study is biased in some way our results may not be representative of the population of interest. For example, volunteers to advertisements for studies often have a personal interest in the area of study. The prevalence of disease or exposures in a volunteer group may be very different from that in the underlying population, hence this may result in either an over- or underestimate of the true prevalence. Therefore, if the estimate of interest is a prevalence then a sample that is not representative of the target population *will* result in an inaccurate estimate which cannot be generalised to the target population. This bias could operate in either direction; for example, healthier individuals may be more able to take part or in contrast individuals with the studied disease will be more interested in the study and hence agree to take part.

In analytical studies, selection bias relates to the estimate of the association between exposure and an outcome. In terms of systematic sampling error, the following distinction can be made in analytical studies:

Nondifferential selection

So long as any systematic errors in the selection of participants occur equally to all groups being compared (e.g. treatment groups in a randomised controlled trial or exposure groups in a cohort study), then whilst the results may not be representative of any groups in the target population underrepresented in the sample, the estimate of the association between exposure and outcome will be unbiased. Hence, in analytical studies an unrepresentative sample does not necessarily lead to selection bias. For example a trial of an antihypertensive drug (versus placebo) recruits patients from an outpatient clinic. It is noted that of all eligible patients, those from ethnic minority groups are less likely to participate in the trial thereby creating an unrepresentative sample and reducing the generalisability of the findings. However, the distribution of ethnic minority patients is the same across treatment and placebo arms, so the overall effect of the drug on lowering blood pressure is likely to be unbiased.

Differential selection

If, however, any systematic bias in the selection of participants occurs differentially across groups, then selection bias may be present and result in either an under- or overestimate of the association between exposure and outcome. Thus if we continue with the above example, if ethnic minority patients were more likely to be allocated to the treatment arm and pharmacologically were less responsive to the treatment, then the estimate of the drug effect would be biased downwards and be an underestimate.

Measurement bias

There will also be errors in the measurement of exposure and/or outcome in any epidemiological study. For example, an individual's blood pressure will vary from day to day or even throughout the day, hence different measurements taken on the same individual will vary around their usual blood pressure at random. Alternatively, the device measuring blood pressure may be imprecise so there again will be random variation in readings. Indeed, there will always be some degree of *random* error in the measurement of exposures and outcomes. If however, the device is inaccurate such that it always under- or overestimates blood pressure, or for example the health care professional using the device always rounds measurements up or down, then there will be some degree of *systematic* error.

Random and systematic errors in such measurements can lead to the misclassification of a participant with respect to the exposure and/or outcome. If the error is random, misclassification will also be random and the proportions classified into each category will be right. However, systematic error will lead to systematic misclassification with the wrong proportions of individuals classified into different groups.

In a cross-sectional study systematic measurement error may lead to an inaccurate estimate of prevalence. In an analytical study, where we are interested in the accuracy of the estimate of the association between an exposure and outcome,

bias can be introduced by both random and systematic measurement error. It is important to ascertain whether errors are likely to be differential across the exposure and outcome groups.

Nondifferential misclassification

Whether measurement errors are random or systematic, if the errors and any resulting misclassification occur equally in all groups we have nondifferential misclassification and the estimate of the association between exposure and outcome will be underestimated (diluted) since the errors will tend to make the groups more similar.

Differential misclassification

If however, measurement error and subsequent misclassification is different across the groups the estimate of the association between exposure and outcome may be either under- or overestimated, and it is often impossible to know which way the bias may have affected the results. For this reason we are generally more concerned with differential misclassification than nondifferential.

Each of these types of bias will be considered in more detail in the context of different analytical study designs throughout the book.

Confounding in epidemiological studies

A crucial issue in interpreting the results of epidemiological studies is whether there is an association with a third variable that provides an alternative explanation for the observed association between exposure and disease. This is known as **confounding**.

Confounding can occur when the exposure (E) under study is also associated with a third factor (confounder) (C), which also affects the chance or amount of disease (D). This is depicted in Figure 3.2. In this case, their association with the confounder may influence the apparent association between exposure and disease.

Depending on the direction of the confounder-disease (C-D) and confounder-exposure (C-E) associations, the observed exposure-disease (E-D) association may be too large or too small. In some cases, an apparent E-D association may be completely explained by the effects of one or more

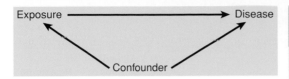

Figure 3.2 Circumstances in which a third factor can bias the association between exposure and disease.

Table 3.2 Association between asthma and social class.

		Asthma		
		Yes	No	Total
Social class	Deprived	33 (9.8%)	303 (90.2%)	336
	Affluent	24 (4.0%)	570 (96.0%)	594

confounding variables. To be a confounder, the third variable must (i) be associated with the exposure, (ii) be a risk factor for the disease, and (iii) must not be on the causal pathway between the exposure and the disease.

The only study design in which confounding should not be a problem (though this assumption needs to be checked) is the randomised controlled trial (see Chapter 11). Because the exposure (treatment) is allocated randomly, no other factors should be associated with it.

Example of confounding

Table 3.1 shows results from a cross-sectional study (see Chapter 5) of 930 adults, which examined whether vitamin C consumption (high or low) is associated with asthma.

The odds ratio (as described in Chapter 2) for the association between vitamin C consumption and asthma is:

$$\text{OR} = \frac{24 \div 518}{33 \div 355} = \frac{24 \times 355}{33 \times 518} = 0.50.$$

Vitamin C appears to be protective against asthma, but we need to consider whether this association could be explained by a factor, which is associated with both asthma and vitamin C consumption. The investigators found that asthma was more common in more deprived social classes, and that vitamin C consumption also varied greatly with social class, as shown in Tables 3.2 and 3.3.

It is therefore possible that social class confounds the observed association between vitamin C consumption and asthma. How can we take account of the effect of social class when we estimate the association between vitamin C consumption and asthma?

Controlling for confounding in the design of a study

As explained above, the process of randomly allocating participants to treatment groups in a randomised controlled trial should remove any possible association between the exposure and the potential confounder as allocation to treatment arm should not be influenced by any known or unknown confounder.

For other epidemiological studies exclusion can be incorporated into the design. The study could recruit all subjects from the same social class. However this would make it harder to find enough subjects and would restrict the generalisability (applicability) of the findings.

Controlling for confounding in the analysis of a study

Standardisation is a method that is sometimes used to control for differences in age groups, when the rates of disease between two populations with different age structures are compared (e.g. the rate of lung cancer in the UK and the rate of lung cancer in Malawi). This method is less common than

Table 3.1 Association between asthma and vitamin C consumption.

		Asthma		
		Yes	No	Total
Vitamin C consumption	High	24 (4.4%)	518 (95.6%)	542
	Low	33 (8.5%)	355 (91.5%)	388

Table 3.3 Association between vitamin C consumption and social class.

		Vitamin C consumption		
		Low	High	Total
Social class	Deprived	279 (83.0%)	57 (17.0%)	336
	Affluent	109 (18.4%)	485 (81.6%)	594

Table 3.4 Analyses of the association between vitamin C consumption and asthma, stratified by social class.

		Deprived Asthma	No asthma				Affluent Asthma	No asthma
Vitamin C consumption	High	5	52		Vitamin C consumption	High	19	466
	Low	28	251			Low	5	104
	OR = 0.86					OR = 0.85		

methods described below, and is usually only used to control for age.

Stratification means that we estimate the association between exposure and disease separately for different levels (strata) of the confounder. We then combine the odds ratios in the different strata to produce an estimated odds ratio for the E-D association that is controlled for the effect of the confounder.

In this example, we stratify the analysis by social class. If the effect of vitamin C is independent of social class then we should see approximately the same association. If social class confounds the association between vitamin C and asthma then the effect will change after stratification. In this study, the association was much reduced (see Table 3.4).

Since the estimates of the vitamin C–asthma association are similar in the two strata, it makes sense to combine the information in the different strata to get a single estimate of the vitamin C–asthma association. This is done using **Mantel-Haenszel** methods or **regression models**. Using these methods provides an estimate of the association between vitamin C consumption and asthma, controlled for the effects of social class. You will also see this referred to as 'adjusted for' social class. Keeping the level of the confounder constant in each stratum is analogous to conducting a laboratory experiment in which we control the environment so that only the factor of interest varies. Occasionally one can find evidence that the effects of exposure on outcome are very different by strata and this is unlikely to be due to chance. This is technically known as **interaction** or **effect modification** as a third factor alters the exposure–disease association. In this case the combined or pooled effect will be misleading and it is better to present the strata-specific associations.

In this example the estimate of the OR is attenuated to 0.86, after controlling for social class. Therefore, after controlling for the confounding effect of social class, there was little evidence that

vitamin C consumption protects against asthma (formal testing of the association found that the results were consistent with chance).

Controlling for the effects of a number of confounders

Often, a number of different factors may confound the exposure-disease association in which we are interested. To control (adjust) for the effects of a number of confounders, we use **regression** models. Models that take account of the effects of a number of different confounders are called **multivariable models.**

In the medical literature, associations with binary disease outcomes are most commonly (but not always) expressed as odds ratios and analysed using a method called **logistic regression**. For example, a research paper might report odds ratios for the association between vitamin C consumption and asthma, controlled for the effects of age, sex, smoking and social class. Each of these variables is likely to be associated with both asthma and with dietary habits, and so each is a potential confounder of the relationship between vitamin C consumption and asthma.

Reporting the results of analyses

When reading a report of any observational study, it is vital to consider whether the authors have accounted adequately for the effects of confounding factors in their analyses. Therefore it is usual to display both the crude association (the estimated association before possible confounding variables are taken into account) as well as the estimated association after controlling for confounding.

For example, Table 3.5 shows the association between (1) hormone replacement therapy and (2) high blood pressure on the incidence of heart disease in a cohort of women aged between 45 and

Table 3.5 Crude and adjusted risk ratios for HRT and blood pressure and IHD in women.

	Crude risk ratio (95% CI)	Adjusted risk ratio, after controlling for socioeconomic status, age and smoking
Reported use of hormone replacement therapy (HRT)	0.57	0.95
High blood pressure at baseline	1.81	1.78

75. We can see that the apparent protective association of hormone replacement therapy (HRT) is explained by the confounding effects of socioeconomic status, age and smoking. On the other hand, whilst it is established that socioeconomic position, age and smoking are associated with both high blood pressure and heart disease, the fact that controlling for these variables makes little difference to the estimated adverse effect suggests that these variables do not confound the association between high blood pressure and IHD.

The degree to which the crude association changes after adjustment for confounding indicates how strongly the crude association was confounded by the variables controlled for in the adjusted analysis.

Are adjusted results perfect?

No! Although adjusting results for potential confounders can remove some or most of the confounding effect of that variable, it rarely is perfect. This is because the confounder itself may be poorly measured, or there may be other potential confounding variables that we have not measured, or do not know about. This is called **residual confounding**.

 FURTHER READING

Webb P, Bain C, Pirozzo S (2005) *Essential Epidemiology: An Introduction for Students and Health Professionals.* Cambridge: Cambridge University Press.

 KEY LEARNING POINTS

- The validity of a sample estimate relates to whether it is an accurate estimate of the true population value and is determined by how representative a sample is of the population and whether any bias has been introduced into the study
- The reliability of a sample estimate relates to how precise it is – how certain we can be of the true population value
- Bias is a systematic error that relates either to the selection of participants into or out of a study or to the measurement of exposure and/or outcome
- Bias is inherent in all epidemiological studies though different types are more or less likely to impact different studies
- A confounding factor is one that may provide an alternative explanation for an observed association between an exposure and outcome and may lead to either an over or underestimate of the true association
- Confounding effects all epidemiological studies with the exception of the randomised controlled trial
- Ways of dealing with confounding include stratification and multivariable regression

4

Statistical inference, confidence intervals and P-values

Kate Tilling, Sara T. Brookes and Jonathan A.C. Sterne
University of Bristol

Learning objectives

In this chapter you will learn:

✓ to estimate a population statistic using a sample statistic;

✓ to calculate and interpret 95% confidence intervals (CIs) for means and proportions;

✓ to interpret the difference between two means or proportions using a 95% confidence interval;

✓ the meaning of a P-value, and to derive P-values for differences in means and proportions;

✓ to interpret P-values and confidence intervals in research findings.

Estimating a population statistic

Research studies are carried out to answer specific questions about the health of a group of people, for example:

(a) What is the mean systolic blood pressure in men aged over 65 in the UK?

(b) What is the prevalence of smoking in men aged over 65 in the UK?

(c) is blood pressure different in smokers compared to nonsmokers?

(d) is the prevalence of smoking different in men compared to women?

In the first case, we say that the **target population**, i.e. the population of interest, is all men aged over 65 in the UK. This can be expanded to include all future men aged > 65 in the UK. However, we clearly can't find all these men, and measure their systolic blood pressures and ask about whether they smoke. Instead, we use a study

---

Epidemiology, Evidence-based Medicine and Public Health Lecture Notes, Sixth Edition. Yoav Ben-Shlomo, Sara T. Brookes and Matthew Hickman.
© 2013 Y. Ben-Shlomo, S. T. Brookes and M. Hickman. Published 2013 by John Wiley & Sons, Ltd.

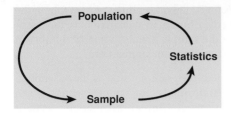

Figure 4.1 Using statistical methods to make inferences about the population, in a research study.

sample to make inferences about the target population (see Figure 4.1).

There are two ways in which a sample can be considered representative of a target population. The first is where we have a list of the people in the target population (e.g. all men in the UK aged > 65, from census or General Practice records) and we randomly select the study sample from this (e.g. randomly select a number of men aged > 65 from census records). The second is to use eligibility criteria for the study sample, and then assume that the study sample represents all people satisfying those criteria. For example, eligibility criteria for a randomised trial of a new treatment for prostate cancer might include the specification of stage of disease, years since diagnosis, response to other treatments, and absence of other comorbidities.

Example: Estimating blood pressure

Suppose we have a target population of 100,000 men aged over 65 in one region of the UK. Hypothetically, we could measure the systolic blood pressure of every one of these men. Assume that if we could do this, the true distribution (shown in Figure 4.2) would have a mean of 140 mmHg and a standard deviation of 15 mmHg. Note that the distribution is not Normal – it is **skewed** to the right, as there are a small number of individuals with very high blood pressures.

In practice we could not measure the blood pressures for everyone in such a large population. So what happens if we measure the systolic blood pressures in a sample from this population? We

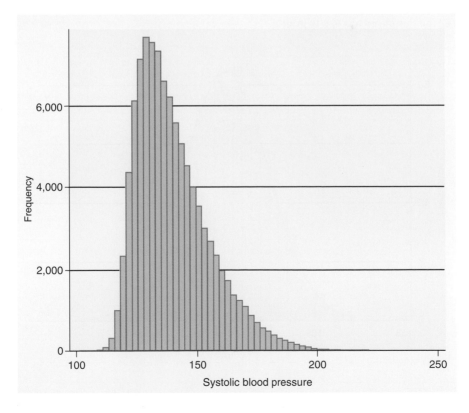

Figure 4.2 Histogram of systolic blood pressure in a population of 100,000 men aged > 65 years.

randomly selected 100 men from this population, and found that they had a mean blood pressure of 139.3 mmHg, with standard deviation 14.8 mmHg. We carried out this process of sampling 100 men nine more times, obtaining 10 samples in total. The means of these 10 samples were:

139.3 138.4 142.2 139.7 136.7 141.3
137.8 139.7 138.9 140.3.

Although none of the sample means is exactly the same as the true population mean (which we know to be 140 mmHg), they are all fairly close to this mean. In order to understand how just one sample can be used to make inferences about the whole population, we need to look at the **sampling distribution**. This is the distribution the sample means follow if we take lots of samples from the same population. To show this, we repeat this sampling 990 more times (obtaining 1,000 samples in total) and draw a histogram of the sample means (Figure 4.3). Note that the horizontal scale of this histogram is much narrower than that for the histogram of values in the entire population (Figure 4.2). The mean of all the sample means shown in Figure 4.3 is 139.8 mmHg and the standard deviation of all the sample means is 1.49 mmHg.

This example illustrates three key facts about the sampling distribution of a mean (that is, the distribution of the sample means in a large number of samples from the same population):

(1) Provided the sample size is large enough (>100 individuals), the sample means have an approximately Normal distribution – even if the population distribution is not Normal.

(2) The *mean* of this distribution is equal to the population mean. Here the mean of the sample means is 139.8 mmHg, which is approximately equal to the population mean which we know to be 140 mmHg.

(3) the *standard deviation* of the sampling distribution of a mean depends on both the amount of variation in the population (measured by the standard deviation) and on the sample size of the samples (*n*). We call this the **standard error** of the mean (to distinguish it from the standard deviation in the population). The formula for the standard error (*SE*) is:

$$SE = \frac{SD}{\sqrt{n}}.$$

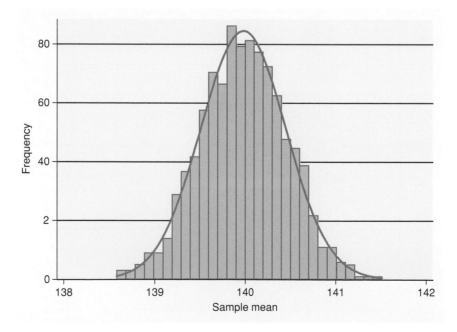

Figure 4.3 Histogram of sample mean systolic blood pressure from 1,000 samples each of 100 men, from a population of 100,000 men aged > 65 years with a mean systolic blood pressure of 140 mmHg and a standard deviation of 15 mmHg, with a Normal curve superimposed.

So as the sample size gets bigger the standard error of the mean gets smaller – it is a more precise estimate of the population mean. Here the standard deviation of the 1,000 sample means (the standard error) was 1.49 mmHg. This is close to the theoretical value of the standard error for samples of size 100, which (from the above formula) is $15/10 = 1.5$ mmHg.

Confidence interval for a population mean

In practice we want to use a mean from a single sample of individuals to make inferences about the value of the true population mean. We know from the example above that the mean of all possible sample means is the true population mean – so we start by using our sample mean as an estimate of the true population mean. We also know from the example above that a single sample mean is unlikely to be exactly the same as the population mean.

Because we know that the distribution of sample means is Normal for large sample sizes, we can say that 95% of the individual sample means are within 1.96 *SE*s of the mean of this distribution, which is the true population mean (see Chapter 2).

If we transpose this sentence we can say that 95% of the time the true population mean is within 1.96 *SE*s of the observed sample mean.

In other words the interval from $\overline{X} - (1.96 \times SE)$ to $\overline{X} + (1.96 \times SE)$ (where $\overline{X}$ is the sample mean) will include the true population mean on 95% of occasions. This interval is known as the **95% confidence interval** for the population mean and the values $\overline{X} - (1.96 \times SE)$ and $\overline{X} + (1.96 \times SE)$ are known as the 95% confidence limits.

The multiplier of 1.96 in the confidence intervals described above was based on the assumption that the sample means follow a Normal distribution. For smaller sample sizes (less than about 50) we have to use a different multiplier, t', which is derived from the *t* distribution.

We can calculate a 99% confidence interval, a 90% confidence interval, and so on, in a similar way, by changing the multiplier from 1.96 to 2.58 (99% CI) or 1.64 (90% CI) – these different multipliers are readily available from statistical tables.

Example: Estimating blood pressure (continued)

Figure 4.4 shows the point estimates and 95% confidence intervals for 20 different random samples of 100 men, taken from a population with mean blood pressure of 140 mmHg and *SD* 15 mmHg. Notice that, although the individual 95% confidence intervals vary, 19 out of 20 (i.e. 95%) contain the true population mean of 140. The confidence interval from the second sample (shown with the red bar) does not contain the true value for the population mean.

In practice, of course, we would base our inference on only one sample: we used repeated samples in the discussion above to illustrate the properties of sampling, distributions and confidence intervals. For example, if we had obtained only the first sample of 100 men, our best estimate of the mean systolic BP for men aged > 65 in the UK would be 138.8 mmHg, with 95% CI 135.9 to 141.7 mmHg. We are 95% confident that the mean systolic BP for men aged > 65 in the UK lies between 135.9 and 141.7 mmHg.

Estimating a population proportion

Another common problem is that of estimating a population proportion. For example, what proportion of men in the general population are smokers? Inference about proportions is based on their sampling distribution, in the same manner as for means. Perhaps surprisingly, the sampling distribution of a proportion is approximately Normal. The mathematical reason for this is beyond the scope of this book but a simple explanation is that a proportion is a mean of zeros and ones ($21/100 = 0.21$ is the average of 21 ones and 79 zeroes). As stated earlier, the distribution of sample means tends to the Normal distribution as the size of the samples increase, even if the underlying population distribution is not Normal.

The standard error of the sample proportion p (denoted $SE(p)$ here) can be shown to be:

$$SE(p) = \sqrt{\frac{p \times (1 - p)}{n}},$$

where n is the sample size.

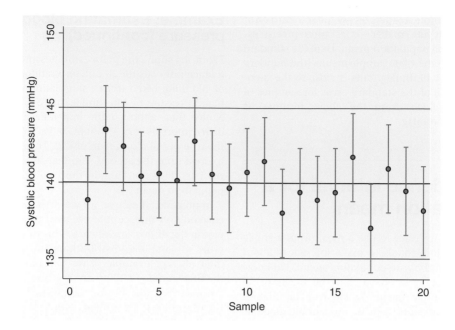

Figure 4.4 Means (dots) and 95% Confidence intervals (bars) for Systolic Blood Pressure (mmHg) from 20 samples of 100 men each, from a population of 100,000 men aged > 65 with a mean systolic blood pressure of 140 mmHg and a standard deviation of 15 mmHg.

Confidence interval for a population proportion

We estimate the population proportion by our sample proportion, p.

The standard error is used to derive a 95% confidence interval in the same way as before:

95% confidence interval $= p - (1.96 \times SE(p))$ to $p + (1.96 \times SE(p))$

Note that for proportions the multiplier is always 1.96; the formula does get unreliable for small samples but there is no straightforward equivalent to the t distribution here.

Example: Estimating the prevalence of smoking

Suppose that we have a population of 100,000 men aged > 65 years, we take one random sample of 100 men of whom 21 are smokers.

The sample proportion is $p = 21/100 = 0.21$, so we estimate the true proportion of smokers among men aged > 65 in the general population to be 21%

The standard error of the proportion is

$$SE(p) = \sqrt{\frac{0.21 \times 0.79}{100}} = 0.041,$$

so the 95% confidence interval is:

$0.21 - (1.96 \times 0.041)$ to $0.21 + (1.96 \times 0.041)$
$= 0.13$ to 0.29,

i.e. 13% to 29%.

Thus we are 95% confident that the proportion of smokers in the population of men aged > 65 in the UK lies between 13% and 29%. Note that this confidence interval is quite wide: we would need many more than 100 men to estimate the population proportion to within (say) 1%.

Comparison of two means

Medical research questions usually relate to the comparison of two (or more) groups, rather than to estimating single means or proportions. For example:

(a) is blood pressure different in smokers compared to nonsmokers?
(b) is the prevalence of smoking different in men compared to women?

Again, we use samples to make inferences about the target population. So, we use the difference between two sample means as our best estimate of the difference in means in the population. Sampling variability means that the true difference in the population will not be exactly the same as the difference in our sample. As before, we can describe the sampling distribution of the differences in means by calculating a standard error of the sample mean difference. The formula for this standard error shows that this is done by adding the squares of the standard errors of the two means:

$$SE(\overline{X}_1 - \overline{X}_0) = \sqrt{SE(\overline{X}_1)^2 + SE(\overline{X}_0)^2}$$
$$= \sqrt{\frac{SD(X_1)^2}{n_1} + \frac{SD(X_0)^2}{n_0}}.$$

Note that $SE(\overline{X}_1 - \overline{X}_0)$ means 'standard error of $(\overline{X}_1 - \overline{X}_0)$', not '$SE \times (\overline{X}_1 - \overline{X}_0)$'. The subscripts 0 and 1 denote the two groups under comparison, commonly 1 denotes the exposed group and 0 the unexposed group.

We then use this standard error to calculate a confidence interval around our estimate of the population mean difference:

$$95\% \text{ C.I. for } \overline{X}_1 - \overline{X}_0 = (\overline{X}_1 - \overline{X}_0)$$
$$- (1.96 \times SE(\overline{X}_1 - \overline{X}_0)) \text{ to } (\overline{X}_1 - \overline{X}_0)$$
$$+ (1.96 \times SE(\overline{X}_1 - \overline{X}_0)).$$

Example: Is blood pressure different in smokers compared to nonsmokers?

To investigate whether smoking is related to blood pressure, systolic blood pressure was measured in 100 men aged > 65, of whom 36 were smokers and 64 nonsmokers. The results are shown in Table 4.1.

The 95% confidence intervals for the population means are: 135 to 143 mmHg in nonsmokers and 140 to 150 mmHg in smokers. There is very little overlap between these confidence intervals, which suggests that there might be a difference in mean systolic blood pressure between smokers and nonsmokers. However, we are interested in the *amount* by which systolic blood pressure differs in smokers compared to nonsmokers.

The sample difference in mean systolic blood pressure comparing smokers with nonsmokers is:

$$\overline{X}_1 - \overline{X}_0 = 145 - 139 = 6 \text{ mmHg.}$$

Thus, our best estimate is that male smokers have a mean systolic blood pressure which is 6 mmHg higher than the mean systolic blood pressure in male nonsmokers. To derive a 95% confidence interval for the mean difference we need to calculate its standard error:

$$SE(\overline{X}_1) = SD(X_1) \Big/ \sqrt{n_1} = 15 \Big/ \sqrt{36} = 2.5, \text{ and}$$
$$SE(\overline{X}_0) = SD(X_0) \Big/ \sqrt{n_0} = 15 \Big/ \sqrt{64} = 1.88,$$

so

$$SE(\overline{X}_1 - \overline{X}_0) = \sqrt{2.5^2 + 1.88^2} = 3.125.$$

We then use the standard error to calculate a 95% confidence interval:

$$95\% \text{ C.I. for } \overline{X}_1 - \overline{X}_0 = 6 - (1.96 \times 3.13) \text{ to}$$
$$6 + (1.96 \times 3.13) = -0.1 \text{ mmHg to } 12.1 \text{ mmHg.}$$

We are 95% confident that in the population of men aged > 65 in the UK, mean blood pressure is between 0.1 mmHg lower and 12.1 mmHg higher in smokers than in nonsmokers. Thus the mean blood pressure could be considerably higher in smokers than nonsmokers, or could be slightly lower.

Comparison of means in small samples

The formula given above is valid for large samples (> 50 individuals in each group). For smaller samples then, as with the confidence interval for a single mean, we have to use:

(1) a multiplier in the confidence interval which is based on the t distribution and is a little greater than 1.96; and
(2) a slightly different formula for the standard error of $\overline{X}_1 - \overline{X}_0$.

Table 4.1 Hypothetical descriptive statistics of SBP amongst smokers and nonsmokers.

Group	Number of men	Mean SBP (mmHg)	SD (mmHg)
0 (nonsmokers)	64	139 ($\overline{X}_0$)	15
1 (smokers)	36	145 ($\overline{X}_1$)	15

Both distributions must be approximately Normal, and the standard deviations of the two distributions must be approximately equal.

Unless the sample sizes are very small or the standard deviations in the two groups are very different then the resulting confidence interval will not change by much in the small sample procedure. In our example, the confidence interval calculated using the small sample procedure is -0.2 to 12.2 mmHg, only slightly wider than the confidence interval of -0.1 to 12.1 calculated above.

Comparison of two proportions

We are often interested in comparing the **proportion** of people with a particular characteristic in two (or more) groups. For example, we might compare the proportion of men who smoke to the proportion of women who smoke. We use an approach that is similar to the comparison of two means described above – we use the sample difference in proportions to estimate the population difference, and use the standard error of the sample difference to calculate a 95% confidence interval around that estimate. Again, the standard error for the difference between two proportions is calculated by adding the squares of the standard errors of the two proportions. If p_0 is the proportion in the baseline (**reference group**) and p_1 the proportion in the comparison group, then:

$$SE(p_1 - p_0) = \sqrt{SE(p_1)^2 + SE(p_0)^2}$$
$$= \sqrt{p_1(1 - p_1)/n_1 + p_0(1 - p_0)/n_0}.$$

Example: What is the difference between the proportion of men and women that smoke?

To estimate the difference between the proportion of men who smoke and the proportion of women who smoke, we selected a (hypothetical) sample of 2,000 people aged > 65 in the UK, and ascertained their sex and smoking habits. Table 4.2 shows the results.

The proportion of women that smoke (p_0) is 15% and the proportion of men that smoke (p_1) is 25%. The 95% confidence interval for the prevalence of smoking among men is 22.6% to 27.4%, while that for women is 12.5% to 17.5%. The difference in

Table 4.2 Hypothetical data from population-based cross-sectional study of 2,000 people aged > 65 in the UK.

	Group	Nonsmoker	Smoker	Total
Male	0	900 (75%)	300 (25%)	1,200
Female	1	680 (85%)	120 (15%)	800
Total		1,580	420	2,000

the prevalence of smokers in men compared to women is:

$$p_1 - p_0 = 0.25 - 0.15 = 0.1 \ (10\%).$$

The standard error is:

$$SE(p_1 - p_0) = \sqrt{\frac{0.25 \times 0.75}{1,200} + \frac{0.15 \times 0.85}{800}}$$
$$= 0.0178 \text{ or } 1.78\%.$$

This gives a 95% confidence interval of:

$$0.1 - (1.96 \times 0.0178) \text{ to } 0.1 + (1.96 \times 0.0178)$$
$$= 0.065 \text{ to } 0.135.$$

With 95% confidence, the difference between men and women in the population prevalence of smoking is between 6.5% and 13.5%. It thus appears that men tend to have a higher prevalence of smoking than women, in people in the UK aged > 65 years.

We might alternatively choose to obtain a relative difference between the proportions by estimating the risk ratio p_1/p_0 (Chapter 2). In this instance the risk ratio would be $0.25/0.15 = 1.67$. There is a 67% relative increase in the prevalence of smoking amongst men as compared to women. Adding and subtracting 1.96 times the standard error to derive a 95% confidence interval does not work well for risk ratios (or odds ratios), because they cannot be less than zero. Whilst confidence intervals for such estimates are calculated in a different way (and are beyond the scope of this book), their interpretation is similar to that for difference in means and proportions, described above.

Investigating hypotheses

Science generally can be thought of as a process of disproving hypotheses. For example, Newton's laws of mechanics were accepted until Einstein showed that there were circumstances in which they did not work.

We can formalise this idea by looking for evidence against a **null hypothesis**. Usually, this states that there is no association between the exposure and outcome variable. Examples of null hypotheses might be:

- mean blood pressure is the same in smokers and nonsmokers;
- there is no difference in the proportion of smokers between men and women.

As with confidence intervals, we use a sample to tell us about the population. In this context, we look for evidence against the null hypothesis about the population. A sample estimate of a statistic (for example, mean, proportion, difference in means or difference in proportions) has a sampling distribution that is Normally distributed with mean equal to the population value, and standard error that we can calculate using the formulae given earlier in this chapter. To test our null hypothesis (often written H_0), we assume that the null hypothesis is the truth, and thus that samples are Normally distributed around that null hypothesis value. We then use standard properties of the Normal distribution to calculate the chance of seeing a sample estimate at least as different from the null hypothesis value as the one we observed – this is called the **P-value**.

We derive the P-value by calculating the *test statistic*:

$$z = \frac{\text{difference between sample estimate and null hypothesis value}}{\text{standard error of sample estimate}}.$$

If the null hypothesis is true, this test statistic is Normally distributed with mean 0 and standard deviation 1. We can use tables of the Normal distribution to estimate the probability of getting a test statistic at least as great as the one we observed – by convention, we also include the possibility of getting a sample estimate at least as different from the null hypothesis value in the other direction, to obtain a 'two-sided' P value

(see Table 4.3). P-values decrease as the z statistic (the number of standard errors away from the null value) gets further away from 0.

Interpretation of P-values

The smaller the P-value, the lower the chance of getting a difference as big as the one observed if the null hypothesis is true. Therefore, the smaller the P-value, the stronger the evidence against the null hypothesis. If the P-value is large (more than 0.1, say) then the data do not provide evidence against the null hypothesis, since there is a reasonable chance of getting the observed difference if the null hypothesis was true. A large P-value does not provide evidence that the null hypothesis is true, it simply tells us that our sample provides little evidence against the null hypothesis). If the P-value is small (less than 0.001, say) then a difference as big as that observed is very unlikely if the null hypothesis is true, and there is strong evidence against the null hypothesis. This is illustrated in Figure 4.5.

Before it became easy to calculate exact P values from statistical computer packages, we used to say that the difference was 'statistically significant' and 'reject' the null hypothesis when the P-value was less than 0.05. The 0.05 threshold was an arbitrary one which became commonly used in medical and psychological research. These days, in reporting the results of medical research, we should report the precise P-value along with the 95% confidence interval, and interpret the results of our analyses in the light of both. (It should be acknowledged that the 95% confidence level is based on the same arbitrary value as the 0.05 threshold – a z value of 1.96 corresponds to a P-value of 0.05.) Interpretation of a confidence interval should not focus on whether or not it contains the null value, but on the range and potential importance of the different values in the interval.

Table 4.3 Two-sided P values for different values of z.

Z	0.2	0.4	0.6	0.8	1.0	1.2	1.4	1.6	1.8	2.0
P value	0.842	0.689	0.549	0.424	0.317	0.230	0.162	0.110	0.072	0.046

Z	2.2	2.4	2.6	2.8	3.0	3.2	3.4	3.6	3.8	4.0
P value	0.028	0.016	0.0093	0.0051	0.0027	0.0014	0.0007	0.0003	0.0001	0.0001

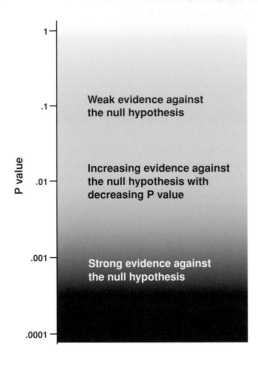

Figure 4.5 Guide to interpretation of P values. *Source*: Kirkwood BR and Sterne JAC (2003) *Essential Medical Statistics*, 2nd edn, Blackwell Science Ltd.

Example: What is the difference between mean systolic blood pressure in smokers and nonsmokers? (continued)

The difference in mean systolic blood pressure between smokers and nonsmokers was 6 mmHg, with a standard error of 3.125.

We now ask whether this study provides evidence against the **null hypothesis** that, in the target population, there is no difference in mean systolic blood pressure between smokers and nonsmokers. Under the null hypothesis, the difference in means is zero. We want to know the P-value – the probability of getting a difference of at least 6 mmHg (in either direction) if the null hypothesis is true. We derive the P-value by calculating the *test statistic*:

$$z = \frac{\text{difference between sample estimate and null hypothesis value}}{\text{standard error of sample estimate}}.$$

In this instance the sample estimate is the difference in means and the null hypothesis value is zero, hence:

$$z = \frac{\text{difference in means}}{\text{standard error of difference in means}}$$
$$= \frac{\overline{X}_1 - \overline{X}_0}{SE(\overline{X}_1 - \overline{X}_0)}$$
$$z = \frac{6}{3.125} = 1.92.$$

The probability of observing a difference at least as great as 1.92, if the null hypothesis of no difference is correct, is greater than 0.046 and less than 0.072 (from Table 4.3 above). We can use a computer to calculate the precise P-value, which is 0.0578. Thus this sample provides some (weak) evidence against the null hypothesis.

P-values and confidence intervals

We have introduced two ways to use statistical methods to make inferences about a target population from a sample (Figure 4.1):

(1) A confidence interval gives us the range of values within which we are reasonably confident that the population statistic lies.
(2) The P-value tells us the strength of the evidence against the null hypothesis.

 KEY LEARNING POINTS

- Whilst research studies are carried out to answer specific questions about a population it is not often possible to measure the entire population
- If a representative sample is obtained inferences can be made about the population of interest
- Estimates obtained from a sample of the population suffer from sampling variation and it is important to take this into account when making inferences through the reporting of confidence intervals
- When investigating associations between an exposure and outcome statistical methods look for evidence against the null hypothesis – that there is no association.
- The calculation and interpretation of a P-value tells us the strength of evidence against the null hypothesis

FURTHER READING

Kirkwood BR, Sterne JAC (2003) *Essential Medical Statistics.* 2nd edn, Blackwell Science Ltd.

Sterne JAC, Davey Smith G (2001) Sifting the evidence: what's wrong with significance tests? Another comment on the role of statistical methods. *BMJ* **322**: 226.1.

5

Observational studies

Mona Jeffreys and Yoav Ben-Shlomo
University of Bristol

Learning objectives

In this chapter you will learn:

✓ the main features of the following study designs: (i) case series; (ii) ecological studies; (iii) cross-sectional studies; (iv) case-control studies; (v) cohort studies;

✓ the strengths and weaknesses of each type of study design;

✓ how to choose a study design for your research question.

Observational vs. intervention studies

Many doctors feel they know which treatments work best from clinical observation or experience. This may be reasonable in some circumstances. For example, when sulphonamides were introduced for the treatment of meningococcal meningitis the effect on mortality was striking. However few treatments have such dramatic effects and research studies are generally required to determine what works best.

The best currently available method of assessing the effectiveness of treatments is the **randomised controlled trial** (**RCT**). This is described in detail in Chapter 11. Other types of study design can also be used for testing hypotheses. These can be listed in the order of the likelihood that they will provide the best quality of evidence. Therefore, we can describe a **hierarchy of evidence** based on study design (see Box 5.1). This ordering, of course, assumes that each study is well-designed and conducted (see Chapter 8 on evidence-based medicine).

In an RCT (also known as an **intervention** or **experimental study**), the investigator tests whether changing something about the patient, or his/her treatment, alters the course of disease. For example, if a random half of smokers were given free nicotine patches and the other half were not, we could determine whether the intervention (i.e. nicotine patches) increased the proportion of participants who quit smoking over the subsequent year. The essence of an interventional study is that we intervene. One of the main advantages of an RCT is that, if randomisation is done properly, the likelihood of both known and unknown **confounders** are balanced across both groups so that any observed differences should be due to a causal effect of the intervention (assuming it isn't due to chance) (see Chapter 3).

On the other hand, **observational studies** investigate whether certain **exposures** (or **risk factors**) are associated with the occurrence or progression of disease, without attempting to interfere with people's life. For example, we could

---

Epidemiology, Evidence-based Medicine and Public Health Lecture Notes, Sixth Edition. Yoav Ben-Shlomo, Sara T. Brookes and Matthew Hickman.
© 2013 Y. Ben-Shlomo, S. T. Brookes and M. Hickman. Published 2013 by John Wiley & Sons, Ltd.

observe whether smokers are more likely to get a heart attack than nonsmokers (smoking status is our exposure and heart attack is the outcome). We do not intervene in any way, we simply observe. There are a variety of reasons why researchers need to conduct studies using observational studies, see Box 5.2.

In this chapter we describe five types of observational study. Each has their own advantages and disadvantages, which are covered at the end of the chapter.

Types of study designs: an overview

Case series

A case series is a report, usually from a specialist, who has observed an unusual occurrence of either a 'new disease' (for example the observation of a rare type of lung infection amongst gay men in the USA heralded the discovery of HIV) or an association between an exposure and disease. In 1961 an Australian obstetrician called William McBride noted an increase in the incidence of around 20% of children born with shortened or absent limbs whose mothers reported taking a drug called thalidomide. This had been promoted as a treatment for morning sickness in 1958. McBride was startled by this much higher than expected incidence of disease. His very brief 100-word report to the Lancet resulted in confirmatory reports from Germany and other countries and subsequently led to the withdrawal of thalidomide (McBride, 1961). In general case reports are hypothesis generating and require higher-quality studies that have information about risk in both exposed and unexposed group as well as data on confounders.

Ecological studies

In most epidemiological studies, we measure exposures and outcomes on an individual level, and analyse these appropriately. An ecological study is a study in which the unit of analysis is a group rather than an individual; instead of measuring, for example, the number of hours of television an individual watches, and relating this to his/her blood pressure, we could analyse the association between the mean number of hours of television watched by people living in different parts of the country (as reported by monitoring of TV behaviour by the national TV broadcaster) and compare this with the average blood pressure measured in a health survey covering the same geographical areas. An advantage of this type of study is that it can often be performed using routinely published data or information found on the internet, so one can provide answers quickly and cheaply. However, the main problem is that on an individual level, the people who are exposed may not be the ones who experience the outcome (e.g. areas with higher TV watching may on

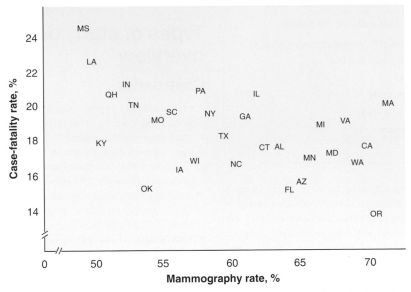

Note. There was a negative association between the two measures (*r* = –.48, *P* = .008, where *r* is the correlation coefficient—a measure of the strength of the linear relationship between mammography and case-fatality rate).

Figure 5.1 Relation between average 1990/91 mammography rates and 2-year case fatality rates for 29 states. *Source*: From Cooper GS, Yan Z, Bowlin SJ *et al.* (1998) An ecological study of the effectiveness of mammography in reducing breast cancer mortality. *Am J Public Health* **88**: 281–4, with permission.

average have higher blood pressure but the people who watch a lot of TV may not be the ones with the high blood pressure). If the associations that are detected on a group level do not hold on an individual level, the study suffers from a type of bias known as **ecological fallacy**.

Example: Mammography use and breast cancer case fatality

To determine the association of mammography with breast cancer case fatality rates, an ecological study of white women aged over 64 years was conducted in the US (Cooper *et al.*, 1998). The exposure variable was the proportion of eligible women in each state who had attended screening mammography. The outcome was the age-adjusted 2-year case-fatality rate for breast cancer. The results are shown in Figure 5.1. The authors conclude, based on these ecological data, that high screening rates are associated with lower breast cancer case fatality rates, presumably as a result of the diagnosis of earlier stage cancers.

Cross-sectional studies

Cross-sectional studies are mainly used to measure the burden of disease in a population, though they can also examine risk-factor associations. It represents a 'snapshot' of disease in a population at one moment in time (e.g. on a pre-specified day – 1 July 2011 – taken as the prevalence day or a period (e.g. over a year – 2011). This is particularly helpful for diseases that do not necessarily present to doctors as patients may be asymptomatic, e.g. high blood pressure, maturity onset diabetes. Thus, if one screens participants, one will identify individuals both known and not known to have the disease. The latter group may often be more common and this phenomenon is referred to as the **clinical iceberg**, as medical services are only aware of the ice above the water line. This is important both for the introduction of any screening programme (see Chapter 16) as well as planning health care services.

To undertake a cross-sectional study one must first define a **target population**. This is the population to which one wants to generalise the study findings (see Figure 5.2). Although one could try to measure disease in the complete target population this is usually not done as it is unnecessary and would greatly add to the cost of the study. Instead one takes a sample of individuals in the target population (**selected sample**). These subjects

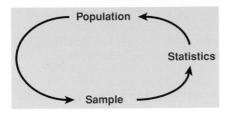

Figure 5.2 Use of statistics to make inferences about the population from the sample.

must be representative of the target population as otherwise the results will be **biased**. This is best done by either randomly sampling areas or individuals within areas. **Random sampling** implies that each individual has equal chance of being selected. These subjects are then invited to take part in the study though inevitably some will not wish to do so leaving you with data on a **study sample**. Again, if those not taking part are more or less likely to have the disease, the results will be biased in either over or under-estimating the **prevalence** of disease especially if the response rate is poor.

One then requires a standardised **case definition** to allow one to classify subjects into normal or disease (see Chapter 1). This may have more than one group such as probable disease and possible disease as some subjects may have some but not sufficient criteria to fulfil the complete case definition. One can then calculate a prevalence risk with a 95% confidence interval (CI), which indicates our degree of uncertainty around the estimate. In addition to classifying subjects as having disease or not one can also measure exposures either by questionnaire, examination or biosamples. As exposure is collected at the same time as disease status, this association needs to be treated with caution as it may reflect a **reporting bias** (e.g. cases of disease may be more aware and report of a positive family history than subjects without disease) or may be secondary to the disease, known as **reverse causality** (e.g. an association between serum inflammatory markers and atherosclerosis may be noncausal and due to damage to the arteries).

Example: The prevalence of diagnosed and undiagnosed diabetes and its association with ethnicity in the USA. (Harris *et al.*, 1998)
NHANESIII is a large (18,825) cross-sectional study of US adults (>20 years) living in their own homes (target population). 81% of the randomly selected sampled population agreed to take part in an interview and examination (study sample). The interview classified subjects into non-Hispanic whites,

African Americans and Hispanic whites. Subjects were also asked if they had a past history of diabetes diagnosed by a physician. Subjects had a blood sample after an overnight fast and some were given a glucose challenge test. 5.1% of subjects were known to have diabetes but 2.7% had undiagnosed diabetes and 6.9% of subjects had impaired glucose tolerance (a pre-diabetes stage that has a high risk of going onto diabetes). African American and Hispanic whites were 1.6 and 1.9 times more likely to have diabetes than non-Hispanic Whites. This could not be due to reverse causation or differential access to health care as both known and unknown cases were ascertained.

Case-control studies

A case-control study compares the frequency of exposure among people with the disease (cases) with that in a comparable group without the disease (controls). Subjects are selected on the basis of the outcome, i.e. whether or not they have the disease, then exposure is measured retrospectively. The exposure data may be reported by each subject, or extracted from records if available, but always are collected after disease status has been ascertained. This is the opposite of a prospective cohort study (see 'Cohort studies' section, below, pp. 40–42). See Figure 5.3.

If the exposure is more common amongst cases than amongst controls, it is associated with an increased risk of disease and may be a causal factor. Similarly, if it is less common amongst cases than controls, it may be protective.

The key principle for selection of controls is that the controls represent the population from which the cases came. Controls must be individuals who would have been designated as cases in the study, if they had developed the disease in question. Typically, control selection can be classified as disease-based or population-based.

(1) Disease-based controls are usually chosen for convenience; they often come from a ward

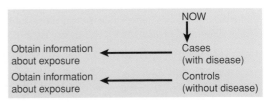

Figure 5.3 Time sequence for exposure measurement in case-control studies.

in the same hospital from which the cases are identified. When using disease-based controls, it is important that the disease that they have is thought not to be related to the exposure under study. This type of control is usually easy to recruit, especially for hospital doctors, and hence such studies are relatively cheap.

(2) Population-based controls may be selected from the electoral register, random digit telephone recruitment or from primary care patient registers; in the UK, these cover about 98% of the population. For convenience, some studies have asked cases to identify family members or friends to act as controls. These are not true population-based controls, as their characteristics are likely to be more similar to the cases than people drawn from the population.

Which type of control is better?

In general, population-based controls are preferable to disease-based ones, because the prevalence of exposure in the control group should not be biased by the presence of another disease. For example, one of the early case-control studies of lung cancer recruited other patients on a respiratory ward to act as controls. Not surprisingly, these controls were also more likely to be heavier smokers than the general population and the results underestimated the association between smoking and lung cancer. This is an example of selection bias, introduced in Chapter 3, and in general may result in either an underestimation or overestimation of the association between exposure and outcome. It is essential that cases and controls be selected irrespective of their exposure status to avoid selection bias. In other words, if the subject has been exposed they should be no more or less likely to be included in the study.

Example: Sleeping position and Sudden Infant Death Syndrome (SIDS)

A case-control study was carried out to investigate the association between sleeping position and SIDS (Fleming *et al.*, 1990). The cases were 72

infants who had died unexpectedly in the study area between 1987 and 1989. For each case, the infant's health visitor was asked to identify the two controls living in the same neighbourhood who were closest in age to the case. The families of babies who had died were visited within 72 hours of the death, and again two to four times over following months. The control families were visited at home as soon as possible after the case's death. A structured medical and social history was taken. Babies who had been put to sleep on their front had over eight times the risk of having died of SIDS compared to those put to sleep in other positions, odds ratio 8.8 (95% CI 7.0 to 11.0). Following this, and other case-control studies, several countries launched a 'back to sleep' campaign in 1991, one of the key messages of which was to advise parents to put babies to sleep on their back. This had dramatic effects on the rates of SIDS, which fell from 1.7 per 1,000 live births in 1990 to 0.6 per 1,000 in 1995.

Cohort studies

Cohort studies are observational studies in which the exposures of interest are measured at the start of the study, among people who have not yet developed the outcome. The subjects are then followed up to see whether those who were exposed develop disease at a different rate than those not exposed (see Figure 5.4). The subjects are defined by some common characteristic, for example people who live in the same area, who were born in the same week, who attend the same University, or who work in the same industry. Such a study is also referred to as a prospective cohort study.

Example: Fruit, vegetables, and colorectal cancer risk in the European Prospective Investigation into Cancer and Nutrition (EPIC) (van Duijnhoven *et al.*, 2009) EPIC is a large, multinational cohort study, designed to investigate the relationships between diet, nutritional status, lifestyle and environmental factors and the incidence of cancer and other chronic diseases. It includes over half a million people in ten European

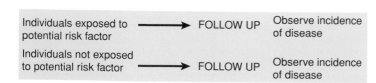

Figure 5.4 Time sequence for exposure measurement in cohort studies.

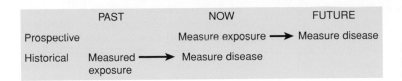

Figure 5.5 Comparison of prospective and historical cohort studies.

countries. In an analysis of 452,755 subjects, after an average follow-up of 8.8 years, 2,819 incident colorectal cancer cases were reported. People who reported a high consumption of fruit and vegetables had a lower risk of colon cancer compared to those who reported less, e.g. comparing the highest to the lowest quintile of consumption, the risk ratio was 0.76; 95% CI: 0.63, 0.91; P-value < 0.01.

A second type of cohort study is the historical cohort study. In this type of study, data on exposure is obtained from pre-existing historical records, and subjects for whom these records are available are followed to see if they have experienced the outcome of interest at any time up to the present (see Figure 5.5). The major advantage of the historical design is in studying long-term effects of exposure, since one does not need to wait for new disease to emerge as in a prospective study. However measurement of exposure is dependent on finding historical records, which may not contain good quality data as they were not collected for the purpose of research. Note that some authors call a historical cohort study 'retrospective'. However, this is misleading, as we are still looking forward in time, unlike in a case-control study. It is just that the follow-up time has already passed.

Example: Childhood energy intake and adult cancer mortality

A historical cohort study was carried out to investigate the association between childhood energy intake and later cancer mortality (Frankel *et al.*, 1998). Between 1937 and 1939, 1,352 families took part in Lord Boyd Orr's Carnegie survey of family diet and health in prewar Britain. Standardised methods were used to weigh and record the food available for the entire family at the beginning of one week. Every purchase of food during the survey week was also recorded and another inventory of all food in the home was made at the end of the week. In addition, the number of meals consumed outside the home and the weight and composition of household refuse were recorded during the week. A note was also made of which family members were present for each meal. In 1997, a total of 3,834 people were followed up through linking the original data with the NHS central register. Cause-specific mortality was available up to June 1996. Fully adjusted models showed a higher risk of cancer mortality (**hazard ratio** 1.15, (95% CI 1.06 to 1.24) per 1 MJ/day) in people with a higher energy intake.

There are several special types of cohort studies, which can be useful for answering particular questions.

(1) A birth cohort typically includes babies born in a particular time-frame. For example, the National Study of Health and Development in the UK includes a sample of all people who were born in England, Wales or Scotland during one week of March 1946.

Example: Socio-economic differences in childhood growth trajectories (Howe *et al.*, 2010)

The Avon Longitudinal Study of Parents and Children (ALSPAC) study is a birth cohort that has followed over 14,000 children since birth. Pregnant women resident in one of three Bristol-based health districts with an expected date of delivery between 1 April 1991 and 31 December 1992 were invited to take part in the study. Of these women, 14,541 were recruited. From these pregnancies, there were 14,062 live born children, 13,988 of whom were alive at 1 year. Follow-up has included parent- and child-completed questionnaires, links to routine data and clinic attendance. The aim of this study was to model growth trajectories from birth to age 10 years, to examine the socio-economic patterning of these trajectories. The authors found a clear gradient in birth length across categories of maternal education; average birth length in boys was 0.41 cm lower and in girls 0.65 cm lower in the lowest maternal education category compared with the highest. Socio-economic differences in childhood growth were small and only resulted in minimal widening of the height inequality with increasing age. By the age of 10 years, the mean difference between children in the lowest and highest maternal education categories was 1.4 cm for boys and 1.7 cm for girls.

(2) An occupational cohort includes people who all work (or have worked) in a particular industry. This method has often been used to demonstrate the hazards associated with occupational exposures. Within an industry, groups of workers may be defined according to job title, to determine how likely it is that they are exposed to a particular substance. Biological measures of the substances of interest can be used to further refine the measurements of exposure.

Example: Trichloroethylene exposure and end-stage renal disease (Radican *et al.*, 2006)
The Hill Air Force Base occupational cohort comprises all civilians employed at the aircraft maintenance facility in Utah for at least 1 year between 1 January 1952, and 31 December 1956. The cohort included 14,455 workers, approximately half of whom had been exposed to trichloroethylene (TCE). The employment records were linked to mortality data and data from the US Renal Data System to determine the incidence of end-stage renal disease. Exposure to TCE was associated with an increased risk of end-stage renal disease, hazard ratio 1.92 (95%CI 1.03 to 3.59). Given the rarity of this exposure in the general population, such a study required an occupational cohort, with higher than normal levels of exposure, to determine this risk.

(3) A clinical cohort (or 'disease cohort') is a group of patients with a particular diagnosis. These types of cohorts are used to study factors which affect prognosis, and may also be known as a survival cohort. Usually, participants are recruited to the cohort as closely as possible to the time of diagnosis. This type of study can also be used to determine the outcomes of patients following a particular procedure, in which case participants would ideally be recruited prior to the procedure.

Example: Socio-economic inequalities in cancer survival in New Zealand: The role of extent of disease at diagnosis (Jeffreys *et al.*, 2009)
A survival cohort of all adults who had a cancer registered on the New Zealand Cancer Registry between 1994 and 2003 was constructed, to investigate the effect of extent of disease at diagnosis on socio-economic inequalities in cancer survival. The relative difference in 5 year survival for colorectal cancer for people living in the most deprived areas compared to the least deprived areas was 10% (95% CI 9% to 10%). Having adjusted for the extent of the disease at presentation, the gap was reduced to 6% (95% CI 2% to 14%).

(4) A nested case-control study is a design that is used to maximise the strengths of a cohort study, while minimising on cost. These sorts of studies are case-control studies by design, but the cases and controls come from a well-defined cohort, in which exposure data have been collected prior to the outcome being diagnosed. These types of studies are most commonly used when blood samples in a cohort have been collected and stored, but the planned biochemical analysis of these, for a specific factor, is expensive. In this instance, people in the cohort who have developed the disease, and a sample of controls from within the cohort are identified, and assays need only be performed on this subset, rather than on the full cohort.

Example: Vitamin D and colorectal cancer (Jenab *et al.*, 2010)
In the EPIC study described above, a nested case-control study was performed to investigate the association between circulating vitamin D levels and colo-rectal cancer risk. The vitamin D was measured in blood samples taken at the start of the cohort study. To avoid performing the vitamin D assay on the whole cohort, the 1,248 cases with colorectal cancer were matched to 1,248 controls without cancer. As shown in Figure 5.6, the mean vitamin D levels were higher in the controls (open squares) compared to the cases (filled diamonds), having adjusted for age, sex and study centre with an obvious seasonal pattern. This suggests that pre-diagnostic vitamin D is associated with a lower risk of colorectal cancer.

Advantages and disadvantages of analytical study designs

We often start with weak evidence (case series or ecological study) that suggests a hypothesis and this is then followed up with more expensive,

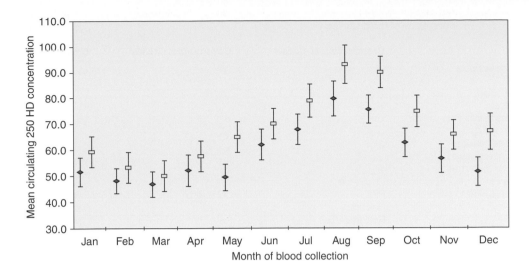

Figure 5.6 Association between case control status and vitamin D levels by months of the year.

time-consuming rigorous designs as it would be premature to launch such a study without at least some supportive evidence. All observational designs still suffer from the problems of confounding, unlike well-conducted RCTs, though there are special observational designs that help reduce this problem (see Chapter 7). Among observational studies, cohort studies provide the best evidence that an exposure–outcome association is causal. In cohort studies, the temporal relationship between exposure and outcome is clear because exposure was measured before the onset of disease. Being able to determine the temporal nature of exposure and outcome is an important indicator (amongst others) of causality (see Chapter 7). In case-control studies, exposure is measured after disease has occurred, so the exposure may have been influenced by disease.

Cohort studies may, however, suffer from other types of bias, in particular **loss to follow-up bias** (selection out of the study). These studies are often conducted over many years, in which time individuals may move and lose contact with the study investigators, or they may become too ill, or simply grow tired of participating in the study. If the loss of participants occurs equally from the exposure groups (nondifferentially) then the estimate of the association between exposure and outcome will be unbiased. If however loss to follow-up occurs differentially across exposure groups and the reason for loss to follow-up is related to the outcome, loss to follow-up bias may

occur, resulting in either an under or overestimate of the association. This is a particular concern if the proportion lost is large (>30%).

In examining evidence for causal relationships, case-control studies are superior to cross-sectional studies, because we *attempt* to ascertain subjects' exposure status before the onset of disease. In cross-sectional studies we measure exposure at the same time as outcome and therefore cannot disentangle whether exposure preceded outcome or outcome influenced exposure. However, case-control studies can be particularly prone to selection bias, as described earlier in this chapter, and whilst all studies might be prone to some degree of measurement bias (Chapter 3), a specific type of measurement bias that effects case-control studies is **recall bias**.

In a study such as a case-control study where subjects have to recall past exposures, there is likely to be an element of error in the measurement of such exposure. If this occurs in the same way amongst cases and controls (nondifferential) then this is likely to bias the estimate of association to the null. What is more problematic is where this recall is differential across cases/controls leading to recall bias. Subjects with a disease may think more carefully about possible exposures than controls. Indeed they may convince themselves of exposure even where there has been none. For example, patients with Parkinson's disease (PD), a neurological disorder, are more likely to report a history of a past head injury than healthy

Table 5.1 Pros and cons of the analytical study designs.

	Cross-sectional studies	Case-control studies	Cohort studies
Timescale / cost	✓	✓✓	✓✓✓
Bias			
Selection	✓✓	✓✓✓	✓
Recall	✓✓	✓✓✓	x
Loss to follow-up	x	x	✓✓✓
Confounding	✓✓✓	✓✓✓	✓✓✓
Reverse causality	✓✓	✓✓✓	x
Multiple exposures	✓✓✓	✓✓✓	✓✓✓
Multiple outcomes	✓✓✓	x	✓✓✓
Measures	Prevalence	–	Incidence
Measure of association	Risk	Odds ratio	Rate ratio
	Risk ratio		Risk ratio
	Risk difference		Risk difference
			Hazard ratio

controls. Is this because a head injury actually causes PD or that they are more likely to remember such an event? Recall bias is a particular problem with case-control studies as subjects are asked about their exposure *after* they have developed the disease and this may alter their response. These strengths and weaknesses are summarised in Table 5.1.

In all observational studies, the possibility that confounding has influenced the results must be considered. Providing that we have measured the appropriate variables, we may control for their effects in the analysis. However, in ecological studies the variables are measured at a group rather than individual level, and so we cannot exclude the possibility of confounding. This can lead to the ecological fallacy, the assumption that the average characteristics of populations are applicable to individuals within the population. The weakest evidence is provided by reports from case series or other clinical anecdotes. This is because the absence of any comparison group makes apparent patterns difficult to interpret.

Of course, this simple guide to study quality should be interpreted with caution; a well-done case-control study may provide more valid evidence than a poorly designed cohort study. However if faced with conflicting evidence between a randomised controlled trial and a case-control study we would usually believe the randomised trial.

 KEY LEARNING POINTS

- There are five different types of observational study designs which differ in their position on the hierarchy of evidence. Cohort studies are regarded as more robust than case control, then cross-sectional studies, ecological studies and finally case series
- Cohort designs can be prospective or historical
- Each study design has different strengths and weaknesses though in general prospective cohort studies are less prone to bias than other designs as well as having a direct measure of incidence
- Recall bias is a particular problem found in case control studies and not found in cohort studies
- Loss to follow-up bias may occur in cohort studies
- One often starts with weaker study designs to explore a hypothesis and then progresses to more rigorous designs to test the hypothesis

 REFERENCES

Cooper GS, Yan Z, Bowlin SJ, *et al.* (1998) An ecological study of the effectiveness of mammography in reducing breast cancer mortality. *Am J Public Health* **88**: 281–4.

Fleming PJ, Gilbert R, Azaz Y, *et al.* (1990) Interaction between bedding and sleeping position in the sudden infant death syndrome: a population based case-control study. *BMJ* **301**: 85–9.

Frankel S, Gunnell DJ, Peters TJ, *et al.* (1998) Childhood energy intake and adult mortality from cancer: the Boyd Orr cohort. *BMJ* **316**: 499.

Harris MI, Flegal KM, Cowie CC, *et al.* (1998) Prevalence of diabetes, impaired fasting glucose and impaired glucose tolerance in US adults. The Third National Health and Nutrition Examination Survey, 1988–1994. *Diabetes Care* **21**: 518–24.

Howe LD, Tilling K, Galobardes B, *et al.* (2010) Socioeconomic differences in childhood growth trajectories: at what age do height inequalities emerge? *J Epidemiol Community Health* doi:10.1136/jech.2010.113068

Jeffreys M, Sarfati D, Stevanovic V, *et al.* (2009) Socioeconomic inequalities in cancer survival in New Zealand: The role of extent of disease at diagnosis. *Cancer Epi Biomarker Prev* **18**(3): 915–21.

Jenab M, Bueno-de-Mesquita HB, Ferrari P, *et al.* (2010) Association between pre-diagnostic circulating vitamin D concentration and risk of colorectal cancer in European populations: a nested case-control study. *BMJ* **340**: b5500.

McBride WG (1961) Thalidomide and congenital abnormalities. *Lancet* ii: 1358.

Radican L, Wartenberg D, Rhoads GG, *et al.* (2006) A retrospective occupational cohort study of end-stage renal disease in aircraft workers exposed to trichloroethylene and other hydrocarbons. *J Occup Environ Med* **48**(1): 1–12.

van Duijnhoven FJB, Bueno-De-Mesquita HB, Ferrari P, *et al.* (2009) Fruit, vegetables, and colorectal cancer risk: the European Prospective Investigation into Cancer and Nutrition. *Am J Clin Nutr* **89**: 1441–52.

6

Genetic epidemiology

David M. Evans and Ian N. M. Day
University of Bristol

Learning objectives

In this chapter you will learn:

✓ what genetic epidemiology is;
✓ some of the major recent advances in genetics;
✓ the major methods for estimating heritability;
✓ the difference between monogenic and complex disease;
✓ the major gene mapping strategies;
✓ how genetic epidemiology can reveal unknown disease pathways;
✓ when it is appropriate to utilize genetic testing;
✓ the problems associated with genomic profiling and direct to consumer genetic testing.

What is genetic epidemiology?

Genetic epidemiology is the study of the role of genetic factors in determining health and disease in families and in populations, and the interplay of these genetic factors with the environment. Early in the field's history, investigators were primarily concerned with estimating the relative importance of **genes** and environment in disease aetiology. Today, the explosion of molecular genetic technology has propelled the field swiftly forward, so that the focus is now on identifying the actual functional genetic variants that predispose to disease. These advances are slowly starting to filter through to clinical practice. Genetic testing has been used increasingly over the past two decades to assist in the screening, carrier testing and/or diagnosis of various conditions. The continued pace of tech-nological advances promises a future in which an individual may be able to access their entire genetic sequence should they wish to, and to understand its implications. In parallel, population and case-based epidemiological studies will continue to reveal mechanisms and pathways underlying disease aetiology, which will become the drug targets of tomorrow.

This chapter outlines the scope of genetic epidemiology as well as some of the major advances that have occurred in the field over the last few years. Genetics contains a plethora of terms which may be unfamiliar to clinicians and students of epidemiology. Whilst a complete treatise on genetic nomenclature is beyond the scope of this text, we have provided the reader with a glossary of terminology that might prove useful. The reader is referred to any of the classic texts in genetics for a fuller explanation of these terms and basic genetics in general (see also the further reading at the end of this chapter and the glossary sections at the end of the book).

Epidemiology, Evidence-based Medicine and Public Health Lecture Notes, Sixth Edition. Yoav Ben-Shlomo, Sara T. Brookes and Matthew Hickman.
© 2013 Y. Ben-Shlomo, S. T. Brookes and M. Hickman. Published 2013 by John Wiley & Sons, Ltd.

What's new in genetics?

A high quality 'finished' sequence of the human genome was completed in 2003 to much fanfare. The *Human Genome Project* was the culmination of thirteen years' painstaking effort from scientists across the globe and millions of dollars of public and private funding. The end result was the ~3 billion base pair genetic sequence of a single reference individual. The importance of the human genetic sequence cannot be overemphasised, but essentially revolves around the simple premise that if the human genetic sequence is known, then its function can begin to be understood.

The focus then shifted to understanding variation in the sequence between different individuals. The human genome sequence is almost exactly the same in all people (i.e. 99.9%), but variation in this sequence between different individuals helps explain why some people are more susceptible to disease than others. The SNP Consortium was established in 1999 to discover and catalogue point mutations in the human genetic sequence called **single nucleotide polymorphisms** (SNPs) which are thought to occur roughly 1 to every 300 base pairs of sequence. Ten years on, there are well over 20 million SNPs in the database, and the focus has again shifted to how best to use this information for the mapping of human disease.

The *International HapMap Project* and its successor the *1000 Genomes Project* have continued SNP discovery efforts but have also focused on documenting the correlation between these genetic markers. Markers in close physical proximity to each other on the genome also tend to be correlated with each other, a phenomenon known as **linkage disequilibrium**. This means that if an individual has one **allele** at a particular locus, they are more likely to have a particular allele at an adjacent locus. The significance is that if the correlation between markers is known, then it is possible to genotype a subsample of markers across the genome (rather than all of them) and obtain approximately the same amount of genetic information, but at far reduced cost.

Monogenic versus polygenic diseases and traits

Monogenic diseases or **Mendelian diseases** are predominantly the result of a single gene. In other words, if an individual has a copy of the risk allele (in the case of a **dominant** disease/phenotype), or

the risk genotype (in the case of a **recessive** disease/phenotype) then they have a high probability of developing the disease. Monogenic diseases are typically transmitted through pedigrees according to simple Mendelian principles. Examples include cystic fibrosis, phenylketonuria, Huntington's Chorea, and sickle cell anaemia. Mendelian diseases (and their associated genetic variants) tend to be rare in populations because of the action of natural selection. That is, individuals who have the disease are often at a disadvantage in terms of survival and or reproduction and are therefore less likely to reproduce and hence pass deleterious variants on to their offspring. Thus the genetic variants that underlie Mendelian traits and diseases tend to be uncommon at the population level, especially diseases transmitted through a dominant mode of inheritance.

Polygenic diseases, as the name suggests, are caused by the combined action of many genes of small effect plus environmental influences. Polygenic diseases are sometimes referred to as *complex diseases* or common diseases. These diseases provide the biggest financial burden to society because of their high prevalence. Examples include asthma, coronary heart disease, hypertension, and types 1 and 2 diabetes. The genetic basis of these conditions is still being determined, but is likely to involve many common variants of small effect and potentially many as yet undiscovered rare variants of small effect also.

Whilst one doesn't think of contagious diseases as being polygenic, many infectious diseases also have a genetic component in that some individuals are more genetically susceptible to the disease than others. A classic example involves the CCR5 chemokine receptor gene mutation and susceptibility to infection with the Human Immunodeficiency Virus (HIV). Individuals who carry two copies of the *CCR5* Δ32 deletion at the locus have nonfunctioning CCR5 receptors. Since some strains of HIV use the CCR5 protein as a co-receptor to gain entry into cells, individuals who are homozygous for the mutation have strong resistance against these varieties of HIV.

Sometimes the distinction between monogenic diseases and complex diseases is not clear cut. Some complex diseases may contain a small proportion of individuals who are affected with the disease primarily because of the action of a single major gene. These forms of disease behave more like monogenic conditions (i.e. the disease often runs in families with a clear pattern of inheritance). For example, the majority of breast cancers are due to environmental factors of unknown aetiology. However, a small proportion of breast cancer cases are due to autosomal dominant mutations in the *BRCA1* and *BRCA2* genes. Both of these genes play an important role in maintaining genomic stability by facilitating the repair of double strand DNA breaks. Women who have deleterious mutations in either of these genes have substantially higher risk of breast and ovarian cancer (particularly early onset cancers) and of recurrent primary tumours. Hence families that carry these mutations tend to have many affected individuals, including males too.

Table 6.1 Heritability of some common diseases.

High heritability (>70%)	Moderate heritability (>30% and <70%)	Low heritability (<30%)
Type I diabetes	Coronary heart disease	Lung cancer
Schizophrenia	Rheumatoid arthritis	Breast cancer
Alzheimer's disease	Anorexia nervosa	
Bipolar disorder		
Ankylosing spondylitis		

Twin studies, adoption studies and migrant studies

Early investigations in genetic epidemiology were focused on determining the relative importance of genetic, shared environmental and unique environmental influences in the aetiology of complex traits and disease. The Classical Twin Design compares the similarity between **monozygotic (identical) twins** and the similarity between **dizygotic (nonidentical) twins**. The rationale is that since monozygotic twins share all their genes in common, whereas dizygotic twins share on average half their genes (i.e. the same as ordinary siblings), any excess similarity of monozygotic twins over dizygotic twins must be the result of genetic factors. The classical twin design enables investigators to estimate the proportion of variance in a trait due to genetic factors. This is called the **heritability** of a trait (Note, the heritability of a trait is actually usually defined as the proportion of variance explained by 'additive' genetic factors but this distinction is beyond the scope of this book).

Studies using the classical twin design have suggested that the vast majority of human traits and diseases are influenced by genetic factors to at least some extent. Table 6.1 shows the heritability of some common diseases as assessed using the Classical Twin Design. The implication is that a family history of disease or the presence of a first degree relative with disease is a potential risk factor for developing that condition. The increase in risk of disease will be proportionally greater for diseases that have high heritabilities.

The degree of similarity between family members may also be quantified by the **relative risk** (λ_R). This measure is different to the risk ratio (relative risk) defined in Chapter 2. The relative risk here is the risk that a relative 'R' of an affected proband will be affected with disease divided by the risk of disease in the general population. For example, it is common to estimate the sibling relative risk (λ_S), and the parent-offspring relative risk (λ_{PO}). If the relative risk equals one (i.e. no difference in risk between related and unrelated individuals), then it is unlikely that there is a genetic component to the condition. A weakness of the relative risk, is that whilst it provides evidence of familiality for a disease, it cannot be used to differentiate between genetic and common environmental sources of similarity between related individuals.

Adoption studies can also be used to estimate the relative contribution of shared environmental and unique environmental influences to a trait of interest. The rationale is that similarity between an individual and their adopted relatives can only be due to shared environment (since these individuals are genetically unrelated). Therefore it is possible to compare the phenotypic similarity between biological relatives and adopted relatives and so estimate the relative importance of shared and nonshared environmental components.

Migration studies compare the risk of disease between individuals in their native country, the risk amongst individuals who have migrated to a new country, the risk amongst second generation migrants and risks amongst the indigenous population. If the risk of disease among migrants and second generation migrants is the same as in their native country, but different from the indigenous group of the country they have migrated to, then this is strong evidence for a genetic component underlying disease.

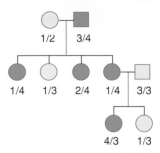

Genotypes for a marker with alleles {1,2,3,4}

Figure 6.1 A pedigree diagram illustrating the principles of linkage analysis.

Genetic mapping of diseases

Linkage analysis examines the co-segregation of genetic markers with a disease or trait of interest in pedigrees of related individuals. Consider the pedigree in Figure 6.1. All of the individuals in the family have been genotyped at a single marker of interest. The fact that the '4' allele appears to be transmitted along with the disease provides evidence that there is a disease causing variant on the chromosome somewhere close to the genotyped marker.

Females are denoted by circles and males by squares. Filled shapes represent affected individuals, and hollow shapes unaffected individuals. A horizontal line between two individuals denotes a mating, whereas a vertical line denotes a parent–offspring relationship. For example, the unaffected mother and the affected father at the top of the diagram have produced four daughters, three of whom have the disease of interest, and one who does not. One of the affected daughters mated with an unaffected male to produce two daughters, one who has the disease, and one who does not. Each individual has been genotyped at a single genetic marker, and their genotype for this marker is provided below them in the diagram. It appears as if the '4' allele at the genetic marker segregates with the disease in this pedigree.

Linkage analysis usually involves analysing several large pedigrees with many affected individuals. It is best suited to identifying genomic locations which harbour rare variants that have large effects – exactly the situation for most Mendelian Diseases. At the time of writing, the molecular basis of over 3,000 Mendelian conditions were known, many a direct result of genetic mapping through linkage analysis. These are all described in the online OMIM database (http://www.ncbi.nlm.nih.gov/omim).

Whilst linkage analysis has been spectacularly successful in elucidating the genetic basis of Mendelian diseases, it has been far less useful in determining the genetic basis of complex traits and diseases. Unlike Mendelian diseases, complex diseases are the result of many genes of small effect. Linkage analysis does not perform well in these situations and lacks power to detect common variants of small effect. Nevertheless linkage identified a handful of genetic variants (of moderately large effect) in several conditions including Crohn's disease and type II diabetes.

Genetic **association analysis** in contrast attempts to find a difference in the frequency of genetic variants (**genotype**) between individuals with disease (cases) and individuals without disease (controls) (**phenotype**). Statistical methods employed in traditional epidemiology are used to determine the significance and strength of the association between the genetic variant and disease. If a variant is more common in case individuals, then it is a risk variant that predisposes to disease. If a variant is less common in cases than in controls, then it is a protective variant that decreases the likelihood of disease. Association analysis is best suited to identifying common variants that convey moderate to high risk of disease (e.g. odds ratios >1.1).

Early applications of the method called **candidate gene association studies** examined one region of the genome at a time that were selected for their perceived functional relevance. Unfortunately, despite being based on quite well understood functional pathways, the vast majority of these early studies were underpowered to detect variants of small effect that underlie the majority of complex traits and diseases. Higher density SNP representation within genes and across the genome, as well as increased sample sizes, were all necessary steps to achieve power to detect effect sizes as small as those now recognised as typical for individual loci underlying complex traits. Perhaps the most notable example during this period was the discovery, through a combination of approaches, of the effect of *APOE* 4 alleles in predisposing late onset Alzheimer's disease (LOAD). Heterozygous carriers have a 2–3-fold increased risk of LOAD, whilst homozygotes have a 10–15-fold increased risk and a substantially decreased chance of reaching age 100 years without developing the disease.

Genome-wide association studies

Since 2005, rapid advances in genotyping technology have enabled researchers to perform **genome-wide association studies** (GWAS) which examine hundreds of thousands of genetic markers simultaneously across the genome, rather than just analysing a few markers in a candidate region (see Figure 6.2). Essentially thousands of individuals are genotyped on genome-wide SNP chips which contain assays for hundreds of thousands of **single nucleotide polymorphisms** (SNPs). SNPs refer to a single mutation in the DNA sequence that can

vary between individuals. Frequency of the genetic variants in cases and controls are compared just as in a candidate gene association study, the only difference being that very strong evidence of association is required to declare a genetic variant truly associated with the disease because of the hundreds of thousands of statistical tests performed (typically $p < 5 \times 10^{-8}$) (this reduces the chance of a *false positive* result also known as a **type I error**). The first such study identified a gene of remarkably large effect, *CFH*, which predisposed homozygotes to a $\sim$7 fold increased risk of age related macular degeneration.

In 2007, one of the very first GWAS, The Wellcome Trust Case Control Consortium (WTCCC), was published in the prestigious journal *Nature*. The WTCCC was a massive collaboration between 26 investigators across the United Kingdom whose aim was to determine the genetic basis of seven different common diseases: bipolar disorder,

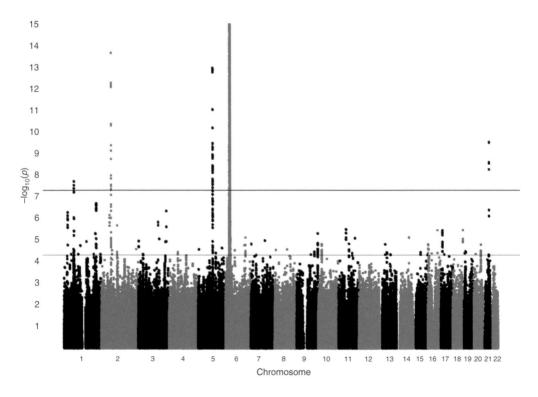

Figure 6.2 A 'Manhattan Plot' of a genome-wide association study of the autoimmune disease Ankylosing Spondylitis. Each point on the graph represents the results of a single statistical test. Position along the genome is plotted along the x axis with the alternating colours reflecting the different chromosomes. A measure of statistical significance is plotted on the y axis (in this case –log10(p-value)). Points above the upper line meet the criteria for 'genome-wide significance'. Points above the lower line are flagged for possible interest. A number of interesting regions are apparent on chromosomes 1, 2, 5, 6 and 21. These regions contain genetic variants which are associated with risk of Ankylosing Spondylitis.

coronary heart disease, Crohn's disease, hypertension, rheumatoid arthritis, and types one and two diabetes. The study was extraordinarily successful identifying genetic variants associated with coronary heart disease, Crohn's disease, rheumatoid arthritis and types I and II diabetes. The WTCCC generated substantial interest amongst the popular media, and paved the way for larger and more detailed genetic studies of these and other complex diseases.

Since this landmark study, genome-wide association studies have led to an explosion in knowledge regarding the genetic aetiology of many different complex traits and diseases. At the time of writing, over 1,200 genetic variants had been associated with 210 complex traits and diseases. This is a particularly impressive achievement given that only a handful of common disease variants had been mapped prior to 2005. Notably this has been the case for many conditions whose aetiology has been largely refractory to other approaches (e.g. bipolar disorder, schizophrenia). In some cases the analyses have identified genes and biological pathways that the scientific community had no idea were involved in aetiology of the condition previously. (See Chapter 7 for an example of how genetic variants are used to study nongenetic exposures using the principles of **Mendelian randomisation**.)

A classic example is Crohn's disease- a form of auto-immune inflammatory bowel disease. Several genome-wide association studies including the WTCCC have shown that genes involved in autophagy (the catabolic process through which the cells own components are degraded through lysosomes etc.) are important in Crohn's disease pathogenesis. Previous to this, the scientific community had not suspected that autophagy played a role in development of Crohn's disease. This result, and many others like it, have generated considerable interest amongst molecular biologists and prompted functional studies into these newly identified biological pathways. It is hoped that some of these pathways will become the drug targets of tomorrow.

Despite the fact that genome-wide association studies have helped identify over a thousand genetic variants underlying complex disease, for the majority of diseases, most of the heritability has yet to be explained. This phenomenon is termed the *missing heritability* and will likely occupy scientists' attention for at least the next decade. The focus of gene mapping is now turning from genome-wide association to *genome-wide sequencing* where individuals' entire genomes are sequenced and subsequently analysed. It is hoped that genome-wide sequencing will enable scientists to examine the effect of rarer genetic variation on health and disease, perhaps explaining some of the missing heritability.

Screening and testing for major genetic diseases

Genetic testing of monogenic diseases is employed in a diverse range of medical applications including prenatal and newborn screening, carrier testing and medical diagnostics. These tests typically have very good clinical validity in that the correlation between genotype and disease is very strong.

In the UK, the neonatal 'heelprick' test currently screens biochemically for five disorders, including four recessive diseases (cystic fibrosis, phenylketonuria, medium chain acyl CoA dehydrogenase deficiency and sickle cell disease). The first three represent mutations prevalent in those of Western European ancestry. The fourth is prevalent in malaria prone regions of the world due to favourable survival of sickle cell carriers infected with malaria, and hence in ethnic subgroups from those regions. In each instance, dietary or other medical interventions can change the course of the disease.

In populations with dominant founder mutations such as specific *BRCA* breast cancer gene mutations, specific mutation screening is offered. In other populations, screening is offered before marriage, for example, sickle cell carrier and thalassaemia carrier tests in regions where these are extremely prevalent. In populations with high consanguinity rates, screening for a wide range of recessive biochemical disorders is undertaken. Screening for Downs syndrome (trisomy of chromosome 21) is also widely used, especially in older mothers whose foetuses are at high risk (up to 1–5%), and involves a combination of biochemical and ultrasound criteria, with genetic follow-up for definitive proof.

Among autosomal dominant disorders, most general practices will have families with monogenic disorders such as hypercholesterolaemia, monogenic cardiomyopathies and cardiac conduction defects, and monogenic cancer risk genes particularly *BRCA1* and *BRCA2*. Each of these can readily claim the lives of young and middle aged adults but in each instance, there is some mix of treatment and surveillance options to mitigate risk. The least tractable disorder is probably Huntington's disease, and following counselling many at risk individuals in such families elect not to take the informative gene test even though pre-symptomatic diagnosis could advise reproductive or other life choices.

Genomic profiling of complex diseases

Whilst genetic testing has been of substantial clinical utility in predicting risk of monogenic disease, there are substantial problems in applying the same approach to complex traits and diseases. A major problem is that the effect sizes of the individual genetic variants underlying complex diseases are small, typically conferring only a small increased risk (i.e. odds ratios < 1.3). The predictive value afforded by genotyping a single variant is therefore likely to be negligible for the vast majority of common diseases. This has led to the idea of testing multiple genetic loci simultaneously, also called **genomic profiling**, which collectively may result in superior prediction of complex disease risk.

The last few years have witnessed a steep rise in the number of private companies attempting to exploit the idea behind genomic profiling by offering customers direct to consumer genetic testing. Companies offering these sorts of service typically advertise online, require their customers to complete an online order and then send off a buccal sample of their DNA for genome-wide SNP genotyping. Consumers are then provided with an online report that purports to indicate whether the individual is at increased risk, average risk or low risk from a number of different diseases. The cost of service is typically in the range of US$200 to US$1,000. Providers include 23andMe, DecodeMe and Navigenics.

At present, the predictive utility of genomic profiling is at best questionable for the vast majority of common diseases. A number of studies have shown empirically that different direct-to-consumer providers can give different predictions of increased, decreased or average risk for the same individual tested. There are even documented examples of instances where a company has postulated that an individual is at low risk of a condition, despite the individual already suffering from the disorder in question!

It is too early to say whether genomic profiling will prove to be clinically useful in the future, but it is worth noting that the predictive utility of any genetic test is bounded by the heritability of the disease by definition. For example, it would be impossible for a genetic test to predict more than 50% of the variance of a trait/disease that had a heritability of 50%. A more pertinent question might be whether genetic testing can add to prediction over and above knowledge of environmental risk factors, or whether genetic testing can offer clinically useful information over and above looking at the medical history of one's first degree relatives (i.e. parents and siblings). Since parents carry half, and siblings on average half a related individual's genetic material, examining one's first degree relatives should be considerably more informative (and far less costly!) than genotyping a few genetic variants which together only explain a small proportion of the overall heritability.

Promising examples of genetic testing in complex diseases

As discussed above, there are few complex diseases where genetic testing is currently of clinical utility. Two possible exceptions are Age-related Macular Degeneration (AMD) and Late onset Alzheimer's Disease (LOAD). Both conditions are unusual for complex diseases, in that genetic variants of largish effect have been identified for both. Several preliminary studies have shown that genotyping these variants can discriminate between affected and unaffected individuals with a moderate degree of accuracy. Nonetheless, clinicians have not yet found any reason to type the AMD risk gene, *CFH*. The predictive power is not high, there is no specific pre-disease preventative measure for which it would be a decision tool, disease diagnosis is clinical and *CFH* genotype offers no value for prognosis or monitoring. Similar arguments currently prevail for *APOE* in LOAD, although at risk individuals for dementia do argue that 'forewarned is forearmed' and that they might plan their lifestyles, spending and family decisions accordingly.

A notable success story has been using genetic testing to strengthen the clinical diagnosis of the auto-immune disease Ankylosing Spondylitis (AS). AS is a common inflammatory arthritis, affecting 4/1,000 white Europeans, which causes pain and stiffness predominantly of the spine, and can lead to inexorable progressive fusion (ankylosis) of the spine and other affected joints. The disease is polygenic, but unlike most other complex diseases, AS is strongly associated with a single genetic variant of large effect, HLA-B27, making it more similar to a Mendelian disease in some respects.

AS is particularly difficult to diagnose in its early stages since radiographic changes to the spine may not be obvious. Diagnosis is usually based on a combination of symptom report, family history, radiographic abnormalities, and in some cases, HLA-B27 testing. HLA-B27 testing in individuals of Northern European ancestry has approximately 90% **sensitivity** (i.e. the probability of a positive test result given the disease) and 90% **specificity** (i.e. the probability of a negative test result given the individual does not have the disease) making it a useful confirmatory tool in diagnosis of the condition. Whilst HLA-B27 testing is currently expensive (roughly £40 per assay), SNPs identified from genome-wide association studies which correlate with HLA-B27 status promise to cut the cost of this diagnostic assay significantly.

carriers of one of the variants in this gene have a ~17-fold increased risk of suffering the side effect implying that there may be some utility in screening individuals for carrying this mutation before commencing statin therapy in order to ensure caution with dosage and aggressive monitoring for side effects.

Another example concerns polymorphisms that affect warfarin metabolism. Warfarin dosing can be challenging given that there is marked variation in the drug response between individuals and it is necessary to maintain a narrow therapeutic range, in that blood levels which are too high can lead to bleeding and levels which are too low, clotting. There are two genes known to be involved in the metabolism of warfarin (*CYP2C9*) and vitamin K epoxide reductase (*VKORC1*). Genetic studies have identified two variants, *2 and *3, in *CYP2C9* that affect drug half-life. Specifically, break down of warfarin is reduced by ~40% in patients with the *2 variant and by ~90% in those with the *3 variant. Likewise, variation in *VKORC1* is responsible for about 20–25% variation in required warfarin dose. If an individual's genotype at these polymorphisms were known a *priori* then this knowledge could conceivably assist in warfarin dosing, helping to ensure that blood levels of the drug were maintained within the narrow therapeutic range, and reducing serious adverse effects of overdosing such as hemorrhagic stroke.

Pharmacogenomics

Pharmacogenomics is the branch of pharmacology which deals with the influence of genetic variation on drug response. Pharmacogenomics is in its early stages, but the ultimate aim is to be able to personally tailor drug choice, dosage and side effect profile according to an individual's genetic profile.

A recent discovery which holds promise in pharmacogenomics concerns genetic variants in the solute carrier organic anion transporter 1B1 (SLCO1B1) gene. Variants in this gene have been found to influence risk of statin-induced myopathy, a rare side effect of statin medication that results in muscle pain and weakness in association with elevated creatinine kinase levels, and in severe cases muscle breakdown, myoglobin release and risk of renal failure and death. Homozygous

Next generation sequencing (NGS) and the future

2009 witnessed the emergence of **next generation sequencing** (NGS) technology. It is now technologically possible to sequence the entire genome of an individual in a matter of days on desktop instrumentation (compare this to the 13 years it took hundreds of investigators from the Human Genome Project to sequence a single genome just a decade ago). Whilst the technology is expensive (~US$20,000 for a single genome), costs continue to fall rapidly, with a near term goal of US$1,000 per genome. While there remain major challenges in the assembly, data handling and interpretation of such data, a number of single gene or syndromic disorders previously uncharacterised by linkage mapping due to their rarity and sporadic or recessive nature, have now had their causal genes identified.

Internationally, there are population-based programmes ongoing both to define the depth of rarer sequence diversity (broadly 0.1–5% minor allele frequency) such as the *1000 Genomes Project* and also to start to relate such sequence diversity to disease phenotypes by resequencing the genome in large disease collections. While considerable challenges lie ahead, even in interpreting sequence differences in the coding region (exome) of the genome, this technology will further accelerate our knowledge of pathways and disease risk variants.

NGS also offers a new and high resolution approach to examine gene expression profiles and the methylation profiles of tissues and cells (methylation refers to the addition of a methyl group to cytosine bases in the DNA genetic sequence). In parallel, the necessary large tissue and cell banks are being built up in order to acquire further insight into the wide picture of genetic diversity and how it functionally relates to disease. In different cancer cell types, different types of mutagenesis have been observed consistent with the known risk factor exposures for that cancer, for example cigarette smoking in lung cancer and ultraviolet light in melanoma. Subphenotyping of cancer types has found diagnostic application, and through earlier approaches even before NGS, a range of markers have emerged into routine practice heralding a new era of stratified medicine in which genotype is being used both to classify diagnostically, for prognosis and to predict drug responses and side effects, and to monitor therapy. The arsenal of knowledge guaranteed to emerge over the next few years at the level of the general population and common diseases, augurs well for the widespread application of genetic epidemiological discovery to many areas of medicine.

> ### 🔑 KEY LEARNING POINTS
>
> - Genetic epidemiology is the study of the role of genetic factors in determining health and disease in families and in populations, and the interplay of these genetic factors with the environment
> - Twin studies, adoption studies and migration studies can be used to estimate the relative importance of genetic, common environmental and unique environmental factors in disease aetiology
> - Monogenic diseases are cause by a single gene, whereas polygenic diseases are typically the result of multiple genes of small effect and the environment
> - Linkage analysis examines the cosegregation between genetic markers and a trait of interest in pedigrees of related individuals. Association analysis examines the difference in frequency of a genetic variant between cases and controls
> - Genetic testing of monogenic diseases is employed in a diverse range of medical applications including prenatal and newborn screening, carrier testing and medical diagnostics
> - Genomic profiling is currently of limited utility because the variants assayed only explain a small proportion of the overall heritability of disease.

FURTHER READINGS

International HapMap Consortium (2005) A haplotype map of the human genome. *Nature* **437**: 1299–1320.

International Human Genome Sequencing Consortium (2001) Initial sequencing and analysis of the human genome. *Nature* **409**: 860–921.

Janssens ACJW, van Duijn CM (2010) An epidemiological perspective on the future of direct-to-consumer personal genome testing. *Investigative Genetics* **1**: 10–15.

Manolio T (2010) Genomewide association studies and assessment of the risk of disease. *N Engl J Med* **363**: 166–76.

Manolio T *et al.* (2009) Finding the missing heritability of complex diseases *Nature* **461**: 747–53.

Strachan T, Read A (2010) *Human Molecular Genetics*, 4th edn. New York: Garland Science Publishing.

Wang L, McLeod HL, Weinshilboum RM (2011) Genomics and drug response. *N Engl J Med* **364**: 1144–53.

Wellcome Trust Case Control Consortium (2007) Genome-wide association study of 14000 cases of seven common diseases and 3000 shared controls. *Nature* **447**: 661–78.

7

Investigating causes of disease

Debbie A. Lawlor and John Macleod
University of Bristol

Learning objectives

In this chapter you will learn:

- ✓ that causal factors are probabilistic and may be neither necessary nor sufficient to ensure a specific outcome;
- ✓ what are the possible noncausal reasons for observing an association between an exposure and outcome;
- ✓ criteria used to guide for considering whether an exposure is causal;
- ✓ analytical methods to help determine causality;
- ✓ special observational designs and the use of genetic instruments to help in making causal inferences;
- ✓ that the population researcher's and physician's perspective of a potential causal exposure may differ.

Epidemiology, association and causality

The nature of causation (or causes) is the subject of extensive philosophical discussion. A pragmatic definition of causation is something that, *of itself*, influences the probability of an outcome. Possible causes are often called **exposures**. Exposures can be something that increases or decreases the incidence of disease but can also include interventions (drugs or lifestyle) that can alter the prognosis once disease has been established. Some causes are *necessary*, i.e. exposure to them is essential if a given outcome is to happen; causes may also be *sufficient*, i.e. exposure to them *alone* is enough to ensure that the relevant outcome happens. Most important causes in epidemiology are, however, *neither necessary nor sufficient* – for example around 90% of lung cancer in the population is attributable to exposure to tobacco smoke but exposure to tobacco smoke is not necessary, nor is it sufficient to cause lung cancer. We, therefore, often are dealing with a probabilistic definition of causes identified by studying groups of many people. Examples of the kinds of

---

Epidemiology, Evidence-based Medicine and Public Health Lecture Notes, Sixth Edition. Yoav Ben-Shlomo, Sara T. Brookes and Matthew Hickman.
© 2013 Y. Ben-Shlomo, S. T. Brookes and M. Hickman. Published 2013 by John Wiley & Sons, Ltd.

causal questions that we would like to answer in epidemiology are:

(1) Will the incidence of heart disease be reduced if people exercise more?

(2) Will treatment with antiretrovirals result in patients with HIV infection living longer on average?

(3) Does screening for Chlamydia infection reduce infertility in women in a population?

When we observe an association between an exposure (A) and an outcome (B), before assuming that this reflects causation we always consider four possible noncausal explanations.

(1) **Chance** – statistical tests provide evidence for or against the null hypothesis (see Chapter 4)

(2) **Bias** – i.e. systematic error in measurement of the exposure or outcome we are investigating (see chapter 3 for more details).

(3) **Reverse causation** – In this case rather than exposure A leading to outcome B the reverse is true (B in fact causally influences A). To reliably conclude that A is a possible cause of B we need information with a longitudinal dimension that allows us to confirm that the occurrence of A precedes the occurrence of B. This rules out cross-sectional or 'snapshot' data (see Chapter 5) and can also be difficult to ascertain in case-control studies (see Chapter 5). Reverse causality can still occur in prospective cohort studies if there are individuals in the cohort with undiagnosed disease at baseline. This is less of an issue in prospective studies that recruit participants very early in their life course (for example, birth-cohort studies) where recruitment and measurement of the relevant factors occurs before the onset of most pathological processes. However, for most diseases there is a **latency period** between pathology and clinical diagnosis, which may last many years and during which patients may experience pathophysiological changes (for example, atherosclerosis prior to a heart attack will increase a variety of inflammatory markers that one can measure in the blood (Timpson *et al.*, 2005)) or symptoms that could affect behaviour. One approach that can be used to reduce this problem is to remove early years of follow-up (when undiagnosed prevalent cases are most likely to occur and generate an association that is possibly due to reverse causality). The value of this was illustrated in data from two large prospective cohort studies that showed removing deaths from the first five years and correctly controlling for masking confounding by smoking increased the strength of association between overweight and obesity and reduced survival in adults (Lawlor *et al.*, 2006). However, to do this requires very large sample sizes or large collaborations (such as the *Emerging Risk Factor Collaboration* (Wormser *et al.*, 2011) that includes several hundreds of thousands of participants and in most publications removes the first 5–10 years of follow-up from analyses) where data are meta-analysed (see Chapter 12) to provide adequate statistical power and precision of estimates.

(4) **Confounding** – i.e. when the association apparent between exposure and outcome is explained by the fact that they are both independently associated with a third factor outside of any common causal pathway (see Chapter 3). For example, greater consumption of fruit and vegetables is associated with lower risk of coronary heart disease. However, it is possible that some or all of the association between fruit and vegetable consumption and coronary heart disease is explained by those who eat more fruit and vegetables being less likely to smoke cigarettes and more likely to exercise a lot than those who eat less fruit and vegetables, and that these risk factors are the 'real' reason why heart disease is less in groups who eat more fruit and vegetables.

Observational studies generally provide clues about causality. The ultimate test of a cause is experiment – if manipulation of a putative causal exposure under controlled experimental conditions leads to a predicted change in an outcome then this is the most convincing evidence of causality as one can control for bias and both known and unknown confounders (see Chapter 11).

Conditions for causality

In 1965 Austin Bradford Hill detailed '*viewpoints*' or 'conditions for causality' (Phillips and Goodman, 2006) for assessing evidence of causation in observational studies. These are listed in Box 7.1. Whilst these are often described as causal criteria (with the implication that they should be used as a checklist to rule causality in or out) it should be noted that Hill did not intend them to

---

Box 7.1 Austin Bradford Hill causal considerations (1965).

(1) **Strength:** 'First on my list I would put the strength of the association.' Although Hill gave useful examples of situations in which strong associations (e.g. sweeping chimneys and scrotal cancer and cigarette smoking and lung cancer) suggested causation he also noted 'We must not be too ready to dismiss a cause-and-effect hypothesis merely on the grounds that the association appears to be slight.'

(2) **Consistency:** 'Has it [the observed association] been repeatedly observed by different persons, in different places, circumstances and times?' If it has, this increases the likelihood the association is causal.

(3) **Specificity:** As a motivating example here, Hill described the increased incidence of lung and nasal cancers in nickel miners. Not only were the age specific incidences considerably greater in nickel miners compared to the general population, but these increased incidences were only present in workers who had started working prior to 1923, when a number of changes had taken place in the refinery. Furthermore, other cancers and causes of death were similar between the miners and the general population. Hill noted: 'the association is limited to specific workers and to particular sites and types of disease and there is no association between the work and other modes of dying, then clearly that is a strong argument in favour of causation'.

(4) **Temporality:** i.e. 'Which is the cart and which the horse? This is a question which might be particularly relevant with diseases of slow development. Does a particular diet lead to disease or do the early stages of disease lead to those peculiar dietetic habits?'

(5) **Biological gradient:** 'If the association is one which can reveal a biological gradient, or dose-response curve, then we should look most carefully for such evidence.'

(6) **Plausibility:** 'It will be helpful if the causation we suspect is biologically plausible. But this is a feature I am convinced we cannot demand.

What is biologically plausible depends upon the biological knowledge of the day.'

(7) **Coherence:** 'On the other hand the cause-and-effect interpretation of our data should not seriously conflict with the generally known facts of the natural history and biology of the disease.' Coherence he suggested could be supported by population (ecological) evidence – for example the emerging sex difference in lung cancer supported a causal role for smoking as this was considerably more common in men than women in the early part of the twentieth century.

(8) **Experiment:** 'Occasionally it is possible to appeal to experimental, or semi-experimental evidence.' This would include randomised controlled trials but also 'natural experiments', where for example an exposure was removed and there was a marked decline in the disease outcome.

(9) **Analogy:** 'In some circumstances it would be fair to judge by analogy.' i.e. He was suggesting that causality was more likely when other similar exposures or risk factors also produced the same or a very similar outcome. 'With the effects of thalidomide and rubella before us we would surely be ready to accept slighter but similar evidence with another drug or another viral disease in pregnancy.'

Comments in quotation marks are taken directly from Hill's original paper (A. B. Hill (1965) The environment and disease:Association or causation? *Proc R Soc Med* **58**: 295–300).

---

be used in this way stating in his paper that 'None of my nine viewpoints can bring indisputable evidence for or against the cause-and-effect hypothesis and none can be required *sine qua non*' (Hill, 1965).

Approaches to examining causality

A number of different analytical approaches have been suggested for testing causality in observational studies, including the use of **Mendelian randomisation** which will be considered later in the chapter. Two other analytical approaches are an examination of sensitivity and specificity of associations.

Sensitivity analyses

Once an association has been examined using conventional multivariable approaches with adjustment for all measured potential confounding factors, a **sensitivity analysis** can be undertaken to address the question – what magnitude of associations between a potential confounder and the risk factor and outcome of interest would be required to explain or reverse the observed (multivariably adjusted) association? Once this has been established the authors of a paper (and the readers) can consider whether it is likely that such a confounder exists. One problem with this approach is that it can fail to take account of the possibility that there may be many unmeasured confounders each with a small effect but jointly producing a very large (due to confounding) association. For example, it has been shown that the combined effects of 15 characteristics that were each independently associated with vitamin C and coronary heart disease, could in combination produce an odds ratio between vitamin C and coronary heart disease of 0.60 that was completely due to these confounding factors, despite the fact that individually each would only produce relatively modest vitamin C-heart disease associations (Lawlor *et al.*, 2004).

Specificity of association

Bradford Hills suggested that the specificity of an association (that is, that the exposure is not associated with multiple outcomes) was a useful criteria for judging causation. Some exposures are likely to be causally related to more than one health outcome. For example, cigarette smoking causes increased risk of lung cancer and cardiovascular disease. However, in large cohort studies where one can look at associations with many outcomes, this is a potentially very powerful and cheap method for exploring causality. This approach involves thinking of an outcome that you would absolutely not expect to be associated with the outcome of interest other than through confounding and then comparing the association of the exposure you are interested in with this new outcome to the main association you think might be causal. This is an underused method in epidemiology. One of the best examples of this approach was a study that tested the hypothesis that hormone replacement therapy (HRT) causally reduced risk of coronary heart disease in women (long before any randomised controlled trials

(RCT) had been done). The researchers argued that if the hormone replacement-cardiovascular disease association was not explained by socioeconomic confounding then one would not expect an association between hormone replacement and deaths due to accidents. Accidental deaths (as are cardiovascular deaths) are more common in individuals from poorer socioeconomic backgrounds but there is no biological reason to consider that HRT protects one from accidents. Instead they found that women who reported using HRT were half as likely to die of cardiovascular disease and accidental deaths (both odds ratios 0.5). They concluded that socioeconomic confounding was a strong candidate for explaining the association with cardiovascular disease (Petitti *et al.*, 1986). This notion was supported by a subsequent large RCT that failed to find any cardiovascular benefit.

Alternative observational methods for determining causality

It is generally accepted that an RCT provides the strongest evidence for a causal association (see Chapter 11). However, there are a number of important causal epidemiological research questions for which it is not feasible or ethical to conduct an RCT. There are a variety of alternative observational approaches that can be used (see Chapter 17 for assessing public health interventions) that go some way to consider residual confounding. We will describe four different methods: parental–offspring comparisons; within and between sibling (including twin) comparisons; cross-cohort comparisons; Mendelian randomisation.

Parental–offspring comparisons

Do maternal exposures during pregnancy have a direct biological effect on offspring outcomes, through influencing the intrauterine environment in which the foetal development of the offspring occurs? Comparing maternal–offspring to paternal–offspring associations is useful for examining whether maternal pregnancy exposures acting via intrauterine mechanisms are causally related to offspring outcomes. If there were a direct biological effect of intrauterine exposure on offspring health status, then the link with offspring health should be much stronger for exposure among mothers than for exposure among fathers. For example, maternal smoking during pregnancy is associated with lower offspring birth-weight, whereas smoking by the father during pregnancy is only weakly associated (and entirely abolished after adjustment for maternal smoking).

Within and between sibling (including twin) comparisons

Examining associations within sibling-pairs is a useful method for controlling for any potential confounding factors that are identical or very similar in siblings (such as socioeconomic position), whether these confounding factors are actually measured in the study or not. For example, in a large record linkage study of 386,485 singleton-born Swedish men from 331,089 families, the association between birthweight and gestational age with blood pressure at age 18 was examined (Lawlor *et al.*, 2007). Lower birth-weight and earlier gestational age were associated with higher systolic blood pressure (measured at age 17–19) both within siblings and between nonsiblings. The similarity in associations within siblings and between unrelated people suggested that this association in general cohorts/populations was equally unlikely to be explained by confounding background socioeconomic position. Twin studies also can control for potential confounding by genetic factors (by comparing within twin pair associations between monozygotic (identical for genetic variation in nucleic DNA) and dizygotic twins) (see Chapter 6). For example, the Swedish Twin Registry (Bergvall *et al.*, 2007) found that in monozygotic (genetically identical) pairs, a 500g lower birth-weight was associated with an odds ratio of hypertension of 1.74 (95% CI 1.13, 2.70), and within dizygotic pairs the equivalent odds ratio was 1.34 (95% CI 1.07, 1.69). The similarity of associations within both types of twins provides evidence that the inverse association of birth-weight with hypertension is independent of genetic and environmental factors shared by twins including maternal and fetal genotype (except foetal mitochondrial DNA), socioeconomic factors and gestation.

Cross-cohort comparisons

This approach is based in part on Bradford-Hill's viewpoint that a consistent association 'observed by different persons, in different places, circumstances and time' increases the likelihood that the association is causal. For example, a large number of cohort studies have suggested that individuals who are breast fed (as opposed to formulae fed) have lower BMI, blood pressure and other cardiovascular risk factors and higher IQ in later life, but these associations could be explained by confounding. In a cross-cohort comparison (one from the UK and one from Brazil), the authors found no association between family income and breastfeeding in the Brazilian cohort, but a strong positive association in the UK cohort, with higher rates of breastfeeding observed in the higher income groups (Brion *et al.*, 2011). Children who were breastfed had higher IQ scores in both studies, with the magnitudes of these associations being similar. By contrast in the UK cohort children who were breastfed had lower BMI and blood pressure even after adjustment for income and other potential confounders, whereas there were no such associations in the Brazilian cohort. These findings suggest that the association of breastfeeding with IQ is causal but those of breastfeeding with BMI and blood pressure are likely to be confounded.

Mendelian randomisation studies

Mendelian randomisation studies have been likened to a 'natural' RCT. Mendelian randomisation is the term that has been given to studies that use genetic variants in observational epidemiology to make causal inferences about modifiable (nongenetic) risk factors for disease and health-related outcomes. Such studies exploit the facts that (a) genetic variants are rarely associated with the wide range of socioeconomic and lifestyle characteristics that confound many nongenetic observational association studies and (b) because genes are allocated at conception their associations with later outcomes cannot be explained by reverse causality.

For example, it is well established that heavy alcohol use by pregnant women has adverse effects on health outcomes in their children, including effects on cognitive development, though such exposure and effects (such as foetal alcohol syndrome) are rare. Many women, however, do drink some alcohol during pregnancy, generally at moderate levels. Current public health advice is conflicting with some official bodies suggesting moderate alcohol use during pregnancy is 'safe' and others advising abstention. In part this is because of inconsistencies in the evidence base: with some studies suggesting that moderate alcohol use during pregnancy was associated with *better* cognitive outcomes in children compared to abstention from alcohol, but such an association may be confounded.

The metabolism of alcohol in the body is influenced by several genes. A particular rare variant of the alcohol dehydrogenase gene (which makes it difficult to break down alcohols that are otherwise toxic) is consistently associated with abstinence from alcohol (compared to moderate use). This genetic variant is not associated with mothers' education or other socioeconomic characteristics and nor is it associated with other lifestyle characteristics such as smoking. This genetic instrument was used to investigate effects of maternal alcohol use on children's cognitive outcome in a large UK based birth cohort study (Fitz-Simon *et al.*, 2010). In this study, in keeping with results from previous studies, the children of mother's reporting moderate alcohol use during pregnancy had higher IQ scores and did better in standard school tests than the children of mothers reporting abstinence from alcohol. Moderate alcohol using mothers however were also more affluent, more educated, less likely to smoke, more likely to take exercise and to have a healthy diet, in other words were confounded by a range of possible influences on their children's cognition.

Adjusting for these factors in statistical models lessened but did not abolish the apparently beneficial effects of alcohol on the cognitive outcomes studied – illustrating the limitations of statistical adjustment and problem of 'residual confounding'. When the children of women whose genotype would predispose them to abstinence from alcohol were compared to children of women without this genotype a completely opposite picture emerged to that seen using the classical epidemiological approach. Children of women with the 'abstinence gene' did better in school tests and had higher IQ scores than women with 'moderate use' genes. This is convincing evidence that maternal alcohol use actually exerts a damaging effect on children's cognitive development, an effect that only became apparent with use of a study design – Mendelian randomisation – able to adequately address the issue of residual confounding. Other examples include studies that have examined the causal role of c-reactive protein, BMI, triglyceride levels and lipoprotein(a) with cardiovascular risk factors and events; the association of fat mass with bone density and of folate acid/homocystein levels with mental health outcomes.

Causality at the level of the population – implications for the doctor-patient relationship

The overall impact of an exposure on disease in the population depends on the size of the risk and the prevalence of the exposure. From a public health/population perspective a rare exposure with a high risk ratio may be less important than a common exposure with a modest or low risk ratio. The population attributable risk (also known as aetiological fraction which is related to the risk difference as explained in Chapter 2) is one measure of the impact of an exposure on disease at the population level.

Epidemiology, however, cannot fully address the question of the cause of an individual's disease. This applies equally for RCTs as for observational epidemiological studies. For clinicians this has important implications. When informing patients about whether a particular treatment or lifestyle change will be beneficial to them we need to be honest and acknowledge that (currently) there is no scientific means of being sure about this. What can be said is, for example, amongst all adults with high blood pressure (hypertension) there will be a greater proportion who have a stroke in the future than amongst all adults without hypertension and that if all those with hypertension are treated with antihypertensive medication the proportion of strokes in that group will be reduced. We can also attach approximate probabilities to these outcomes given different scenarios based on epidemiological evidence.

Patients are not unfamiliar with notions of probability and chance. For example, in our clinical experience it is actually unusual for patients to invoke the apocryphal 'Uncle Norman' who smoked 60 cigarettes a day till he was run over by a bus at the age of 90 as evidence that smoking is harmless. Patients appear to accept, as we regularly remind them, that 50% of lifelong smokers die from a smoking related cause but they also seem to realise that this means 50% of smokers will not die from a smoking related cause and that the difference between the two groups may be substantially a product of chance. Uncle Norman was clearly lucky in relation to the consequences of his smoking, if unlucky with regard to the fatal bus.

Clinicians have often struggled with the question of how best to use epidemiological evidence to inform conversations with patients. For example, in relation to treatment discussions an approach popularised by the Evidence Base Medicine movement involves use of the 'number needed to treat' (see Chapter 11) the reciprocal of the absolute risk difference. This metric, within certain assumptions, tells a patient how many people have to take a particular treatment – typically for a year – for one of them to avoid the adverse outcome the treatment is intended to avert. How helpful patients find this information in relation to their own treatment decisions is unclear. In our experience, one of the most frequent questions asked of doctors by patients is still, 'What would you do if you were me?'

The wider issue here is perhaps the fact that there are many things patients would like us to be certain about that we cannot know and we have to be honest that we cannot know whether they will fall into the group who do not die because of their smoking or not. We also cannot know if they will be the one (amongst the number needed to treat) who will avoid the adverse outcome if they all took a particular treatment. Acknowledging and discussing uncertainty is a fundamental part of both clinical medicine and public health. For more discussion of this idea visit the understanding uncertainly website http://understandinguncertainty.org/.

KEY LEARNING POINTS

- It can be difficult to decide whether an observational association truly reflects causation and one must consider chance, bias, confounding and reverse causation
- Being able to test causation in observational studies is important because for many possibly important risk factors it is not possible to do an RCT. Even where it is possible to do an RCT, these costly experimental studies are best done where there is good prior support for the intervention being likely to be causal
- There are a number of criteria that can help weigh up the evidence around causality
- Sensitivity analyses and the specificity of an association may help determine if associations are causal or are due to residual confounding
- Various epidemiological designs such as parent-offspring, within and between sibling designs, cross-cohort comparisons and Mendelian randomisation can be helpful in controlling for unmeasured confounders and testing causality
- Mendelian randomisation studies use our new knowledge about genetics so that genetic variants are used as instruments to test causal associations similar to an RCT
- Translating probabilities of risk to an individual patient consultation can be challenging and highlights the degree of uncertainty behind clinical decision making

📖 REFERENCES

Bergvall N, Iliadou A, Johansson S, *et al.* (2007) Genetic and shared environmental factors do not confound the association between birth weight and hypertension: a study among Swedish twins. *Circulation* **115**(23): 2931–8.

Brion MJA, Lawlor DA, Matijasevich A (2011) What are the causal effects of breastfeeding on IQ, obesity and blood pressure? Evidence from comparing high-income with middle-income cohorts. *International Journal of Epidemiology* **40**: 670–80.

Fitz-Simon N, Lewis SJ, Davey Smith G, *et al.* (2010) Alcohol consumption during pregnancy and children's cognitive development: Mendelian randomization study using the ADH1B genotype. *Reproductive Sciences.* **17**(3 supplement): 99A.

Hill AB (1965) The environment and disease: association or causation? *Proc R Soc Med* **58**: 295–300.

Lawlor DA, Hart CL, Hole DJ, Davey Smith G (2006) Reverse causality and confounding and the associations of overweight and obesity with mortality. *Obesity* **14**: 2294–2304.

Lawlor DA, Hübinette A, Tynelius P, *et al.* (2007) Associations of gestational age and intrauterine growth with systolic blood pressure in a family-based study of 386 485 men in 331,089 families. *Circulation* **115**(5): 562–8.

Lawlor DA, Davey Smith G, Bruckdorfer KR, *et al.* (2004) Observational versus randomized trial evidence. *Lancet* **364**: 755.

Petitti DB, Perlman JA, Sidney S (1986) Post-menopausal estrogen use and heart disease. *N Engl J Med* **315**: 131–2.

Phillips CV, Goodman KJ (2006) Causal criteria and counterfactuals; nothing more (or less) than scientific common sense. *Emerg Themes Epidemiol* **3**: 5.

Timpson NJ, Lawlor DA, Harbord RM, *et al.* (2005) C-reactive protein and metabolic syndrome: Mendelian Randomization suggests associations are non-causal. *Lancet* **366**: 1954–9.

Wormser D, Kaptoge S, Di Angelantoinio E, *et al*; the Emerging Risk Factor Collaboration (2011) Separate and combined associations of body-mass index and abdominal adiposity with cardiovascular disease: Collaborative analysis of 58 prospective studies. *Lancet* **28**: 23–30.

 ## FURTHER READING

Davey Smith G, Ebrahim S (2003) 'Mendelian randomisation': can genetic epidemiology contribute to understanding environmental determinants of disease? *International Journal of Epidemiology* **32**: 1–22.

Davey Smith G, Ebrahim S (2005) What can mendelian randomisation tell us about modifiable behavioural and environmental exposures? *BMJ* **330**(7499): 1076–9.

Davey Smith G, Lawlor DA, Harbord R, Timpson N, Day I, Ebrahim S (2008) Clustered environments and randomized genes: a fundamental distinction between conventional and genetic epidemiology. *PloS Medicine* **4**: e352-doi:10.1371/journal.pmed.0040352.

Lawlor DA, Leary S, Davey Smith G (2009) Theoretical underpinning for the use of intergenerational studies. In: Lawlor DA, Mishra GD (eds), *Family Matters. Designing, Analysing and Understanding Family-based Studies in Life Course Epidemiology*. Oxford: Oxford University Press, pp. 13–38.

Strully KW, Mishra GD (2009) Theoretical underpinning for the use of sibling studies in life course epidemiology. In: Lawlor DA, Mishra GD (eds), *Family Matters: Designing, Analysing and Understanding Family-based Studies in Life Course Epidemiology*. Oxford: Oxford University Press, pp. 39–56.

 ## MORE ADVANCED READING

Greenland S (1996) Basic methods for sensitivity analysis of biases. *International Journal of Epidemiology* **25**: 1107–16.

Lawlor DA, Harbord RM, Sterne JAC, Timpson NJ, Davey Smith G (2008) Mendelian randomization: using genes as instruments for making causal inferences in epidemiology. *Statistic in Medicine* **27**:1133–63.

Ripatti S (2009) Random effects models for sibling and twin-based studies in life course epidemiology. In: Lawlor DA, Mishra GD (eds), *Family Matters. Designing, Analysing and Understanding Family-based Studies in Life Course Epidemiology*. Oxford: Oxford University Press, pp. 229–50.

 ## WEBSITES

Useful websites for finding out more about how to assess and think about causality:

Understanding uncertainty – http://understandinguncertainty.org/

Bad Science – http://www.badscience.net/

Self-assessment questions – Part 1: Epidemiology

Q1 The following are haemoglobin levels (in 100 g/L) for six women: 106, 114, 119, 121, 122, 131. If the observed value of 131 is mistakenly recorded as 1,311 g/L, what will be the effect on the summary measures for this study? (Select one or more answers.)
  (a) an increase in the median
  (b) an increase in the mode
  (c) an increase in the mean

Q2 The prevalence of asthma is widely thought to be increasing, but reasons for this are unclear. An epidemiologist undertook a cross-sectional study of asthma in Bristol by measuring the current frequency of doctor diagnosed asthma as well as nocturnal cough and wheeze in a sample of 11-year-old children attending private schools. The questionnaire also included questions on a family history of asthma as well as other sociodemographic variables. Which of the following statements about the study are true? (Select one or more answers.)
  (a) By knowing what percentage of all children currently have asthmatic symptoms one can calculate the incidence of asthma.
  (b) The results can be generalised to all 11-year-olds living in Bristol
  (c) The researchers should have randomly selected the study sample from the study population.
  (d) The data can be used to examine whether there is an association between asthma symptoms and a family history
  (e) The prevalence was calculated as 5 per 100 or 5%. This means for every 100 11-year-olds in this sample, 5 currently have symptoms.

Q3 The width of a confidence interval will get smaller when which of the following changes occur? (Select one or more answers.)
  (a) The desired level of confidence increases
  (b) The sample size 'n' increases
  (c) The between-subject variation in the outcome variable increases
  (d) The standard error gets larger
  (e) None of the above

Q4 Which of the following statements about P values are true? (Select one or more answers)
  (a) The 'P' stands for Possible value
  (b) The P value measures the strength of the evidence against a null hypothesis
  (c) The larger the P value the stronger the evidence against the null hypothesis
  (d) A P value can be as large as infinity
  (e) The P value is the probability of getting a difference at least as big as the one in our study, if the null hypothesis is true.

Q5 Which of the following is NOT a Mendelian disease?
  (a) Sickle-cell anaemia
  (b) Huntington's chorea
  (c) Hypertension
  (d) Cystic fibrosis

Q6 Which of the following is *not* a reason why genetic testing of complex diseases is likely to be limited?
  (a) The predictive utility of genetic testing is limited by the disease's heritability
  (b) Most genetic loci underlying complex diseases are of small effect

Epidemiology, Evidence-based Medicine and Public Health Lecture Notes, Sixth Edition. Yoav Ben-Shlomo, Sara T. Brookes and Matthew Hickman.
© 2013 Y. Ben-Shlomo, S. T. Brookes and M. Hickman. Published 2013 by John Wiley & Sons, Ltd.

Table QA.1 Numbers of patients receiving seasonal flu vaccine.

	A/H1N1 patients (n = 60)	Other patients (n = 180)	Odds ratio (95% CI) adjusted for socio-economic status	P value
Received seasonal flu vaccine	8	53	0.27 (0.11 to 0.66)	P < 0.001

(c) Many genetic loci typically underlie complex diseases

(d) Technology is not yet sufficiently advanced to assay genetic polymorphisms

Q7 Which of these study designs provides investigators with the *best* estimate of a complex trait's heritability?
(a) Classical twin design
(b) Migration study
(c) Adoption study
(d) Genome-wide association study

Q8 What is the difference between a standard deviation and a standard error?

Q9 What is the difference between a reference range and a confidence interval?

Q10 Seasonal influenza vaccination and risk of influenza A/H1N1 (swine flu)
(modified from Garcia-Garcia L, Valdespino-Gomez JL, Lazcano-Ponce E *et al.* (2009) *BMJ* **339**: b3928)

In 2009, a new strain of influenza A virus subtype H1N1, was reported in the southwestern United States and Mexico. In the absence of a specific A/H1N1 vaccine, researchers in Mexico investigated whether vaccination with the 2008–9 seasonal influenza vaccine was associated with the risk of influenza A/H1N1. The study identified all people who had attended the National Institute of Respiratory Diseases in the preceding two months who had tested positive for influenza A/H1N1. People were also selected

who had received medical care at the Institute for a diagnosis other than influenza during the study period. The administration of seasonal flu vaccination for the 2008–9 winter season was investigated by face to face or telephone interviews with the patients or close relatives.
(a) What is the study design employed here? Is it the best design for this research question?
(b) What is the null hypothesis?
(c) What is measurement bias and what type commonly affects this type of study design?
(d) What is meant by selection bias in the context of this study? Might this be present here?
(e) From Table QA.1, interpret the odds ratio, confidence interval and P value. Would you recommend the use of the seasonal flu vaccine to reduce the risk of A/H1N1?

Q11 Risk assessment for respiratory complications in paediatric anaesthesia
(modified from von Ungern-Sternberg BS, Boda K, Chambers NA *et al.* (2010) *The Lancet* **376**: 773–83)

Respiratory adverse events in children are one of the major causes of morbidity and mortality during paediatric anaesthesia. The aim of this study was to determine whether there is an association between a family history of asthma and occurrence of

Table QA.2 Perioperative respiratory events amongst children with a family history of asthma compared to those without.

	Unadjusted risk ratio (95% CI)	P value	Adjusted risk ratio* (95% confidence interval)	P value*
History of asthma	2.93 (2.21 to 3.89)	<0.001	1.86 (1.41 to 2.46)	<0.001

*Adjusted for age and sex of child and smoking status of parents.

Table QA.3 Differences in ultrasound markers of atherosclerosis.

	Least Deprived	Most Deprived	Difference in means, adjusted for age and sex (95% CI)	P value
Mean (SD) carotid intima-media thickness (mm)	0.68 (0.10)	0.70 (0.10)	−0.02 (−0.03 to −0.01)	<0.001

perioperative (during anaesthesia or recovery) respiratory adverse events. 9,297 children who had general anaesthesia for surgical or medical interventions at a hospital in Perth, Australia, between February 2007 and January 2008 were included in the study. Before surgery a questionnaire was completed based on the medical history of the patient, including whether there was a family history of asthma. Children were monitored during anaesthesia and time in the recovery room, for any respiratory event including laryngospasm, bronchospasm, airway obstruction, oxygen desaturation (<95%), and severe or sustained cough.

(a) What is the exposure variable and primary outcome variable? What types of variable are they?

(b) What is the study design employed here? Is it the most appropriate design for this research question?

(c) From Table QA.2, describe and interpret the effect of a having a family history of asthma on risk of perioperative adverse events. Interpret the risk ratio, confidence interval and P-value for the unadjusted analysis.

(d) In the adjusted analysis the authors control for age and sex of the child and smoking status of the parents. Choose one of these variables and explain why it has been adjusted for. What effect did the adjustment have on the results and why?

Q12 Differences in atherosclerosis according to area level socioeconomic deprivation (adapted from Deans KA, Bezlyak V, Ford I *et al.* (2009) *BMJ* **339**: b4170)

Ill health is more prevalent in areas of relative social deprivation, as exemplified by the higher incidence of coronary heart disease in such areas. The aim of this study was to examine the relationship between social deprivation and ultrasound markers of atherosclerosis (thickening of the artery walls), which is a sign of coronary heart disease. Participants were randomly selected from the UK electoral roll. Based on their address (postcode), individuals were assigned a deprivation level of 1 to 5, using a national system. Carotid intima-media thickness was measured via ultrasound (the thicker the intima-media, the higher the amount of atherosclerosis).

(a) From Table QA.3, interpret the results for the relationship between carotid intima-media thickness and socioeconomic deprivation.

(b) What other explanations for the association between socioeconomic deprivation and atherosclerosis seen in this study should be considered before concluding that the relationship is causal? How likely is each of these?

Part 2

Evidence-based medicine

8

An overview of evidence-based medicine

Yoav Ben-Shlomo and Matthew Hickman
University of Bristol

Learning objectives

In this chapter you will learn:

- ✓ what is meant by the term evidence-based medicine (EBM);
- ✓ common misperceptions about EBM;
- ✓ the existing evidence behind EBM;
- ✓ the EBM domains;
- ✓ the stages of EBM practice.

One of the major changes in the teaching and practice of medicine has been the rapid growth in **evidence-based medicine (EBM)**, which is reflected in this new edition by now having its own subsection. As Paul Glasziou and colleagues have argued 'a 21st century clinician who cannot critically read a study is as unprepared as one who cannot take blood pressure or examine the cardiovascular system' (Glasziou *et al.*, 2008). Evidence-based medicine, previously referred to as **clinical epidemiology**, has grown rapidly over the last 20 years, partially as a result of better-quality research, systematic methods to accumulate and summarise these data, and easy access to high-quality databases such as the Cochrane collaboration or EBM-based guidelines that allow health professionals to quickly access evidence when considering patient management.

What is evidence-based medicine?

There are several different definitions of EBM but we favour a modified version of what was proposed by David Sackett and colleagues as 'the conscientious, explicit and judicious use of current best evidence in making decisions about the care of individual patients *and improving the health of populations*' (words in italics have been added by us to incorporate a broader public health dimension). EBM uses the **hierarchy of evidence** (see Chapter 5, Box 5.1) to help weigh up the relative importance of different types of evidence. It is common today to usually use evidence from more than one study by systematically collating and

---

Epidemiology, Evidence-based Medicine and Public Health Lecture Notes, Sixth Edition. Yoav Ben-Shlomo, Sara T. Brookes and Matthew Hickman.

synthesising data across all studies using the technique of meta-analysis (see Chapter 12 for more details). In general, randomised trials are placed above clinical experience but EBM does not ignore such experience especially in the absence of good-quality trials. When applying the hierarchy of evidence it is important to appreciate that the ordering only applies if the evidence from each type of design comes from well-conducted studies as otherwise this may be misleading. For example, a poorly conducted trial may be less valid than data from a high-quality cohort study.

This definition of EBM counters some common misperceptions about EBM highlighted in Box 8.1. Listening to patients' preferences is an essential aspect of good medical practice and these can be formally used in EBM by allocated scores (**utilities**) to different outcomes or side effects so that a treatment may appear to have more benefit than harm in one patient than another (see Chapter 13 on health economics). This prevents a cookbook approach and at the end of the day the health professional may choose to follow a different management path than that promoted by a guideline, though they should be able to justify this, especially if this goes against national or international evidence-based guidelines. For example the National Institute for Health and Clinical Excellence in March 2012 had guidance covering 363 interventional procedures, 249 technology appraisals, 147 clinical guidelines and 36 Public Health guidance documents. It also provides an evidence-based portal through its own website NHS Evidence (https://www.evidence.nhs.uk/).

One of the biggest criticisms about practising EBM is that it is simply not practical in a busy clinic. This is a valid point though electronic access to high-quality summary reports (e.g. critically appraised topics CATs) is making this less relevant and enthusiasts such as Paul Glasziou have demonstrated how they can practice EBM in 'real time' as long as one has internet access and access to key databases and journals.

One of the key terms in the above definition is the word *explicit*. This means that EBM compared to non-EBM practitioners should use quantitative data to help them and patients decide on management options. Whilst both types of practitioners may recommend the same drug treatment, the EBM doctor is more likely to explain the harms and benefits by using information on the *number needed to treat* or the probability or risk of an event. This *probabilistic* way of thinking can be difficult for some doctors (see Chapter 7) as it describes an average effect which may not reflect the experience of the patient in front of them. Variation (also known as heterogeneity) in the potential benefits of treatment has been used as a criticism of EBM, but it is possible to take this into account to some degree by translating the relative benefits of treatment (e.g. relative reduction in mortality 20%) into absolute benefits taking into account individual patient characteristics. For example, after a myocardial infarction, the benefits of aspirin in terms of preventing future cardiovascular events outweigh any harm from bleeding side effects. This is because the absolute risk of another cardiovascular event is high in this population. However, in a younger healthier patient with a much lower absolute risk, the harm from aspirin may now outweigh the potential benefits, even if in relative terms the benefits are the same. Advice concerning aspirin is constantly under review as new evidence emerges. For example, recent research suggests that aspirin may now also reduce the risk of cancer and metastatic spread.

Box 8.1 Misperceptions about EBM.

- EBM denigrates clinical experience
- Ignores patient values
- Promotes an unthinking cookbook approach to medicine
- A cost-cutting tool
- An ivory tower research exercise not suited to everyday clinical practice
- Leads to therapeutic nihilism in the absence of evidence from randomised controlled trials

Source: Modified from Straus SE, McAlister FA (2000) Evidence-based medicine: a commentary on common criticisms. *CMAJ* 163: 837–41.

The EBM Domains

Any clinical encounter can result in a number of issues that are amenable to an EBM approach. These are grouped into the five domains as listed in Table 8.1. These will all be covered in the subsequent chapters other than aetiology which we have addressed in the epidemiology section.

Table 8.1 EMB domains.	
Patient or commisioner/ policy-maker	**EBM domain**
What is making me feel unwell?	Diagnosis
Will this have any long term consequences?	Prognosis
Why did I get ill?	Aetiology
What can you do to help me?	Treatment
Are any interventions worth paying for? (commissioners, policymakers)	Cost-effectiveness

For example on a paediatric ward round you may encounter a child who has recently been admitted with their first episode of shortness of birth which was subsequently diagnosed as asthma. One could consider the following questions: what is the most useful diagnostic test (or set of tests) to differentiate asthma in a child from other causes of shortness of breath? Will this child have persistent asthma symptoms in adulthood and will this have any long term functional limitations? Did exposure to allergens or chemicals in childhood have a role in their development of asthma? Will maintenance of inhaled steroids reduce the likelihood of future admissions and are they cost-effective?

What is the evidence that EBM changes the way we practise?

Paradoxically, the evidence behind the benefits of EBM is limited mainly because it is very hard to undertake research to evaluate EBM teaching. A **systematic review** (see Chapter 11) undertaken in 2004, on postgraduate training found 23 articles but most were either before and after comparisons, or nonrandomised comparison studies with only two being randomised controlled trials. Not surprisingly, most assessed knowledge and found that some form of teaching (workshop, journal club, seminars) improved understanding and knowledge and critical appraisal skills. Some studies, but not all, found that those taught EBM had more positive attitudes to EBM and behaviour change but when this was integrated with clinical practice. None of the studies measured changes in health outcomes but they were not designed to do this.

Stages of EBM

There are several steps in being a EBM practitioner. These are (a) formulate a clear question, (b) search for the evidence, (c) critically appraise the evidence, (d) apply the evidence (or not) to the individual patient or population as appropriate.

Sackett coined the acronym PICO (**P**atient, **I**ntervention, **C**omparator, **O**utcome) as a helpful tool in formulating EBM questions. For aetiological and prognostic questions the intervention is equivalent to the risk or prognostic factor and for diagnostic questions this would be a diagnostic test. Table 8.2 gives two examples.

The process of finding evidence is becoming simpler as more databases are being developed that synthesize the evidence though it may be necessary to go back and read the original primary studies. To undertake a full bibliographic database search (e.g. Medline) can be very time-consuming and will identify many irrelevant papers as well as potentially missing some important

Table 8.2 Two examples of EBM questions.	
Prognostic question	
Patient	A 77-year-old woman with hypertension, and moderate left ventricular enlargement
Intervention	Presence of nonrheumatic atrial fibrillation
Comparator	Absence of nonrheumatic atrial fibrillation
Outcomes	Risk of stroke risk over a specific time period (5 or 10 years) (both as relative risk and absolute risk difference)
Therapy question	
Patient	A 77-year-old woman with nonrheumatic atrial fibrillation, hypertension, and moderate left ventricular enlargement
Intervention	Warfarin therapy
Comparator	No therapy or aspirin
Outcomes	Reduction in stroke risk versus increase in bleeding complications (relative and absolute risks)

Source: Modified from Rosenberg W, Donald A (1995) Evidence based medicine: an approach to clinical problem solving. *BMJ* **310**: 1122.

ones depending on the quality of the search strategy. Databases such as the Cochrane collaboration (http://www.cochrane.org/) are extremely valuable though are mainly limited to intervention studies. In the United Kingdom, the NHS evidence website (https://www.evidence.nhs.uk/) provides a portal to other sources of evidence including EBM guidelines as produced by the National Institute for Health and Clinical Excellence (http://www.nice.org.uk/). Other databases are focussed on certain disciplines or settings such as BestBets (http://www.bestbets.org/) that was initially designed for emergency room or on-call problems (http://www.eboncall.org/).

Having found some evidence, it will be necessary to appraise it to some degree. The subsequent chapters should provide you the knowledge and skills to undertake such an appraisal but like most things you only get good by constant practice. If one is fortunate, then there will already be a published high-quality meta-analysis or highly respected guideline that cites the evidence. It should be noted that much 'evidence' is based on expert or consensus opinion which may or may not be evidence-based and even in the presence of evidence can be biased. For example a comparison of 24 Cochrane reviews with industry sponsored or other reviews found that the industry sponsored reviews were more likely to recommend the therapy and with fewer reservations than the Cochrane reviews even though the cited evidence was essentially the same (Jorgensen *et al.*, 2006).

Different groups of experts may produce different guidelines and this may reflect cultural attitudes or financial incentives to patient management. Even apparently neutral evidence should be read with some caution. For example a review of 53 Cochrane reviews highlighted some problems with the reviews in almost a third with about a fifth where the authors felt that the conclusions of the review were not supported by the evidence (Olsen *et al.*, 2001). There are now a myriad of methodological checklists (see http://www.unisa.edu.au/cahe/CAHECATS/ such as CONSORT (single trials), STROBE (observational studies), PRISMA (systematic review and meta-analysis of trials) MOOSE (meta-analysis of observational studies), STREGA (genetic association studies. Such checklists are a useful tool to remind you of what key aspects of design, analysis and interpretation can go wrong but should not be applied blindly as there is a danger of rejecting evidence on the basis of some methodological problem even when this

may mean the real benefit could actually be even more substantial.

Finally there is the issue of **generalisability** and whether the evidence is relevant to the individual patient that generated the question in the first place. There will always be an element of subjectivity in such a decision and in some cases one will need to apply external knowledge such as pharmacology to decide whether the findings in one population should or should not apply to another. For example, many therapeutic trials do not include many ethnic minority patients so a benefit seen in a Caucasian population may or may not apply to South Asian patients. In this case a judgement has to be made about whether it is reasonable or not to generalise such findings and a discussion about the uncertainty with the patient should be undertaken.

Often an EBM search can highlight the absence of evidence or only the presence of poor quality evidence. For example a review of 109 inpatients seen in Oxford for one month found that for 53% of primary treatments there was trial evidence to support therapy. In an additional 29% there was convincing nonexperimental evidence and in 18% there was no evidence that therapy was better than no therapy (Ellis *et al.*, 1995). This figure is likely to be less good for some other specialties e.g. primary care. Such *absence of evidence does not mean evidence of absence* and should act as a stimulus for future research to help fill such evidence-based gaps.

 KEY LEARNING POINTS

- Study designs should be evaluated according to the hierarchy of evidence

- EBM tries to use evidence in an explicit fashion by quantifying benefits and harms using concepts such as the numbers need to treat

- The five EBM domains are diagnosis, prognosis, aetiology, treatment and cost-effectiveness

- PICO is a useful acronym to help formulate clear EBM questions

- EBM is undertaken according to the following stages: formulating a question, search for evidence, appraising evidence and applying the evidence, if appropriate

- Generalisability of evidence as well as considering patients' preferences is important in applying evidence to individuals

REFERENCES

Ellis J, Mulligan I, Rowe J, *et al.* (1995) Inpatient general medicine is evidence based. *Lancet* **346**: 407–10.

Glasziou P, Burls A, Gilbert R (2008) Evidence based medicine and the medical curriculum. *BMJ* **337**: a1253.

Jørgensen AW, Hilden J, Gøtzsche PC (2006) Cochrane reviews compared with industry supported meta-analyses and other meta-analyses of the same drugs: systematic review. *BMJ* **333**: 782–5.

Olsen O, Middleton P, Ezzo J, Gøtzsche PC, Hadhazy V, Herxheimer A, *et al.* (2001) Quality of Cochrane reviews: assessment of sample from 1998. *BMJ* **323**: 829–32.

Rosenberg W, Donald A (1995) Evidence based medicine: an approach to clinical problem solving. *BMJ* **310**: 1122.

Straus SE, McAlister FA (2000) Evidence-based medicine: a commentary on common criticisms, *CMAJ* **163**: 837–41.

 FURTHER READING

Sackett DL, Strauss SE, Scott Richardson W, Rosenberg W, Brain Haynes R (2000) *Evidence-based Medicine: How to Practice and Teach EBM*, 2nd edn. London: Churchill Livingstone.

9

Diagnosis

Penny Whiting and Richard M. Martin
University of Bristol

Learning objectives

In this chapter you will learn:

- ✓ what is meant by diagnosis;
- ✓ to understand the need for evidence-based diagnosis;
- ✓ to define and calculate measures of accuracy;
- ✓ to recognise potential biases in diagnostic test accuracy studies;
- ✓ to decide if the results will be clinically useful for future patient management.

What is diagnosis?

When a patient develops a new set of symptoms he/she generally wants to know 'What is wrong with me?' Making an accurate diagnosis is essential to ensure that a patient receives appropriate treatment and correct information regarding their prognosis. There are also other less tangible effects of an accurate diagnosis, including relief and reassurance if the diagnosis is mild, and the start of the process of coming to terms with the condition if a more severe diagnosis is made. For example, in the area of multiple sclerosis, there is some evidence that patients benefit emotionally from receiving an early diagnosis (Koopman and Schweitzer, 1999; Mushlin *et al.*, 1994).

What is a diagnostic test?

Tests are defined very broadly to include any procedure, or test, that tries to confirm or identify the presence or absence of a target condition. This includes what we traditionally think of as tests, for example, biochemical measurements, imaging, but also taking a patient's history, doing a physical examination and administering questionnaires. Tests are ordered for a variety of reason (a) detection/exclusion of disease (to rule in or rule out a potential diagnosis), (b) **screening**, (c) to make decisions regarding treatment and/or prognosis e.g. an angiogram will confirm diagnosis of heart disease but may also help decide if surgical intervention is required, (d) patient reassurance,

---

Epidemiology, Evidence-based Medicine and Public Health Lecture Notes, Sixth Edition. Yoav Ben-Shlomo, Sara T. Brookes and Matthew Hickman.
© 2013 Y. Ben-Shlomo, S. T. Brookes and M. Hickman. Published 2013 by John Wiley & Sons, Ltd.

(e) following a protocol, (f) medico-legal or financial reasons. Sometimes it is easier to order a test than think about why we are doing it but inappropriate testing can lead to a waste of money that could be better used elsewhere, pain and discomfort and wasted time for patients, possible distress and anxiety as a result of a false positive test, and wrongly reassured patients with false negative tests.

Why study evidence-based diagnosis?

New diagnostic tests may be introduced into practice if they

(1) reduce the risk to the patient (for example, MRI scan rather than brain biopsy);
(2) are less invasive or painful for the patient (for example, ultrasound scan rather than venogram for diagnosing deep vein thrombosis);
(3) are cheaper, quicker or easier to perform;
(4) or are more accurate than existing tests.

Before introducing a new test into clinical practice we need to evaluate it to determine whether it works: i.e. does it distinguish patients with and without the disease and does it benefit the patient? Diagnostic research can be considered to follow the following stages:

- **Stage I – development**
  Do patients with the target condition have different results from 'normal' individuals? Is it safe?
- **Stage II – testing**
  In an appropriate group (spectrum) of patients, does the test accurately distinguish between those with and without the target condition?
- **Stage III – clinical effectiveness**
  Do patients who undergo the test have better health outcomes than similar patients who do not?

Evaluating test accuracy

Classical diagnostic test accuracy studies compare the results of the test of interest, the **index test**, to those of a **reference standard** (also referred to as gold standard), which should be the best available method of determining disease status. Imagine you see a patient with a possible diagnosis of rheumatoid arthritis (RA) but are not sufficiently confident to make the diagnosis based on their clinical features alone. You decided to find out whether there are any studies reporting on new diagnostic tests for RA. You search PubMed (http://www.ncbi.nlm.nih.gov/pubmed) using the term 'rheumatoid arthritis' combined with PubMed's inbuilt clinical query for diagnosis studies (see 'Finding evidence on diagnostic accuracy studies', p. 82, below). You identify a study that evaluated the accuracy of anti-cyclic citrullinated peptide (anti-CCP) antibodies for making an early diagnosis of RA (van Gaalen *et al.*, 2005) and are considering ordering this test to help with the diagnosis.

The results of the anti-CCP test (index test) are compared to the results of the American College of Rheumatology (ACR) criteria after a period of follow-up (reference standard) and the results are cross-tabulated to produce a 2×2 table of results (Figure 9.1). Based on this, estimates of the accuracy of the anti-CCP test can be calculated. These can be expressed as statistics such as **sensitivity**, **specificity**, **predictive values** and **likelihood ratios**.

Sensitivity and specificity

Sensitivity refers to the proportion of those with the condition who have a positive test result (better sensitivity lower percentage with false negative rate). Specificity refers to the proportion of those without the condition who have negative test results (better specificity lower percentage with false positive result).

Sensitivity	TP/(TP + FN)	82/(82 + 71) = 54%
Specificity	TN/(FP + TN)	301/(13 + 301) = 96%

Sensitivity and specificity measures are computed along the columns of the 2×2 table.

A problem with these measures is that they are not directly clinically relevant – they tell us the likelihood of a patient having a positive/negative test result given that they do/do not have the condition (this may sometimes only be found out at death). What we want to know is how likely the person is to have the target condition based on their test results, before we are sure of the final diagnosis. As a

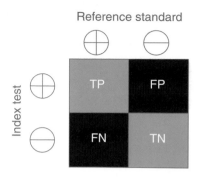

	Reference standard	
	⊕	⊖
Index test ⊕	TP	FP
Index test ⊖	FN	TN

	Final diagnosis	
	RA present	RA absent
Anti-CCP result ⊕	82	13
Anti-CCP result ⊖	71	301

True positives (TP)	Correct positive test result – number of diseased persons with a positive anti-CCP test result
True negatives (TN)	Correct negative test results – number of nondiseased persons with a negative anti-CCP test result
False positives (FP)	Incorrect positive test result – number of nondiseased persons with a positive anti-CCP result
False negatives (FN)	Incorrect negative test result – number of diseased persons with a negative anti-CCP result

Figure 9.1 2 × 2 tables showing the cross-classification of index test and reference standard results. (a) General table. (b) Table based on example of anti-CCP for diagnosing RA.

general rule, tests with high sensitivity can be used to rule out the target condition (because the proportion of false negative tests is low), while those with high specificity can be used to rule in the target condition (because the proportion of false positive tests is low). Useful acronyms for remembering how these apply in practice are SpPin and SnNout (Pewsner *et al.*, 2004) (see Figure 9.2).

Consider our example of anti-CCP for diagnosing RA. We can see that specificity is very high at 96% whereas sensitivity is less good at 54% suggesting that anti-CCP may be useful for ruling in a diagnosis of rheumatoid arthritis as only 4% of patients without RA will have a misleading positive result but is not good for ruling out the diagnosis as 46% of patients with RA will have a misleading negative result.

The best diagnostic test will be one with a very high sensitivity and specificity but there is usually a trade-off, like a see-saw, between sensitivity and specificity, so improving specificity reduces sensitivity and vice versa. However, both high sensitivity and specificity is not always essential depending on how the test will be used in practice.

High sensitivity – In a screening programme (see Chapter 19) the focus of the initial screening test will be on ruling out rather than ruling in disease. A test with a very high sensitivity is therefore required to avoid falsely reassuring patients by telling them they do not have the disease of interest. For example within the breast cancer screening programme, false positives are more acceptable, though this can cause patient anxiety, as those who are test positive on the initial screening

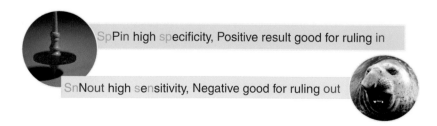

SpPin high specificity, Positive result good for ruling in

SnNout high sensitivity, Negative good for ruling out

Figure 9.2 SpPin and SnNout.

test will be referred for more definitive tests to diagnose breast cancer (7 of every 8 women recalled after a positive mammogram do not have breast cancer).

High specificity – If a test result will be used to decide on initiating treatment that is expensive, invasive and/or toxic, it is important that the diagnostic test (often a definitive test) is highly specific so that one does not treat patients who are subsequently found to not have disease. For example, only women with histologically proven breast cancer after a needle biopsy are offered major breast surgery, potentially toxic chemotherapy or radiotherapy.

Pre-test probability of the target condition

The **pre-test probability** of the target condition can be defined either at the population or the patient level. At the population level it corresponds to the prevalence of the target condition. For a diagnostic cohort study (a study that enrols patients with suspected disease rather than patients whose disease status is known), it can be obtained from the 2 × 2 results table. The pre-test probability of the target condition for an individual patient can be estimated based on their clinical history, results of physical examination, and clinical knowledge and experience. This corresponds to the expected prevalence of the condition in a series of similar patients.

Consider our example: we can estimate the prevalence of RA (population-level pre-test probability) in the population in which the study was carried out as 33%. However, based on the history and physical examination combined with our clinical knowledge and experience we estimate that the patient we have seen has a 45% probability of having RA (individual-level pre-test probability).

test result has the target condition, while the Negative Predictive Value (NPV) is the probability that a patient with a negative test result does not have the target condition. Predictive values are thus directly clinically relevant. However they are strongly dependent on the population pre-test probability, as well as the test's sensitivity and specificity. For example, the prevalence of the target condition is likely to be higher in hospital than general practice settings, and the positive predictive value will be correspondingly higher in hospital settings, even if test sensitivity and specificity are the same. For this reason, the PPV and NPV estimated from a primary diagnostic test accuracy study should not be assumed to apply in other settings, for which the pre-test probability of disease may be very different.

For a given pre-test probability (population or individual), it is possible to calculate the post-test probability of disease if data on the sensitivity and specificity of the test are available. A convenient way to do this is via likelihood ratios – this is discussed further below. When evaluating a diagnostic test it can be helpful to think about how the test modifies the probability of the target condition. By considering how the pre-test probability is modified to give a post-test probability of the target condition, for either a positive or negative test, we can assess the clinical usefulness of the test.

Based on our example, in which the population pre-test probability was 33%, the PPV is 86%, so that patients who test positive have an 86% probability of having RA. The negative predictive value is 81%, so that patients who test negative have a 19% probability of having RA. This supports the conclusions above, based on test sensitivity and specificity, that anti-CCP is more useful for ruling in than ruling out a diagnosis of RA. In this population, its accuracy may not be sufficient to either confirm or exclude RA. However, because

Population pre-test probability (prevalence)	(TP + FN)/ (TP + FP + FN + TN)	(82 + 71)/ (82 + 13 + 71 + 301) = 33%

Positive and negative predictive values and prevalence/pre-test probability of disease

our patient's pre-test probability of having RA is 45% we cannot apply these PPV and NPV estimates directly to him. However as we shall see, we can

Positive predictive value (PPV)	TP/ (TP + FP)	82/ (82 + 13) = 86%
Negative predictive value (PPV)	TN/(FN + TN)	301 / (71 + 301) = 81%

The Positive Predictive Value (PPV) is the (post-test) probability that a patient with a positive

calculate the predictive value for our specific patient using other methods.

Likelihood ratios

A **likelihood ratio** (LR) describes how much more likely a person with the target condition is to receive a particular test result than a person without the target condition. Thus positive LRs describe how much more likely a person with the condition is to receive a positive test than a person without the condition, and negative LRs how much more likely a person with the condition is to receive a negative test than a person without the condition. A positive LR is usually a number greater than 1 up to infinity and a negative LR usually lies between 0 and 1. Thus a LR of 1 is equivalent to making a diagnosis by tossing a coin as you will correctly identify 50% of patients with disease but wrongly diagnose 50% of those without disease.

Likelihood ratios have some powerful properties which make them more clinically useful than other measures of accuracy (Deeks and Altman, 2004) as they can be combined with any estimate of the pre-test probability of disease to give an estimate of the post-test probability of disease. This is done using the mathematical relationship known as Bayes' theorem. The pre-test probability of disease is transformed into the pre-test odds of disease. It is then multiplied by the likelihood ratio to give the post-test odds of disease which can then be transformed into the post-test probability of disease.

The statistical equations used to do this, given a positive test result, are shown in Box 9.1. There are also more simple methods of doing this than working out the calculation by hand. There are online

Positive likelihood ratio (LR +)	$(TP/(TP + FN))/ (FP/(FP + TN))$ or sensitivity / (1 −specificity)	$0.54 /(1−0.96) = 13.5$
Negative likelihood ratio (LR−)	$(FN/(TP + FN))/ (TN/(FP + TN))$ or (1 − sensitivity)/specificity	$(1−0.54)/0.96 = 0.48$

In our example of the anti-CCP test, a likelihood ratio of a positive test result of 13.5 means that a person with RA is 13.5-fold more likely to receive a positive test result than a person without RA; in contrast, a likelihood ratio of a negative test result of 0.48 means that a person with RA is only half as likely to receive a negative test result than a person without RA. The further away the value is from 1 (in either direction) the more useful the test. Table 9.1 summarises the interpretation of different values of likelihood ratios and shows where the anti-CCP test lies in relation to other well known diagnostic 'tests' (including symptoms elicited during clinical history taking).

These examples highlight that clinical histories often have the highest likelihood ratios (e.g. a typical history of angina). The likelihood ratios indicate that a CT scan (likelihood ratio = 26) is better than an ultrasound scan (likelihood ratio = 5.6) for diagnosing pancreatic disease, although the greater accuracy of CT scans needs to be weighed against the fact that they are more expensive. A negative sputum for TB is associated with only a small reduction in the likelihood ratio – this is because many cases with TB often fail to grow the TB bacillus (*Mycobacterium tuberculosis*) in bacterial culture.

calculators (e.g. http://www.dokterrutten.nl/collega/LRcalcul.html) where you simply enter the pre-test probability of disease and the likelihood ratio, the post-test probability of disease is then calculated. Alternatively, there is a tool known as the Fagan's nomogram which can be used to easily obtain estimates of the post-test probability of disease for any given combination of the pre-test probability of disease and likelihood ratio. Fagan's nomogram is shown in Figure 9.3; electronic versions are also available online (e.g. http://www.cebm.net/index.aspx?o=1161). Using the nomogram you simply select a pre-test probability of disease and likelihood ratio, join these via a straight line and extrapolate the line to find the post-test probability of disease. The pre-test probability of disease is the prevalence of disease, or the probability of the disease before the test is carried out. For any particular patient, this can be estimated based on clinical knowledge and experience in a particular setting.

Now consider our example. Based on our 2 × 2 table the positive likelihood ratio is 13.5 and the negative likelihood ratio is 0.48. If we believed that our patient had a pre-test probability of disease of 45% based on their clinical presentation and the results of the physical examination (different

Table 9.1 Interpretation of likelihood ratios with some examples.

LR	Effect on likelihood of disease	Example	Value
>10	Strong increase	CAGE questionnaire, 3 positive responses (alcohol dependency)	250
		Typical history of angina (coronary heart disease)	115
		Positive sputum (TB)	31
		Abnormal CT scan (pancreatic disease)	26
		Positive anti-CCP (RA)	13.5
5–10	Moderate increase	Abnormal ultrasound scan (pancreatic disease)	5.6
2–5	Small increase	Chest radiograph (known lung cancer)	3.5
1–2	Minimal increase	Prostate specific antigen test > 4 ng/ml (prostate cancer)	1.3
		Mammogram (occult breast cancer)	1.2
1	No change		
0.5–1.0	Minimal decrease	Negative sputum (TB)	0.79
0.2–0.5	Small decrease	Negative anti-CCP (RA)	0.48
<0.2	Strong decrease	Normal ventilation-perfusion scan (pulmonary embolus)	0.1
		White blood cell count $<7 \times 10^9$ cells/L (appendicitis)	0.1
		Negative renal sonogram (gross hydronephrosis)	0.02

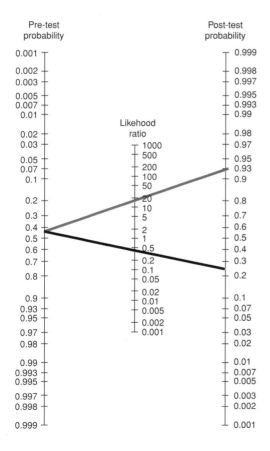

Figure 9.3 Fagan's nomogram.
Note: blue line indicates a positive test result; dark red line indicates a negative test result.

clinicians may have different opinions on this probability), then if his anti-CCP result was positive his post-test probability would have increased to 92% whilst if it was negative it would have decreased to 28% (see Figure 9.3 or Box 9.1 which calculates the post test probability for a positive test result). Our conclusions based on the predictive values obtained directly from the 2×2 table, differed from those that we obtained by tailoring our calculations specifically to our individual patient based on their pre-test probability of disease highlighting the importance of not relying on predictive values reported in primary studies.

> **Box 9.1 Calculation of post-test probabilities using likelihood ratios.**
>
> Pre-test probability $= p = 0.45$
> Pre-test odds $= p/(1 - p) = 0.45/0.55 = 0.82$
> Post-test odds $=$ pre-test odds $\times$ likelihood ratio
> Post-test odds $= o = 0.82 \times 13.5 = 11.07$
> Post-test probability $= o/(1 + o) = 11.07/12.07$
> $= 0.92$

Can I trust the results of a study?

If a study is not well designed, estimates of diagnostic accuracy can differ from the true accuracy,

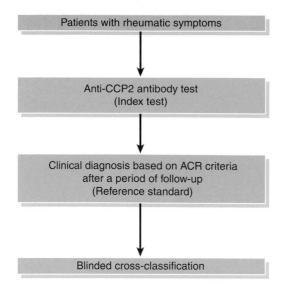

Figure 9.4 Ideal diagnostic accuracy study, based on anti-CCP for the diagnosis of rheumatoid arthritis.

and so you may not be able to trust the results of the study. Figure 9.4 illustrates the ideal diagnostic accuracy study, based on our example of anti-CCP for the diagnosis of rheumatoid arthritis.

Deviations from this design can lead to biased estimates of accuracy. When evaluating the potential for **bias** there are four key areas to consider: *patient selection, test execution, the reference standard,* and *patient flow* (Whiting *et al.,* 2010).

Patient selection

In an ideal study, all consecutive patients, or a random sample (*spectrum*) of patients, with suspected disease should be enrolled and criteria for enrolment should be clearly stated. For our example, a good diagnostic accuracy study will enrol a group of consecutive patients with rheumatic symptoms suggestive of RA but in whom the diagnosis cannot yet be confirmed – this is known as a **diagnostic cohort** design (Figure 9.5a). Studies that avoid inclusion of 'difficult to diagnose patients' or 'grey cases' may result in overoptimistic estimates of accuracy. For example, in the extreme case, if a study evaluating the accuracy of anti-CCP enrols patients with definite RA and a control group of healthy people and uses these patients to derive estimates of accuracy this may lead to overoptimistic estimates of both sensitivity and specificity. This is known as **diagnostic**

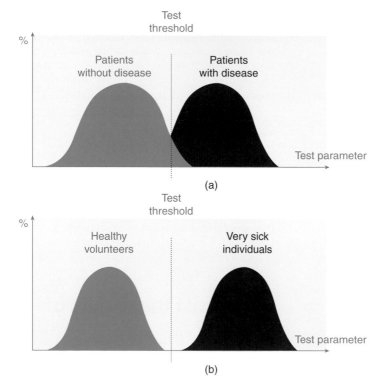

Figure 9.5 Distribution of test results in patients with and without disease: (a) Diagnostic Cohort Study (unbiased design); (b) Diagnostic Case-Control Study (potentially biased design).

case-control design (Figure 9.5b) and results in spectrum bias.

Index test

Ideally, the results of the index test should be interpreted without knowledge (**blind**) to the results of the reference standard. If the person interpreting the index test is influenced by knowledge of the results of the reference standard this may lead to inflated measures of diagnostic accuracy. The extent to which this may affect test results will be related to the degree of subjectivity in the interpretation of the test result. The sequence of testing will also affect the potential for bias. In our example, the anti-CCP test is a biochemical test and so the potential for bias is less than had it been a test with more subjective interpretation such as an X-ray. As the reference standard (ACR criteria) is applied after a period of follow-up the anti-CCP test result will most likely be interpreted before knowing whether or not the included patients have RA, reducing the potential for bias.

Reference standard

The reference standard is the method used to determine the presence or absence of the target condition. Estimates of diagnostic accuracy are based on the assumption that the reference standard is 100% sensitive and specific. If there are any disagreements between the reference standard and the index test, then it is assumed that the index test is incorrect. The use of an appropriate reference standard is therefore very important. In our example there is no definite test for making an early diagnosis of RA and so the best available reference standard is the application of the ACR criteria after a period of follow-up. Interpretation of the results of the reference standard may be influenced by knowledge of the results of the index test. Similar to the issue of blinding for the index test, the extent to which this may affect test results will be related to the degree of subjectivity in the interpretation of the reference standard result and the order of the tests. With our example, the ACR criteria (reference standard) are applied some time after the anti-CCP test and could therefore be influenced by knowledge of the test results, especially as the ACR criteria are compound criteria based mainly on subjective clinical criteria. An unbiased diagnostic study will ensure that those applying

the ACR criteria are blind to the results of the index test.

Patient flow

Ideally all patients who were enrolled into the study should undergo both the index test and a single reference standard at the same time and all are included in the analysis. If the number of patients who were enrolled in the study differs from the number of patients included in the 2×2 table then there is the potential for bias. One reason for withdrawals is **verification bias** (also known as **work-up bias, (primary) selection bias**, or **sequential ordering bias**). This occurs when not all of the study group receive confirmation of the diagnosis by a reference standard, or if some patients receive a different reference standard. If the results of the index test influence the decision on whether to perform the reference standard, or on which reference standard to use, this may result in biased estimates of accuracy. For example, a study evaluating the accuracy of the D-dimer test for the diagnosis of pulmonary embolism (PE) carried out the reference standard of ventilation perfusion scans in those testing positive and used clinical follow-up to determine whether or not those testing negative had a PE. This may result in misclassifying some of the false negatives as true negatives as some patients who had a PE but were index test negative may be missed by clinical follow-up. This misclassification will make both sensitivity and specificity appear better than they really are but if the pre-test probability is less than 50%, it will have a greater effect on over-estimating the sensitivity of the D-dimer test.

Tests may produce indeterminate and/or intermediate test results with varying frequencies. It is important that such results are reported, as this will affect the clinical utility of the test, and omission of some patients from the 2×2 table may bias results. If there is a delay between the application of the index test and reference standard, misclassification due to recovery or progression to a more advanced stage of disease may occur. This is known as **disease progression bias**. The length of time which may cause such bias will vary between conditions. In some situations, such as our example, the reference standard can incorporate a period of follow-up. In such situations a minimum rather than maximum period between the index test and reference standard is required. In our example, all patients should undergo both the anti-CCP test and be evaluated using the ACR criteria. Any indeterminate test results, both on the anti-CCP test and the ACR criteria, should be reported and taken into account in the analysis. If there are any reasons why any of the patients do not undergo both the anti-CCP test and ACR criteria then these should also be clearly reported.

Finding evidence on diagnostic accuracy studies

The most reliable source of evidence regarding the accuracy of a diagnostic test comes from diagnostic systematic reviews. These can be found by searching the Database of Abstracts of Reviews of Effects (DARE) database (www.crd.york.ac.uk/crdweb). By searching the DARE database using the terms 'rheumatoid arthritis' and 'diag*' you can find a recent systematic review that evaluates the accuracy of anti-CCP for the diagnosis of RA (Whiting *et al.*, 2010). The Cochrane Library has also recently started including diagnostic systematic reviews. Although there are currently only a very small number of such reviews published in the Cochrane Library, in the future this will be a useful resource for identifying good quality diagnostic reviews (www.thecochranelibrary.com). Primary studies can be found using PubMed which has a number of inbuilt clinical queries, including ones for diagnosis, that have been designed to help clinicians run more efficient searches. These can be helpful for quickly identifying diagnostic accuracy studies but it is important to note that these are not comprehensive, and use of these filters can results in missing relevant studies.

Can I apply the results to my patients?

Differences in demographic and clinical features or differences in the index test may produce measures of diagnostic accuracy that vary considerably. Reported estimates of accuracy, although possibly unbiased, may have limited applicability to your clinical question if the patients in the study differ from your patient or if the test methods vary, for example in terms of test technology, how the test was conducted, or how the test was interpreted. Imagine you have a 50-year-old patient with rheumatic symptoms of a couple of weeks duration presenting to you in general practice. You should consider whether the study was conducted in general practice, enrolled patients presenting with similar symptoms of a similar duration, included patients of a similar age and involved patients who had undergone a similar pattern of prior testing. For the results of that study to be directly applicable to your patient, the specific details of the anti-CCP test that you are considering ordering for him should also match those evaluated in the study. For example, there are different generations of anti-CCP test which differ biochemically from one another, there are different techniques used to conduct the anti-CCP tests (e.g. ELISA) and different commercial manufacturers. These all have the potential to alter the accuracy of the anti-CCP test.

Acknowledgements

We would like to thank Yoav Ben-Shlomo, David Gunnell and Marie Westwood for sharing relevant lecture slides which contributed to this chapter.

 KEY LEARNING POINTS

- Diagnosis is an essential part of clinical practice, but every 'test' can lead to false positive and false negative diagnoses, with potentially devastating consequences

- Various measures of accuracy can be calculated from a 2 × 2 table

- Likelihood ratios are the most clinically relevant measures, as they can be combined with estimates of the pre-test probability of disease to give the post-test probability of disease

- Various sources of bias covering patient selection, index test, reference standard and patient flow should be considered when evaluating the results of a diagnostic accuracy study

- When determining whether the results are applicable to your patient you need to consider whether the patients, setting, test technology and test interpretation in the study are similar to those for your patient

📖 REFERENCES

Deeks JJ, Altman DG (2004) Diagnostic tests 4: likelihood ratios. *BMJ* **329**: 168–9.

Klareskog L, Catrina AI, Paget S (2009) Rheumatoid arthritis. *Lancet* **373**: 659–72.

Koopman W, Schweitzer A (1999) The journey to multiple sclerosis: a qualitative study. *J Neurosci Nurs* **31**: 17–26.

Mushlin AI, Mooney C, Grow V, Phelps CE (1994) The value of diagnostic information to patients with suspected multiple sclerosis. Rochester-Toronto MRI Study Group. *Arch Neurol* **51**: 67–72.

Pewsner D, Battaglia M, Minder C, Marx A, Bucher HC, Egger M (2004) Ruling a diagnosis in or out with 'SpPIn' and 'SnNOut': a note of caution. *BMJ* **329**: 209–13.

van Gaalen FA, Visser H, Huizinga TW. A comparison of the diagnostic accuracy and prognostic value of the first and second (CCP1 and CCP2) autoantibody tests for rheumatoid arthritis. *Annals of the Rheumatic Diseases* **64**: 1510–12.

Whiting P, Rutjes AWS, Westwood ME, Mallett S, Leeflang M, Reitsma JB, *et al.* (2010) QUADAS-2. www.quadas.org . 6-12-2010.

Whiting PF, Smidt N, Sterne JA, Harbord R, Burton A, Burke M, *et al.* (2010) Systematic review: accuracy of anti-citrullinated Peptide antibodies for diagnosing rheumatoid arthritis. *Ann Intern Med* **152**: 456–64.

10

Prognosis

Yoav Ben-Shlomo and Matthew Hickman
University of Bristol

Learning objectives

In this chapter you will learn:

✓ what prognosis is and what one can use to measure it;

✓ what a prognostic risk factor is;

✓ what methods we use to display and quantify prognostic risk factors;

✓ what makes a good prognostic study and what biases are important.

What is prognosis

Prognosis begins at diagnosis. It concerns 'the expected course of a disease' – derived from the Greek 'knowledge beforehand' or 'foretelling'. Prognosis is an essential activity of medicine – as outlined by Sir James Mackenzie in his book *Diseases of the Heart* (1913):

> *I am rather afraid that our profession as a body does not recognize sufficiently its responsibility in regard to prognosis. When an individual submits himself for an opinion he does so with such implicit confidence that the verdict given may alter the whole tenor of his life (cited in White, 1953)*

What outcomes can be used for prognosis?

The outcome of interest will be disease specific – depending on the natural history of the disease and potential alternative outcomes that may arise or develop. For instance, prognosis could relate to the likelihood of:

- mortality/ risk of death – survival;
- recovery or clearance of symptoms of disease or infection – that may be measured clinically or through other investigations (serological, biochemical or radiological);
- recurrence or relapse of disease;
- **quality of life** – a summary measure based on a quantitative scale that attempts to capture the impact of illness on both physical, psychological and social aspects of well-being;
- physical or other complication of disease – such as disability, dependency and loss of physical/ mental function.

For example, as a doctor you may be presented with the following:

Patient	What will happen
An 18-year-old student who develops schizophrenia	What is the likelihood of recovery or relapse – will she be able to complete her degree?

Epidemiology, Evidence-based Medicine and Public Health Lecture Notes, Sixth Edition. Yoav Ben-Shlomo, Sara T. Brookes and Matthew Hickman.
© 2013 Y. Ben-Shlomo, S. T. Brookes and M. Hickman. Published 2013 by John Wiley & Sons, Ltd.

Patient	What will happen
A 62-year-old man has moderately severe rheumatoid arthritis	How long will it be before he is bedridden?
A 65-year-old woman has localised breast cancer	How long will she live for? Will she die of her cancer or some other cause?

What is a prognostic risk factor?

Whether the course of disease is accelerated, worsened, or improved may depend on other factors – **prognostic risk factors**. This is not to be confused with aetiological risk factors (often just called risk factors) that are factors that may increase or decrease the risk of developing disease onset. The key difference is that prognostic factors influence disease progression – whether or not an outcome (outlined above) associated with the disease occurs – and may guide or interact with management; whereas aetiological factors influence whether disease itself occurs. In some diseases risk factors may operate both on disease progression and onset e.g. age, sex, persistent smoking and obesity can influence onset and progression of heart disease; alcohol can cause liver disease and hasten the progression of liver disease in people with chronic hepatitis infections; cannabis is known to increase the risk of relapse in patients with schizophrenia and is hypothesised to increase the risk of schizophrenia like illness developing.

Other risk factors may influence only one of these dimensions e.g. unprotected sexual intercourse effects HIV disease onset but not progression and CD4 count at diagnosis effects progression only.

Displaying, summarising and quantifying prognostic factors

Time is a critical component of prognosis. Therefore, the outcome may be described in terms of a risk over a specified period of time. For example, in cancer epidemiology the risk of death or survival is often described in terms of the proportion of people with a specific cancer that survive or die over a five-year period. This is called either the **case fatality** rate or the **survival rate**. These are essentially the same measure so if the annual case fatality rate is 10% then the equivalent survival rate is 90%. This measure should not be confused with the **mortality rate** which is calculated as the number of deaths from a specific cause divided by the number of individuals at risk of dying (whether or not they already have the cancer). Hence the case fatality rate will always be greater than the mortality rate which is a function of both the incidence of the disease (risk of developing it unless you can present with sudden death) multiplied by the risk of dying.

Displaying and comparing time to event data – such as survival or mortality, recovery or relapse – involves a special set of techniques (often collectively known as **survival analysis**) that take account of how the risk of an event develops and may vary over time. A **Kaplan-Meier** graph is a traditional method of displaying time to event or survival data and follows a **step function** – where if there is no outcome at a specific time the line is horizontal and whenever there is a change in survival this is shown as a vertical drop (see Figure 10.1). The advantage of a Kaplan-Meier graph is that patients lost to follow-up (or **censored**) can also contribute information (up to the point in time they are no longer in the study). This means they are included in the denominator (patients at risk) up to that point. Survival time data are often highly skewed, so conventionally median rather than mean survival is a better summary central measure. The median survival is time by which 50% of the sample has achieved the outcome (survival, recovery, relapse). In Figure 10.1, 50% of the most malnourished sample with heart failure have died by 10 months after discharge; whereas survival for patients assessed as of adequate nutritional status was 89% at 12 months and 74% at 32 months.

Whilst mean and median survival may often be very similar, the former is very sensitive to outliers (extreme values). For example, Stephen Hawkings the eminent physicist has had motor neurone disease, a rapidly fatal neurological disorder, for over 40 years, despite the fact that survival after 5 years is usually very rare. Including his data in any analysis would make the mean survival appear much better than the median survival.

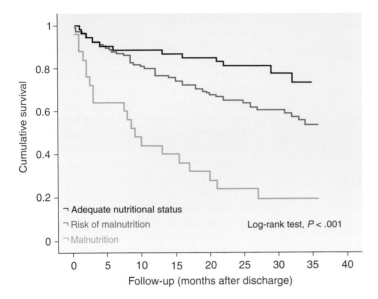

Figure 10.1 Kaplan-Meier survival curves for patients diagnosed with heart failure according to nutritional status.
Source: Bonilla-Palomas JL, Gámez-López AL, Anguita-Sánchez MP *et al.* (2011) Impact of malnutrition on long-term mortality in hospitalized patients with heart failure. *Rev Esp Cardiol* **64**: 752–8.

In studies where 50% of the sample are unlikely to experience the outcome other summary measures are used – e.g. 80% survival or survival at 5 or 10 years. For example, a study may report that at 5 years 70% of the cohort are still alive or 30% have died. To represent uncertainty around these estimates one can present ranges such as the interquartile range (25th–75th percentile) or best case and worst case scenarios (minimum to maximum).

Figure 10.2 shows results from Early Breast Cancer Trialist's collaborative group subdividing mortality risk by duration of Tamoxifen treatment and nodal status (whether cancer extends to lymph nodes). The figure shows that survival of early breast cancer is worse if axillary nodes are involved, and that Tamoxifen improves survival. In this case the researchers have presented differences in survival by prognostic factors (node status, tamoxifen therapy) in absolute terms though as you will see below it is usually more common to express this in relative terms. Hence the absolute benefit of tamoxifen therapy compared to control was larger (4.5% or 4.5 women for every 100 treated) if you had a positive lymph node than if you didn't (3.4%). Though overall node positive women are more likely to die.

Kaplan-Meier and survival curves can illustrate differences in prognosis but do not provide a relative effect estimate. In order to test whether survival differs by a prognostic factor and to adjust for confounders requires a form of regression modelling called **Cox proportional hazard regression**. This will generate a **hazard ratio** with 95% CIs and

P-values – which is similar and can be interpreted in the same way as risk ratios and odds ratios explained in Chapter 2. Although survival rates are allowed to vary over time (as seen in Figure 10.1) – Cox regression assumes that the difference in survival by exposure to the prognostic factor (the hazard ratio) is the same over time – which is known as the **proportional hazards** assumption. This may not always be the case. For example patients with diabetes undergoing major surgery may have a far greater relative hazard of dying in the immediate post-operative period, but if they survive the first month the hazard ratio after this time may be only modestly elevated. (For further information see Kirkwood and Sterne.)

Prognostic study design

To understand prognosis we also need to undertake cohort studies (covered in Chapter 5). However, for a prognostic study these have the major distinction that to be enlisted into the cohort you must already have the disease at the beginning of the study (baseline). This is the opposite of the conventional cohort study where by definition subjects should not have the disease at baseline (**exclusion**) as we are interested in estimating the incidence of disease and risk factors for disease. The conventional cohort studies are **aetiological** cohorts, (though we don't usually specify the term aetiological) because we are

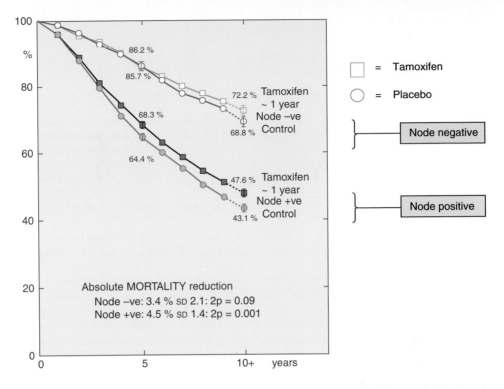

Figure 10.2 Kaplan-Meier graph for women with breast cancer stratified by whether they had a positive lymph node and whether they received tamoxifen from randomised controlled trials.
Source: From Anon. (1998) Tamoxifen for early breast cancer: an overview of the randomised trials. Early Breast Cancer Trialists' Collaborative Group. *Lancet* (1998) **351**: 1451–67, with permission from Elsevier.

trying to elucidate causes of disease in contrast to **prognostic** cohorts where we are trying to understand and predict which patients will have a mild or more aggressive course of disease.

It is important that subjects are recruited as soon as possible after disease onset, though this is usually done after diagnosis, so there may or may not be some delay. For example patients with a heart attack may be recruited within hours of symptom onset whilst patients with dementia may not be diagnosed for several years. We want to recruit **incident** patients rather than any patient with the disease of interest which would mix both incident and **prevalent** cases (see Chapter 2). For some disorders e.g. multiple sclerosis (MS), prevalent cases may have already had the disease for decades. Thus their survival from entry will appear artefactually shorter. In addition, their disease experience will be different from patients who have just been diagnosed. For example a patient with a 20-year history of MS would not have received disease modifying therapies when they first presented but may today. Using their data to

predict future prognosis will therefore be misleading for new patients due to secular differences in care. Even in the absence of new therapies, there may be secular differences in disease severity, so it is believed that cases of MS have a milder form of the disease today than in the past.

Generalisability and bias

When reviewing prognostic studies two important issues to consider are (i) the representativeness or **generalisability** of the **study sample** and (ii) **loss to follow-up bias**.

Generalisability

As previously discussed (see Chapter 5) a representative sample will allow one to generalise findings to appropriate new populations. If the sample is not representative then the results can be very misleading. For example, parents whose children experience a febrile convulsion are keen

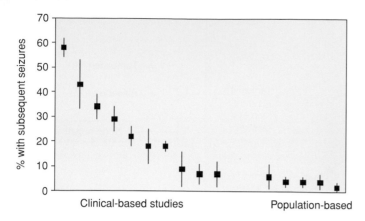

Figure 10.3 Risk of recurrent seizure after a febrile convulsion from either clinical or population-based studies. *Source*: Modified from Ellenberg JH, Nelson K (1980) Sample selection and the natural history of disease: studies of febrile seizures. *JAMA* **243**: 1337.

to know if their child is likely to have future seizures or will be diagnosed with epilepsy. Figure 10.3 shows the future risk, as a percentage, of a second seizure from 15 studies (vertical lines are the 95% confidence intervals). What can you see from this graph?

There is a large degree of variability (**heterogeneity**) in the results ranging from as high as 60% to as low as 2–3%. Why should this be?

Some of this reflects different time periods and definitions used by the studies but there is a clear pattern that results from clinical-based series (paediatric departments, often from specialist hospitals) show much higher risks than those from population-based studies that try to identify all cases regardless of whether they have or have not been seen by a specialist. This is because children seen at specialist centres are usually referred and general practitioners are more likely to do this for more severe or atypical cases that are more likely to have a second seizure (**referral bias**). Thus the risk from clinical series are not representative of all cases or those seen in primary care and parents would be given an overly pessimistic impression of their child's future risk if these data were used to counsel them.

Loss to follow-up bias

It is inevitable in any longitudinal study that some of the original participants do not take part in any future follow-up for the following reasons: death, emigration or no longer willing to stay in the study (refusal). The greater this loss, the more likely that any subsequent results may be biased or misleading. Loss to follow-up bias occurs when those who remain in the study are different from those who have dropped out either in relation to

the outcome or in the relation between the prognostic risk factor and the outcome. This bias could operate in either direction so the results may appear overly optimistic or pessimistic.

Murray and colleagues undertook a 16-year follow-up study of 2,268 patients who had a total hip replacement. Patients who failed to attend had worse pain, range of movement and radiological features at their last assessment than those who stayed in the study. All these factors are predictors for having a future revision. The observed failure risk of the hip procedure was around 20% at 16 years for those who remained in the study but it is likely that those who were lost would have a higher risk given their clinical features. A worst case scenario, assuming that all those lost had to have a revision would make the revised risk around 37%. The true risk would be somewhere between these two estimates.

However, there may be further problems if the strength of a prognostic factor is **differential** between the observed and unobserved cohort (those lost to follow-up).

Let us define failure of a hip prosthesis as either having to have a second procedure (revision) or having severe functional limitations. In the following hypothetical example (Table 10.1), we find that those subjects who have been observed have an overall 20% failure rate and this is greater for older patients, with a **relative risk** of 1.50. Amongst those lost to follow-up there is a higher overall failure rate (40%) and there is also a greater proportion of older patients (60% versus 40%) than in the observed cohort. If we had been able to follow-up all the subjects we would have found a relative risk of failure of 2.0. Thus we have underestimated the prognostic effect of being over 75 years of age in the observed cohort.

Table 10.1 Effects of differential loss to follow-up on estimating the effect of age group of prosthesis failure.

| | Observed cohort | | | |
	Implant failure	Implant success	Total	Risk
Subjects followed up				
> 75 years	100	300	400	25.0
≤ 75 years	100	500	600	16.7
Relative risk				1.5
Subjects lost to follow-up				
> 75 years	300	300	600	50.0
≤ 75 years	100	300	400	25.0
Relative risk				2.0
All subjects (followed up and lost)				
> 75 years	400	600	1000	40.0
≤ 75 years	200	800	1000	20.0
Relative risk				2.0

When appraising any prognostic study it is essential to ascertain how many of the original cohort have not been traced. Ideally a paper should report this in a **flow diagram** and provide reasons as to why subjects have been lost to follow-up. In some countries, such as the United Kingdom, we are fortunate that we can track study participants, with their consent, anywhere in the country through the National Health Service. If a participant develops cancer or dies we can get clinical information such as the type of cancer or cause of death without having to make direct contact with them. This reduces the problem of follow-up bias. Whilst the lower the loss to follow-up the better, even small losses can produce serious bias if the reason for the loss is directly associated with the outcome or is differentially associated with the prognostic factor, such as age in the example above. Whilst more advanced statistical methods, such as **imputation** may sometimes be helpful, the best solution is to try and get some outcome data, if only indirectly, on as many subjects as possible.

Examples of short- and long-term prognostic studies

Short-term prognosis

An extreme example of short-term prognosis is triage in the emergency department where staff may focus their energies on those who are most likely to benefit. Another example would be peri-operative death after surgery. Figure 10.4 below shows the results of prognostic modelling of peri-operative death after colorectal surgery amongst 8000 patients in the United Kingdom and Republic of Ireland. A multivariable model was developed based on age, co-morbidity, Duke's stage, elective or emergency surgery and type of surgical procedure. The model was developed on 60% of the data and then validated on the remaining 40%. In Figure 10.4 you can see how the model predicts the mortality rates very accurately for procedures such as right hemicolectomy and anterior resection. For rarer procedures, such as palliative bypass, there is a greater mismatch but as you can see the 95% confidence intervals are wide. This illustrates how clinicians can give sensible estimates of peri-operative mortality risk, at least in this population, that can help patients and families make informed decisions about care.

Long-term prognosis

These are most commonly used by oncologists in relation to cancer survival. So as we have already seen above (Figure 10.2) one can advise patients on the five-year survival by cancer type (breast, colorectal) and other parameters such as nodal status, histology (e.g. Gleason score for prostate cancer) or biochemistry (e.g. prostate specific antigen for prostate cancer). Prognostic data on cancers are routinely collected on all patients in most developed countries by cancer

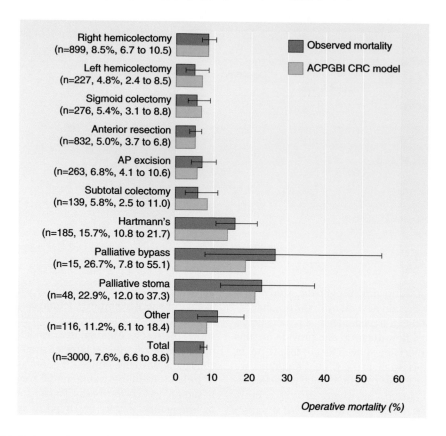

Figure 10.4 Peri-operative mortality risks (and 95% CIs) for surgery in patients with colorectal cancer comparing a predictive model with actually observed results.
Source: Tekkis PP, Poloniecki JD, Thompson MR *et al*. (2003) Operative mortality in colorectal cancer: prospective national study. *BMJ* **327**: 1196–1201 doi:10.1136/bmj.327.7425.1196.

 KEY LEARNING POINTS

- Understanding prognosis and prognostic risk factors is important for doctors and patients to help plan management and their future life
- Prognostic data can be summarised graphically (Kaplan-Meier graph) or using measures such as median or 5-year survival
- A wide variety of outcome measures can be used such as mortality, recurrence, disability, dependency and quality of life
- Prognostic risk factors can be expressed in relative or absolute terms
- Hazard ratios, equivalent to risk ratios, are usually calculated to determine if a prognostic factor is important
- Multivariable prognostic models can be used clinically to guide management decisions

registries. This allows patients and clinicians to get regular up-to-date information on prognosis. Unfortunately many other diseases do not have such data so information on these conditions need to be obtained from research studies that are often expensive and may not be representative of all cases.

 REFERENCES

Anon. (1998) Tamoxifen for early breast cancer: an overview of the randomised trials. Early Breast Cancer Trialists' Collaborative Group. *Lancet* **351**: 1451–67.

Bonilla-Palomas JL, Gámez-López AL, Anguita-Sánchez MP, *et al*. (2011) Impact of malnutrition on long-term mortality in hospitalized patients with heart failure. *Rev Esp Cardiol* **64**: 752–8.

Ellenberg JH, Nelson K (1980) Sample selection and the natural history of disease: studies of febrile seizures. *JAMA* **243**: 1337.

Tekkis PP, Poloniecki JD, Thompson MR, *et al.* (2003) Operative mortality in colorectal cancer: prospective national study. *BMJ* **327**: 1196–1201 doi:10.1136/bmj.327.7425.1196.

 FURTHER READING

Kirkwood BR and Sterne JAC (2003) *Essential Medical Statistics*, 2nd edn. Blackwell Science Ltd.

Moons KGM, Royston P, Vergouwe Y, Grobbee DE, Altman DG (2009) Prognosis and prognostic research: what, why and how? *BMJ* **338**: b375.

White PD (1953) Principles and practice of prognosis with particular reference to heart disease. *JAMA* **153**: 75–9.

11

Effectiveness

Sara T. Brookes and Jenny Donovan
University of Bristol

Learning objectives

In this chapter you will learn:

✓ why randomised controlled trials provide the best evidence of effectiveness of treatment;

✓ the possible sources of bias in a randomised controlled trial;

✓ the reasons for randomisation, blinding and the use of an intention to treat analysis;

✓ the ethical dimensions of trials: clinical equipoise, informed consent;

✓ how qualitative methods can help in the design of randomised controlled trials.

Clinical experience as a guide to the effect of treatments

Many doctors feel they know which treatments work best from clinical observation or experience. This may be reasonable in exceptional circumstances. For example, when sulphonamides were introduced for the treatment of meningococcal meningitis the effect was striking. Whereas before, mortality was very high, it was reduced to almost nil. Other examples of very effective treatments include anaesthesia for surgery and insulin for diabetes. However few treatments have such dramatic effects, and observational evidence from clinical experience alone can be misleading, for several reasons:

- Sick people tend to get better even without treatment. It is difficult to know what would have happened if no treatment, or a different treatment, had been given.
- Doctors do not follow up all of their patients after treatment, and so it is hard to be sure whether they got better or worse.
- Each doctor treats a limited number of patients so apparently dramatic benefits or failures of treatment could be due to chance. Most treatment effects are modest and you need very large studies to demonstrate this.

What we really want to know is what would happen to a patient if they received or did not receive a specific treatment. Ideally we would observe someone who was treated and then using a time machine replay their life without treatment to see if treatment made a difference (this is technically known as the **counterfactual**). However this is

---

Epidemiology, Evidence-based Medicine and Public Health Lecture Notes, Sixth Edition. Yoav Ben-Shlomo, Sara T. Brookes and Matthew Hickman.
© 2013 Y. Ben-Shlomo, S. T. Brookes and M. Hickman. Published 2013 by John Wiley & Sons, Ltd.

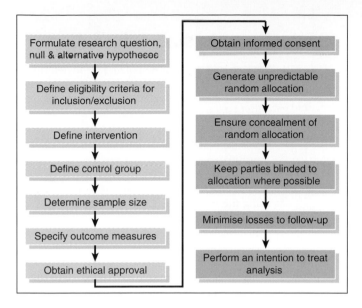

Formulate research question, null & alternative hypotheses	Obtain informed consent
Define eligibility criteria for inclusion/exclusion	Generate unpredictable random allocation
Define intervention	Ensure concealment of random allocation
Define control group	Keep parties blinded to allocation where possible
Determine sample size	Minimise losses to follow-up
Specify outcome measures	Perform an intention to treat analysis
Obtain ethical approval	

Figure 11.1 Essential steps of an RCT.

impossible (though see below for **crossover** studies) so instead we use an experimental approach known as a **randomised controlled trial** (**RCT**).

The essential steps of the RCT

An RCT is the next best thing as subjects are randomly allocated either to (i) an active treatment (or new treatment) arm or (ii) a control arm (comparison group). The control treatment may be a **placebo**, or the current standard treatment. Random allocation means that every patient has the same probability of ending up in one or other group under comparison. This is critical as we want everything to be identical in the two arms except the intervention. Thus, any difference in outcome must reflect the causal effect of the intervention. Provided that enough patients are included in the study and that random allocation is truly random, groups will be comparable for both known and unknown **confounders** (Chapter 3). This is why the RCT is regarded as the best evidence of causality and the best single study design in the **hierarchy of evidence** (see Box 5.1 in Chapter 5). At the end of the twentieth century it was estimated that there were half a million published RCTs (Lau *et al.*, 1998). Whilst the RCT has become widely accepted as the gold standard study design for the evaluation of the effectiveness of

treatments in medicine and health care, poor quality trials continue to frequent the literature (Moher, 2004). Treatment effect may be over- or underestimated because of a number of different forms of bias that may be inherent in an RCT. The steps, outlined in Figure 11.1 and described below, are essential to the design and conduct of RCTs to ensure robust findings.

 Case study *The effects of tamoxifen and raloxifene on the risk of invasive breast cancer – the STAR study* (Vogel *et al.*, 2006)

Tamoxifen is an oestrogen receptor blocker and there is RCT evidence to suggest that healthy women, who are at high future risk of developing breast cancer, have a 49% reduction in risk of developing breast cancer if given tamoxifen compared to placebo (**primary prevention**). However, the drug can have some serious side effects, such as increasing the risk of other cancer, thromboses and the development of cataracts in the eye. Raloxifene, a more selective anti-oestrogen drug, is regarded as having fewer side effects. At the end of the 1990s the STAR study (Study of Tamoxifen And Raloxifene) was set up to directly compare these two treatments amongst women with an increased risk of breast cancer in terms of risk reduction and side effect profiles. The null hypothesis (see Chapter 4) was that 'there is no difference between raloxifene and tamoxifen in terms of their relative effects on the risk of invasive breast cancer'.

Eligibility criteria for inclusion/exclusion

It is important in any RCT (and indeed, any observational study) to have clear **inclusion** and **exclusion** criteria so that the study sample is representative of the population of interest and this aids **generalisability**. If eligibility criteria are too restrictive, the generalisability of the study will also be restricted.

Reasons for exclusion are (i) risky to give them the new treatment (contraindications) (ii) unethical to deny them the conventional treatment or already on new treatment (iii) unable to follow the study requirements, e.g. mental illness, dementia or live far from study sites.

In the STAR RCT, women from 200 clinical centres throughout North America were recruited to the study between July 1999 and November 2004. To be eligible for participation, women had to be at least 35 years of age, be postmenopausal and have an increased 5-year predicted breast cancer risk (>1.66%). Exclusions included (i) those currently taking tamoxifen, raloxifene and other medications that could interact (ii) past medical history of certain disease e.g. deep vein thrombosis (DVT) and (iii) a psychiatric condition that would interfere with adherence.

Definition of intervention and control groups

A clear definition of both the intervention and control is essential so that people reading the results know exactly what was evaluated. There may be more than one control group, for example, comparing new treatment with conventional treatment and placebo.

In the STAR RCT, women received either 60 mg per day of raloxifene (intervention) or 20 mg per day of tamoxifen (control) for a maximum of 5 years. Interventions evaluated in RCTs are often far more complex than this, consisting of many different components. For example, individuals attending a stroke unit may have contact with numerous different health professionals and receive a series of drugs.

Sample size calculation

It is essential in the design of an RCT to determine how many subjects need to be included. In order to do a sample size calculation the investigators need to determine four things:

- the expected level of outcome in the control group;
- the smallest difference in outcome they wish to detect (clinically important) when comparing the two groups (in an equivalence RCT investigators will determine the largest difference in outcome that would still be considered clinically equivalent);
- the strength of evidence that they wish to find (the P-value). In sample size calculations this is often set at 5%, although arguably it should be smaller;
- the probability that they will detect a difference with the specified P-value, if the true difference is of the size they expect. This is called the power of the study and is often set at 80% or 90%.

Many RCTs do not demonstrate strong evidence against the null hypothesis because the sample size is too small (underpowered). When interpreting studies with weak evidence against the null hypothesis, you should always ask whether the sample size was large enough to detect an important difference as *absence of evidence is not the same as evidence of absence* (see Chapter 12 on meta-analysis).

In the STAR RCT the investigators focussed on demonstrating equivalence between the two treatments. They required a 95% probability of correctly concluding that the two treatments were equivalent, if they really were so, with P = 0.05. A sample size calculation determined that 327 events were required (formulae for such calculations can be found elsewhere (Matthews, 2002)). With knowledge of overall rates of invasive breast cancer in the population, the investigators were able to calculate the number needed to participate in the study to obtain 327 or more events. Whilst this may not sound like a lot, they had to screen 184,460 women to identify 20,168 eligible women from whom 19,747 women were randomised (421 not wishing to participate).

Outcome measures

An RCT should always pre-specify its primary outcome measure (this is used for the sample size calculation) but it can have a number of secondary outcomes. The primary outcome measure is often chosen as the most important research question and of greatest clinical benefit. The interpretations of secondary outcomes are likely to be less conclusive due to chance findings or lack of power. All outcome measures should have an explicit definition and time-point stated in the RCT protocol. All pre-specified outcomes should be reported. There are different types of outcome that may be measured in any single RCT.

(1) **Clinical outcomes** are defined, measured and reported by RCT investigators or health professionals. Such outcomes would include, for example, survival, remission, admission to hospital, cholesterol levels.
(2) **Patient reported outcomes (PROs)** are reported by the patient or RCT participants themselves. They provide a patient's perspective and usually **generic** or **disease-specific** questionnaires or a **symptom-specific** measure such as a pain score are used. For example, in an RCT comparing curative treatments for oesophageal cancer, a consultant may be primarily interested in five-year survival; however, a patient may feel that their emotional function is just as important. Whilst PROs may appear to be more subjective they are just as valid.
(3) **Health-care economic outcomes** to determine the relationship between the cost of a specific treatment and its outcomes (see Chapter 13).

A **composite outcome** combines multiple endpoints. An RCT may combine coronary deaths with nonfatal coronary events and surgical interventions such as by-pass grafting. This is often done to increase the power of a trial but may complicate the interpretation of the results.

A **surrogate outcome** refers to a measure that whilst may not be of direct practical importance, is associated with an outcome that is important. For example, a trial of a treatment to prevent dementia may use MRI scans to look at differences in brain atrophy, a surrogate for Alzheimer's disease.

Using such a surrogate outcome will reduce the required length of follow-up, may reduce the cost due to fewer participants and potentially increase the power of the RCT. However they are harder to interpret as patients, clinicians and policymakers are not interested in differences in brain volumes but in dementia risk.

The primary outcome for the STAR RCT was invasive breast cancer identified through pathology and mammography reports. Secondary endpoints included adverse events such as endometrial cancer and quality of life.

Biases

A number of different forms of bias may impact on the findings of an RCT. As described in Chapter 3, **bias** can be classified as relating either to the selection of participants into (or out of) a study or to the measurement of exposure and/or outcome and can be **differential** or **nondifferential**.

Selection bias and allocation concealment

Selection bias occurs in an RCT when individuals allocated to the treatment and control groups differ in some characteristic associated with outcome. For example, a health-care professional who is recruiting participants to a trial of treatments for depression, may systematically allocate those that are more severely depressed to the treatment group and those that are less severe to the control group as they feel it is unethical to deprive patients of what may turn out to be an effective therapy. In this instance any treatment effect is likely to be underestimated, but in general selection bias can affect the estimate in either direction.

In an RCT selection bias can be avoided if proper randomisation is carried out (usually using a computer generated sequence) and the random allocation sequence is concealed or hidden from the investigators enrolling patients so that it is impossible for her/him to have any influence over what treatment is allocated.

Examples of adequate **allocation concealment** include sequentially numbered sealed, opaque envelopes, drug containers prepared by an independent pharmacy and numbered in advance or **central randomisation** at a site remote from the trial location. As the clinicians are unaware of what is the next treatment, they cannot manipulate the randomisation process. Investigators' knowledge of treatment allocation can result in them either knowingly or unknowingly adjusting allocation based on prognostic factors which would mean that allocation is no longer random. The STAR RCT reports that randomisation was computer generated but there is insufficient detail to determine allocation concealment.

If randomisation has been successful, the two groups should be similar. The investigators can reassure themselves of this by brief **baseline comparisons** of factors such as age, sex and disease severity. If there are differences between groups, there are two possible explanations. The first is that random allocation was not truly random and that is was biased in some way, perhaps because of inadequate concealment. The other possibility is that only a few subjects were randomised and important differences between the treatment groups occurred by chance.

Measurement bias and blinding

As described in Chapter 3, both differential and nondifferential misclassification bias can lead to an inaccurate estimate in an analytical study. We are generally more concerned with differential misclassification because the impact of such bias is harder to predict. Two types of differential misclassification bias that can affect RCTs are **performance bias** and **detection bias**.

Performance bias relates to the unequal provision of care between the treatment and control group, apart from the treatment under evaluation. For example, if a health care professional knows that an individual is receiving a placebo or other control they may offer additional therapies. Alternatively, if the patient knows what they are receiving they may change other health behaviours.

Detection bias refers to the biased assessment of outcome, where the outcome assessor or the participant is more or less likely to report a specific outcome in the treatment or control group depending on their beliefs or preferences.

Differential measurement bias in RCTs can be avoided through **blinding** of different parties depending on the nature of the treatments and the outcome assessment. For example, if patients and health care providers are unaware of the treatment allocation no performance or detection bias can be introduced. It should be noted that

when reporting RCTs investigators sometimes write 'single' (either participants or assessors) or 'double blinding' (both participants and assessors) to mean different things. Reports of RCTs should always spell out exactly who has and has not been blinded from treatment allocation.

It is not always possible to blind subjects or health-care providers (such as in most surgical RCTs) and care must be taken in interpreting the results. A blinded RCT (patients and health professionals unaware of allocation) of cannabis for spasticity in multiple sclerosis patients showed patients who received cannabis tablets were more likely to correctly guess their treatment than the placebo arm even though the medications looked identical (presumably because of the effects of cannabis on mood) (Zajicek *et al.*, 2003). Sometimes great effects are made to maintain blinding by the use of '*sham*' procedures. An RCT of foetal grafts for Parkinson's disease randomised patients to active treatment or a sham procedure that involved drilling a burr hole in the skull but not inserting the grafts so that patients and clinical assessors (but not the neurosurgeons) remained blinded to treatment (Olanow *et al.*, 2003).

The STAR RCT reports that it was 'double-blinded' and provides enough information to ascertain that this relates to the participants, clinicians and outcome assessors who were all blinded to allocation. Hence, in this instance performance and detection bias should not be an issue.

Loss to follow-up bias and intention to treat analysis

In RCTs bias may also be introduced in the way in which participants come out of the study. Participants may be 'lost to follow-up' before the end of the study. It is usual to show this in a figure (see Figure 11.2 for STAR study) as part of the **CONSORT** reporting guidelines. If there is differential loss of participants between the treatment and control group and losses are *related to outcome*, then loss to follow-up bias may be introduced into the study and the estimate of the association between treatment and outcome may be either under- or overestimated. For example, suppose for a particular treatment side-effects are more likely amongst older participants who are also more likely to have a worse outcome. If those experiencing the side-effect withdraw from the RCT and are not followed up, then the

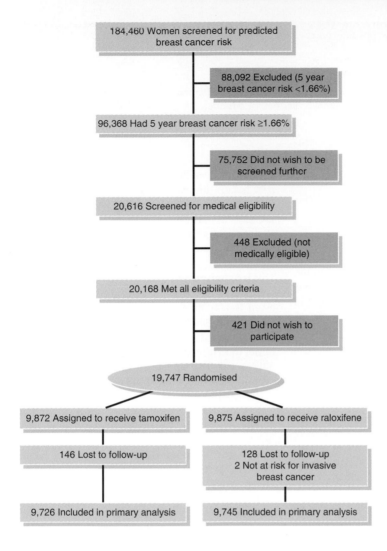

Figure 11.2 STAR study flow diagram.

treatment would appear more beneficial than it really is.

In a RCT the impact of loss to follow-up bias can be reduced by performing an **intention to treat analysis (ITT)** in which patients are analysed in the groups to which they were randomised, regardless of whether they actually received or adhered to their allocated treatment and regardless of whether they remained in the study. This is because only the groups defined by the randomisation are truly comparable: people who do not adhere to the prescribed treatment tend to be systematically different from those that do, in ways that relate to their prognosis. An analysis including only those patients who adhered to their allocated treatment is known as an **on treatment** or **per-protocol** analysis. If ITT analysis is not employed, the results may be biased.

If individuals withdraw from an RCT there may be missing outcome data. In such instances the only way to perform a full ITT analysis is to **impute** values for the missing data and there are methods available for this (Little & Rubin, 2002).

In the STAR study an ITT analysis was undertaken in that women were analysed in the groups to which they were randomised, however, a small percentage of women (1.4%) were lost to follow-up and had no recorded outcome data. Since this percentage is small any potential bias is likely to be small.

Table 11.1 Real (from STAR) and hypothetical data on the risk of a thromboembolic event.

| | Risk of thromboembolic event per 1,000 woman years | | | | | |
	Tamoxifen R_0 per 1,000	Raloxifene R_1 per 1,000	Risk ratio (R_1/R_0)	Risk difference (R_1-R_0)	Risk difference per 1,000	NNTB $(1/|R_1-R_0|)$
Hypothetical results	370	260	0.70	−0.11	−110	9.1
Actual results	3.7	2.6	0.70	−0.0011	−1.1	909.1

Risk ratio and numbers needed to treat

After the results of an RCT have been obtained, it is useful to express the benefits of (or harm from) the treatment as a **risk ratio** (RR) and/or a **risk difference** (RD). One of the secondary outcomes in the STAR RCT was thromboembolic events, a known side-effect of tamoxifen. It was hypothesised that the use of raloxifene would reduce the risk of such complications.

Table 11.1 considers both real and hypothetical risks of a thromboembolic event amongst those allocated to raloxifene and tamoxifen.

From the table we see that in both scenarios, patients randomised to raloxifene were less likely to go on to experience a thromboembolic event. The risk ratios are identical (0.70) and patients on raloxifene were 30% less likely to develop this complication.

However another way of quantifying the benefits is to know how many patients would need to be treated with raloxifene rather than tamoxifen to prevent one thromboembolic event. This is more useful for patients and clinicians in deciding on the merits of treatment. This is known as the **number needed to treat to benefit (NNTB)**. It is extremely easy to calculate, as it is simply the inverse of the risk difference:

$$NNTB = 1/|RD|$$

The vertical signs in this formula indicate that we take the absolute (positive) value of the risk difference, that is, a negative risk difference is treated as positive.

The NNTB will vary by different patient populations, assuming the risk of events vary, even if the RR remains constant. In the hypothetical data, we have made the risk of a thromboembolic event common and so for every 1,000 women treated with raloxifene, we would expect to prevent 110 of the 370 cases that would have occurred among patients on tamoxifen. Thus the risk difference is −0.11 or 110 per 1,000 women and the NNTB = 1/0.11 = 9.1. The interpretation is that for every 10 patients (we round the NNTB up to the nearest integer) treated with raloxifene rather than tamoxifen we would prevent one thromboembolic event. This is an impressive success rate.

However, the actual risk of a thromboembolic event is 1/100th that of the hypothetical data. It follows that NNTB = 1/0.0011 = 909.1. We would therefore need to treat 910 patients with raloxifene rather than tamoxifen to prevent one thromboembolic event. This appears less convincing and the overall cost-effectiveness will depend on the costs of the treatment as well as other potential benefits.

It is important to remember that in medicine almost everything we do to help patients also has the potential to harm them. We can express this as the **number needed to treat to harm (NNTH)**. In the STAR RCT the risk of invasive breast cancer (the primary outcome) was slightly higher amongst those receiving raloxifene: 4.41 per 1,000 as opposed to 4.30 per 1,000 in the tamoxifen group. Hence, the number needed to treat to harm is 1/|0.00441-0.0043| = 1/0.00011 = 9090.9 patients. It is standard practice to round the NNTH down to the nearest integer. Therefore, we need to treat 910 patients with raloxifene rather than tamoxifen to prevent one case of thrombosis and 9090 patients to precipitate one case of invasive breast cancer favouring the balance of benefit to harm.

Qualitative methods in RCTs

Qualitative research methods in health research are used to assess detailed experiences of groups of people and can also be used to observe aspects of the conduct of studies, and have recently started to be included in RCTs. Increasingly, funding bodies are expecting that RCTs will include in their assessments the aspects that most matter to patients, in addition to the usual clinical information. RCT participants' views can be collected by in-depth interviews with groups of participants, selected to cover the range of ages, gender and illness severity of those included in the RCT. The findings from these interviews might indicate that particular symptoms should be measured, and these may be obtained from existing published and validated questionnaires, or a new measure may need to be developed.

There has been considerable interest in what it is like to be involved in participating in an RCT, and several studies using qualitative interviews have shown that it can be confusing if the concepts of equipoise (see below) and randomisation are not presented clearly to patients (Featherstone & Donovan, 1998). Qualitative research has also been used to improve levels of recruitment levels to RCTs (Donovan et al., 2002).

Qualitative research methods also include ways to observe naturally occurring events, to promote better understanding of what actually happens in real life situations, rather than relying on accounts of what may have happened. In RCTs, these methods can be useful for investigating the fidelity of an RCT intervention – that is whether and how the intervention was actually given to RCT participants. This can be particularly important in interpreting the results of the RCT. For example, in an RCT investigating the effectiveness of a leaflet given out by midwives in reducing smoking among pregnant women, qualitative research methods were used to explore with patients whether the leaflets were useful and how they were given them. Interviews with midwives were also undertaken. The intention was that midwives would work through the leaflet in the clinic with currently smoking pregnant women to reduce smoking levels. When the RCT was reported, there was no difference in the smoking quit rate between the group who receive the leaflet and 'usual practice' without the leaflet. The conclusion that could be drawn is that the leaflet was not effective. However, interviews with RCT participants indicated that the leaflets were simply handed out in an envelope and so were not always read. Midwives explained that they found it difficult to tackle an issue as difficult as smoking when they had only just met the women and had other clinical duties to perform. Thus, the qualitative research showed that it was not appropriate to conclude that the leaflet itself was ineffective, and

that the method of delivering the information had been suboptimal (Moore et al., 2002).

Qualitative methods can thus be used to answer important research questions about the design and conduct of an RCT.

Ethical issues in RCTs

All research studies raise ethical issues, such as participant confidentiality. However RCTs involve more difficult issues than observational studies, because they mean that the choice of treatment is not made by patients and clinicians but is instead devolved to a process of random allocation. This means that a patient in an RCT may receive a new untested treatment, or not be able to choose a new active treatment if allocated to the placebo group. In addition there is the issue of 'sham' procedures.

More detailed information on ethical issues, in general, is covered in Chapter 14. Two issues that are specific or slightly different for RCTs are **clinical equipoise** and **informed consent**. It is only ethical to randomise someone to different treatments if there is a lack of evidence about whether one treatement is superior to another. This is even true for placebo-controlled trials as an active treatment may have more adverse events without any benefit. Until such evidence exists, hence the need for the RCT in the first place, we have enough uncertainty to randomise. Informed consent is essential for all studies, but in this case, participants must understand that they have no choice concerning what intervention they receive, as this is randomly allocated. If they feel strongly about either getting or not getting a specific treatment, it is better that they do not take part rather than withdraw after they have been randomised. Independent research ethics committee must review and approve studies before they are undertaken.

Other types of RCTs

The type of RCT that we have described above, which is the most commonly used RCT, is referred to as a parallel group RCT. Frequently used alternative designs include the **cluster randomised trial** and the **crossover trial**.

In some instances the intervention being evaluated may apply at the group (or cluster) level, for example altering the practice of a health professional or team. In such a situation intervention allocation would be by health professional or team rather than by individual patients. Cluster trials are dealt with in more detail in Chapter 17 which considers ways of evaluating public health and complex interventions generally delivered at a group level. Other indications for a cluster trial include logistics and contamination. Imagine a teacher-led intervention to encourage hand washing in schools – allocating individual pupils within a school to either receive the intervention or not would be logistically difficult and may lead to contamination where pupils allocated to control receive some or part of the intervention. Cluster trials must incorporate the clustered nature in both their design and analysis (Donner & Klar, 2000).

Another alternative to the parallel group RCT is the crossover trial, in which all participants receive both the intervention and the control. Participants are randomly allocated to the order in which they receive the treatments, so half will receive intervention followed by control and half control followed by intervention. The advantage of this design is that smaller sample sizes tend to be required since there is less variation in outcome within participants than between participants. Such trials are only appropriate for the evaluation of treatments with short-term effects for stable conditions (generally chronic disease).

🔑 KEY LEARNING POINTS

- The RCT is the gold standard study design for the evaluation of the effectiveness of treatments in medicine and health care
- The key features of the RCT are the presence of a control and random allocation to treatment groups
- Randomisation ensures comparable groups in terms of all known and unknown confounding variables
- There are many essential steps to an RCT including sample size calculation, clear definitions of treatments, careful selection of outcome measures, consideration of ethical issues
- Selection and measurement bias can be minimised in RCTs through adequate randomisation and allocation concealment, blinding of participants, health care providers and outcome assessors, and performing an intention to treat analysis
- Qualitative research methods can be used to explore participants' perspectives of being involved in RCTs, recruitment levels and the fidelity of interventions

📖 REFERENCES

Donner A, Klar N (2000) *Design and Analysis of Cluster Randomization Trials in Health Research*. London: Arnold.

Donovan JL, Mills N, Smith M, Brindle L, Jacoby A, Peters TJ, Frankel SJ, Neal DE, Hamdy FC (2002) Improving design and conduct of randomised trials by embedding them in qualitative research: ProtecT (prostate testing for cancer and treatment) study. *BMJ* **325**: 766–70.

Featherstone K, Donovan JL (1998) Random allocation or allocation at random? Patient perspectives of participation in a randomised controlled trial. *BMJ* **317**: 1177–80.

Lau J, Ioannidis JP, Schmid CH (1998) Summing up evidence: one answer is not always enough. *Lancet* **351**: 123–7.

Little RJA, Rubin DB (2002) Statistical analysis with missing data, 2nd edn. New Jersey: John Wiley & Sons Inc.

Matthews JNS (2002) *An Introduction to Randomized Controlled Clinical Trials*. London: Arnold.

Moher D, Altman DG, Schulz KF, et al. (2004) Opportunities and challenges for improving the quality of reporting clinical research: CONSORT and beyond. *CMAJ* **171**(4): 349–350.

Moore L, Campbell R, Whelan A, Mills N, Lupton P, Misselbrook L, Frohlich J (2002) Self-help smoking cessation in pregnancy: cluster randomised controlled trial. *BMJ* **325**; 1383–6.

Olanow CW *et al.* (2003) A double-blind controlled trial of bilateral fetal nigral transplantation in Parkinson's disease. *Ann Neurol* **54**: 403–14.

Vogel VG, Costantino JP, Wickerham DL, Cronin WM, Cecchini RS *et al.*, for the National

Surgical Adjuvant Breast and Bowel Project (NSABP) (2006). Effects of Tamoxifen vs Raloxifene on the risk of developing invasive breast cancer and other disease outcomes: The NSABP Study of Tamoxifen and Raloxifene (STAR) P-2 Trial. *JAMA* **295**(23): 2727–41.

Zajicek J, Fox P, Sanders H, Wright D, Vickery J, Nunn A, Thompson A, on behalf of the UK MS Research Group (2003) Cannabinoids for treatment of spasticity and other symptoms related to multiple sclerosis (CAMS study): multicentre randomised placebo-controlled trial. *Lancet* **362**: 1517–26.

12

Systematic reviews and meta-analysis

Penny Whiting and Jonathan Sterne
University of Bristol

Learning objectives

In this chapter you will learn to:

- ✓ define a systematic review, and explain why it provides more reliable evidence than a traditional narrative review;
- ✓ succinctly describe the steps in conducting a systematic review;
- ✓ understand the concept of meta-analysis and other means of synthesising results;
- ✓ explain what is meant by heterogeneity;
- ✓ critically appraise the conduct of a systematic review.

What are systematic reviews and why do we need them?

Systematic reviews are **studies of studies** that offer a systematic approach to reviewing and summarising evidence. They follow a defined structure to identify, evaluate and summarise all available evidence addressing a particular research question. Systematic reviews should use and report clearly-defined methods, in order to avoid the biases associated with, and subjective nature of, traditional narrative reviews. Key characteristics of a systematic review include a set of objectives with pre-defined inclusion criteria, explicit and reproducible methodology, comprehensive searches that aim to identify all relevant studies, assessment of the quality of included studies, and a standardised presentation and synthesis of the characteristics and findings of the included studies.

Systematic reviews are an essential tool to allow individuals and policy makers to make evidence-based decisions and to inform the development of clinical guidelines. Systematic reviews fulfil the following key roles: (1) allow researchers to keep up to date with the constantly expanding number of primary studies; (2) critically appraise primary studies addressing the same research question, and investigate possible reasons for conflicting results among them; (3) provide more precise and reliable effect estimates than is

---

Epidemiology, Evidence-based Medicine and Public Health Lecture Notes, Sixth Edition. Yoav Ben-Shlomo, Sara T. Brookes and Matthew Hickman.
© 2013 Y. Ben-Shlomo, S. T. Brookes and M. Hickman. Published 2013 by John Wiley & Sons, Ltd.

possible from individual studies, which are often underpowered; and (4) identify gaps in the evidence base.

How do we conduct a systematic review?

It is essential to first produce a detailed protocol which clearly states the review question and the proposed methods and criteria for identifying and selecting relevant studies, extracting data, assessing study quality, and analysing results. To minimise bias and errors in the review process, the reference screening, inclusion assessment, data extraction and quality assessment should involve at least two independent reviewers. If it is not practical for all tasks to be conducted in duplicate, it can be acceptable for one reviewer to conduct each stage of the review while a second reviewer checks their decisions. The steps involved in a systematic review are similar to any other research undertaking (Figure 12.1).

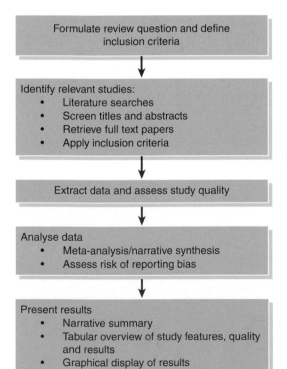

Figure 12.1 Steps in a systematic review.

Define the review question and inclusion criteria

A detailed review question supported by *clearly defined inclusion criteria* is an essential component of any review. For a review of an intervention the inclusion criteria should be defined in terms of patients, intervention, comparator interventions, outcomes (PICO) and study design. Other types of review (for example, reviews of diagnostic test accuracy studies) will use different criteria.

> *Example:* We will use a review by Lawlor and Hopker (2001) on the effectiveness of exercise as an intervention for depression to illustrate the steps in a systematic review. This review aimed 'to determine the effectiveness of exercise as an intervention in the management of depression'.

Inclusion criteria were defined as follows:

Patients:	Adults (age > 18 years) with a diagnosis of depression (any measure and any severity)
Intervention:	Exercise
Comparator:	Established treatment of depression. Studies with an exercise control group were excluded.
Outcomes:	Depression (any measure). Studies reporting only anxiety or other disorders were excluded.
Study design:	Randomised controlled trials

Identify relevant studies

A comprehensive search should be undertaken to locate all relevant published and unpublished studies. Electronic databases such as MEDLINE and EMBASE form the main source of published studies. These bibliographic databases index articles published in a wide range of journals and can be searched online. Other available databases have specific focuses: the exact databases, and number of databases, that should be searched is dependent upon the review question. The Cochrane CENTRAL register of controlled trials, which includes over 640,000 records, is the best single source for identifying reports of controlled trials (both published and unpublished). A detailed search strategy, using synonyms for the type of patients and interventions of interest, and combined using logical AND and OR operators should be used to help identify relevant studies.

There is a trade-off between maximising the number of relevant studies identified by the searches whilst limiting the number of ineligible studies in order that the search retrieves a manageable number of references to screen. It is common to have to screen several thousands of references. Searches of bibliographic databases alone tend to miss relevant studies, especially unpublished studies, and so additional steps should be taken to ensure that all relevant studies are included in the review. For example, these could include searching relevant conference proceedings, grey literature databases, internet websites, handsearching journals, contacting experts in the field, screening the bibliographies of review articles and included studies, and searches for citations to key papers in the field. Online trial registers are of increasing importance in helping identify studies that have not, or not yet, been published. Search results should be stored in a single place, ideally using bibliographic software (such as Reference Manager or EndNote).

Selecting studies for inclusion is a two-stage process. First, the search results, which generally include titles and abstracts, are screened to identify potentially relevant studies. The full text of these studies is then obtained (downloaded online, ordered from a library, or copy requested from the authors) and assessed for inclusion against the pre-specified criteria. Retrieved papers are then assessed for eligibility against pre-specified criteria.

Example: The Lawlor and Hopker (2001) review conducted a comprehensive search including Medline, Embase, Sports Discus, PsycLIT, Cochrane CENTRAL, and the Cochrane Database of Systematic Reviews. Search terms included 'exercise, physical activity, physical fitness, walking, jogging, running, cycling, swimming, depression, depressive disorder, and dysthymia.' Additional steps to locate relevant studies included screening bibliographies, contacting experts in the field, and handsearching issues of relevant journals for studies published in 1999. No language or publication restrictions were applied. Three reviewers independently reviewed titles and available abstracts to retrieve potentially relevant studies; studies needed to be identified by only one person to be retrieved.

Extract relevant data

Data should be extracted using a standardised form designed specifically for the review, in order to ensure that data are extracted consistently across different studies. Data extraction forms should be piloted, and revised if necessary. Electronic data collection forms and web-based forms have a number of advantages, including the combination of data extraction and data entry in one step, more structured data extraction and increased speed, and the automatic detection of inconsistencies between data recorded by different observers.

Example: For the Lawlor and Hopker (2001) review two reviewers independently extracted data on participant details, intervention details, trial quality, outcome measures, baseline and post intervention results and main conclusions Discrepancies were resolved by referring to the original papers and through discussion.

Assess the quality of the included studies

Assessment of study quality is an important component of a systematic review. It is useful to distinguish between the risk of bias (internal validity) and the applicability (external validity, or generalisability) of the included studies to the review question. Bias occurs if the results of a study are distorted by flaws in its design or conduct (see Chapter 3), while applicability may be limited by differences between included patients' demographic or clinical features, or in how the intervention was applied, compared to the patients or intervention that are specified in the review question. Biases can vary in magnitude: from small compared with the estimated intervention effect to substantial, so that an apparent finding may be entirely due to bias. The effect of a particular source of bias may vary in direction between trials: for example lack of blinding may lead to underestimation of the intervention effect in one study but overestimation in another study.

The approach that should be used to assess study quality within a review depends on the design of the included studies – a large number of different scales and checklists are available. Commonly used tools include the Cochrane Risk of Bias tool for RCTs and the QUADAS-2 tool for diagnostic accuracy studies. Authors often wish to use summary 'quality scores' based on adding points that are assigned based on a number of aspects of study design and conduct, to provide a single summary indicator of study quality. However, empirical evidence and theoretical considerations suggest that summary quality scores should not be used to assess the quality of trials in systematic reviews. Rather, the relevant methodological aspects should be identified in the study protocol, and assessed individually.

At a minimum, a narrative summary of the results of the quality assessment should be presented, ideally supported by a tabular or graphical display. Ideally, the results of the quality assessment should be incorporated into the review for example by stratifying analyses according to summary risk of bias or restricting inclusion in the review or primary analysis to studies judged to be at low risk of bias for all or specified criteria. Associations of individual items or summary assessments of risk of bias with intervention effect estimates can be examined using **meta-regression analyses** (a statistical method to estimate associations of study characteristics ('moderator variables') with intervention effect estimates), but these are often limited by low power. Studies with a rating of high or unclear risk of bias/concerns regarding applicability may be omitted, in **sensitivity analyses**.

> *Example:* The Lawlor and Hopker (2001) review assessed trial quality by noting whether allocation was concealed, whether there was blinding, and whether an intention to treat analysis was reported. They conducted meta-regression analyses (see 'Heterogeneity between study results' section, pp. 106–108, below) to investigate the influence of these quality items on summary estimates of treatment effect.

How do we synthesise findings across studies?

Where possible, results from individual studies should be presented in a **standardised format**, to allow comparison between them. If the endpoint is binary (for example, disease versus no disease, or dead versus alive) then risk ratios, odds ratios or risk differences may be calculated. Empirical evidence shows that, in systematic reviews of randomised controlled trials, results presented as risk ratios or odds ratios are more consistent than those expressed as risk differences.

If the outcome is continuous and measurements are made on the same scale (for example, blood pressure measured in mm Hg) then the intervention effect is quantified as the mean difference between the intervention and control groups. If different studies measured outcomes in different ways (for example, using different scales for measuring depression in primary care) it is necessary to standardise the measurements on a common scale to allow their inclusion in meta-analysis. This is usually done by calculating the **standardised mean difference** for each study (the mean difference divided by the pooled standard deviation of the measurements).

> *Example:* In the Lawlor and Hopker (2001) review, the primary outcome of interest, depression score, was a continuous measure assessed using different scales. Standardised mean differences were therefore calculated for each study.

Meta-analysis

A **meta-analysis** is a statistical analysis that aims to produce a single summary estimate by combining the estimates reported in the included studies. This is done by calculating a weighted average of the effect estimates from the individual studies (for example, estimates of the effect of the intervention from randomised clinical trials, or estimates of the magnitude of association from epidemiological studies). Ratio measures should be log-transformed before they are meta-analysed: they are then back-transformed for presentation of estimates and confidence intervals. For example, denoting the odds ratio in study i by OR_i and the weight in study i by w_i, the weighted average log odds ratio is

$$\frac{\sum w_i \times \log(OR_i)}{\sum w_i}$$

Setting all study weights equal to 1 would correspond to calculating an arithmetic mean of the effects in the different studies. However this would not be appropriate, because larger studies contribute more information than smaller studies, and this should be accounted for in the weighting scheme. Simply pooling the data from different studies and treating them as one large study is not appropriate. It would fail to preserve the randomisation in meta-analyses of clinical trials, and more generally would introduce confounding by patient characteristics that vary between studies.

The choice of weight depends on the choice of meta-analysis model. The **fixed effect** model assumes the true effect to be the same in each study, so that the differences between effect estimates in the different studies are exclusively due to random (sampling) variation. **Random-effects** meta-analysis models allow for variability between the true effects in the different studies. Such variability is known as **heterogeneity**, and is discussed in more detail below.

In fixed-effect meta-analyses, the weights are based on the **inverse variance** of the effect in each study:

$$w_i = \frac{1}{v_i}$$

where the variance v_i is the square of the standard error of the effect estimate in study i. Because large studies estimate the effect precisely (so that the standard error and variance of the effect estimate are small), this approach gives more weight to the studies that provide most information. Other methods for fixed-effect meta-analysis, such as the Mantel-Haenszel method or the Peto method are based on different formulae but give similar results in most circumstances.

In a random-effects meta-analysis, the weights are modified to account for the variability in true effects between the studies. This modification makes the weights (a) smaller and (b) relatively more similar to each other. Thus, random-effects meta-analyses give relatively more weight to smaller studies. The most commonly used method for random-effects meta-analysis was proposed by DerSimonian and Laird. The summary effect estimate from a random-effects meta-analysis corresponds to the mean effect, about which the effects in different studies are assumed to vary. It should thus be interpreted differently from the results from a fixed-effect meta-analysis.

Example: The Lawlor and Hopker review used a fixed effect inverse variance weighted meta-analysis when heterogeneity could be ruled out, otherwise a DerSimonian and Laird random effects model was used.

Forest plots

The results of a systematic review and meta-analysis should be displayed in a **forest plot**. Such plots display a square centred on the effect estimate from each individual study and a horizontal line showing the corresponding 95% confidence intervals. The area of the square is proportional to its weight in the meta-analysis, so that studies that contribute more weight are represented by larger squares. A solid vertical line is usually drawn to represent no effect (risk/odds ratio of 1 or mean difference of 0). The result of the meta-analysis is displayed by a diamond at the bottom of the graph: the centre of the diamond corresponds to the summary effect estimate, while its width corresponds to the corresponding 95% confidence interval. A dashed vertical line corresponding to the summary effect estimate is included to allow visual assessment of the variability of the individual study effect estimates around the summary estimate. Even if a meta-analysis is not conducted, it is often still helpful to include a forest plot without a summary estimate, in which case the symbols used to display the individual study effect estimates will all be the same size.

Example: Figure 12.2 shows a forest plot, based on results from the Lawler and Hopker (2001) review, of the effect of exercise compared to no treatment on change in depressive symptoms, measured using standardised mean differences. The summary intervention effect estimate suggests that exercise is associated with an improvement in symptoms, compared to no treatment.

Heterogeneity between study results

Before pooling studies in a meta-analysis it is important to consider whether it is appropriate to do so. If studies differ substantially from one another in terms of population, intervention, comparator group, methodological quality or study design then it may not be appropriate to combine their results. It is also possible that even when the studies appear sufficiently similar to justify a meta-analysis, estimates of intervention effect differ to such an extent that a summary estimate is not appropriate or should accommodate these differences. Differences between intervention effect estimates greater than those expected because of sampling variation (chance) are known as 'statistical heterogeneity'. As part of the process of conducting a meta-analysis, the presence of heterogeneity should be formally assessed. The first step is visual inspection of the results displayed in the forest plot. On average, in the absence of heterogeneity, 95% of the confidence intervals around the individual study estimates will include the fixed-effect summary effect estimate. The second step is to report a measure of heterogeneity, and a p-value from a test for heterogeneity.

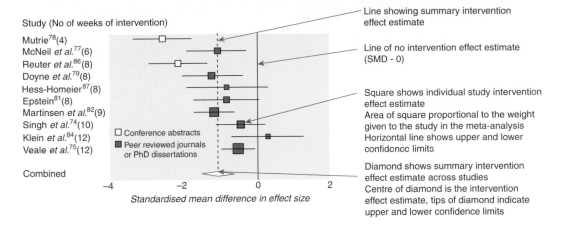

Figure 12.2 Forest plot showing standardised mean difference in size of effect of exercise compared with 'no treatment' for depression.

Heterogeneity can be quantified using the τ^2 or I^2 statistics. The τ^2 statistic represents the between-study variance in the true intervention effect, and is used to derive the weights in a random-effects meta-analysis. A disadvantage is that it is hard to interpret, although it can be converted to provide a range within which we expect the true treatment effect to fall (for example a 90% range for the mean difference). The I^2 **statistic** quantifies the percentage of total variation across studies that is due to heterogeneity rather than chance. I^2 lies between 0% and 100%; a value of 0% indicates no observed heterogeneity, and larger values show increasing heterogeneity. When $I^2 = 0$ then $\tau^2 = 0$, and vice-versa.

A statistical **test for heterogeneity** is a test of the null hypothesis that there is no heterogeneity, i.e. that the true intervention effect is the same in all studies (the assumption underlying a fixed-effect meta-analysis). A test for heterogeneity proceeds by deriving a **Q-statistic**, whose value is not in itself of interest but which can be compared with the χ^2 distribution in order to derive a p-value. As usual, the smaller the p-value the stronger is the evidence against the null hypothesis. Hence, a small p-value from a test for heterogeneity suggests that the true intervention effect varies between the studies. Tests for heterogeneity should be interpreted with caution, because they typically have low power.

If heterogeneity is present then a small number of (ideally pre-specified) subgroup and/or sensitivity analyses can be conducted to investigate whether the treatment effect differs across subgroups of studies (for example, those using high versus low dose of the intervention or those assessed as at high compared to low risk of bias). However, typical meta-analyses contain fewer than 10 component studies, which severely limits the potential for these additional analyses to provide definitive explanations for heterogeneity. If heterogeneity remains unexplained but pooling is still considered appropriate, a **random effects analysis** can be used to accommodate heterogeneity, though its results should be interpreted in the light of the underlying assumption that the true intervention effect varies between the studies. Alternatively, it may be appropriate to present a narrative synthesis of findings across studies, without combining the results into a single summary estimate.

Example: There was substantial variability between the results of the studies of exercise compared with no treatment for depression that were located by Lawlor and Hopker (2001) (Figure 12.2). Four of the 10 confidence intervals around the study effect estimates did not include the summary effect estimate. This visual impression was confirmed by strong evidence of heterogeneity (Q = 35.0, P < 0.001). The estimated value of the between-study variance was $\tau^2 = 0.41$. Lawlor and Hopker reported results from a random-effects meta-analysis, and used meta-regression analyses to investigate heterogeneity due to quality features (allocation concealment, use of intent-to-treat analysis, blinding), setting, baseline depression severity, type of exercise, and type of publication. As shown in Figure 12.2, intervention effect estimates were greater in two studies that were published only as conference abstracts than in the studies published as full papers.

Reporting biases

The dissemination of research findings is a continuum ranging from the sharing of draft papers among colleagues, presentations at meetings, publication of abstracts, to availability of full papers in journals that are indexed in the major bibliographic databases. Not all studies are published in full in an indexed journal and therefore easily identifiable for systematic review. Reports of large externally funded studies with statistically significant results are more likely to be published, published quickly, published in an English-language journal, published in more than one place, and cited in subsequent publications and so their results are more accessible and easy to locate. Reporting biases are introduced when the publication of research findings is influenced by the strength and direction of results. **Publication bias** refers to the nonpublication of whole studies, while **language bias** can occur if a review is restricted to studies reported in specific languages. For example, investigators working in a non-English-speaking country may be more likely to publish positive findings in international, English-language journals, while sending less interesting negative or null findings to local-language journals. It follows that restricting a review to English-language publications has the potential to introduce bias. Even when a study is published, *selective reporting of outcomes* has the potential to lead to serious bias in systematic reviews.

Reporting biases may lead to an association between study size and effect estimates. Such an association will lead to an asymmetrical appearance of a funnel plot – a scatter plot of a measure of study size against effect estimate (the lighter circles in the upper panel of Figure 12.3 are the results of unpublished studies that will be missing in the funnel plot). Therefore **funnel plots** (Figure 12.3), and statistical tests for funnel plot asymmetry, can be used to investigate evidence of reporting biases. However, it is important to realise that funnel plot asymmetry can have causes other than reporting biases: for example that poor methodological quality leads to spuriously inflated effects in

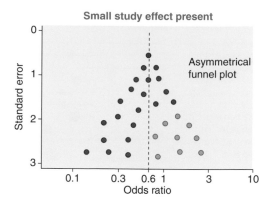

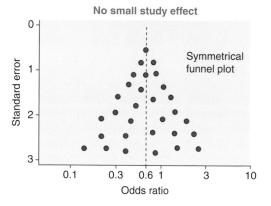

Figure 12.3 Funnel plots showing evidence and no evidence of small study effect.

smaller studies, or that effect size differs according to study size because of differences in the intensity of interventions.

Presenting the results of the review

A systematic review should present overviews of the characteristics, quality and results of the included studies. Tabular summaries are very helpful for providing a clear overview. Types of data that may be summarised include details of the study population (setting, demographic features, presenting condition details), intervention (e.g. dose, method of administration), comparator interventions, study design, outcomes evaluated and results. Depending on the amount of data to be summarised it can be helpful to include separate tables for baseline information, study quality,

Table 12.1 Extract from summary of studies table from the Lawlor and Hopker (2001) review.

	Participants				Intervention			Study quality		
Study	No	Type	Mean age (range or SD)	% female	Details	Duration (weeks)	Main outcome results (95% CI)	Concealment	ITT	Blinded
Singh et al., 1997	32	Volunteers from two community registers of people interested in research	70 (61–88)	63	Nonaerobic exercise: progressive resistance training 3 times a week. Control: seminars on health of elderly people twice a week. Depression not discussed in either group.	10	Mean difference in BDI between exercise and control groups −4.0 (−10.1 to 2.1)	Yes	Yes	No
McNeil et al. 1991	30	Nonclinically depressed elderly people referred by religious and community organisations	72.5	N/A	1. Exercise: walking near home (accompanied by experimenter) 3 times a week for 20–40 minutes. 2. Control: 1 home visit by psychology student, for 'chat,' twice a week. 3. Waiting list control group.	6	Mean difference in BDI between exercise and waiting list control groups −3.6 (−6.6 to −0.6); no significant difference between exercise and social contact groups	No	No	No

and study results. The narrative discussion should consider the strength of the evidence for a treatment effect, whether there is unexplained variation in the treatment effect across individual studies, and should incorporate a discussion of the risk of bias and applicability of the included studies. If meta-analysis is not possible, for example because outcomes assessed in the included studies were too different to pool, then the narrative discussion is the main synthesis of results across studies. It is important to provide some synthesis of results across studies, even if this is not statistical, rather than simply describing the results of each included study.

Example: Table 12.1 shows an extract from the study details table reported in the Lawlor and Hopker (2001) review. This table allows the reader to quickly scan both the characteristics of individual studies (rows) and the pattern of a characteristic across the whole review (columns).

Critical appraisal of systematic reviews

When reading a report of a systematic review the following criteria should be considered:

(1) Is the search strategy comprehensive, or could some studies have been missed?
(2) Were at least two reviewers involved in all stages of the review process (reference screening, inclusion assessment, data extraction and quality assessment)?
(3) Was study quality assessed using appropriate criteria?
(4) Were the methods of analysis appropriate?
(5) Is there heterogeneity in the treatment effect across individual studies? Is this investigated?
(6) Could results have been affected by reporting biases or small study effects?

If a systematic review does not report sufficient detail to make a judgment on one or more of these items then conclusions drawn from the review should be cautious. The PRISMA statement is a 27-item checklist that provides guidance to systematic review authors on what they should report in journal articles. It is not a critical appraisal checklist, but reports following PRISMA should give enough information to permit a comprehensive critical appraisal of the review.

 KEY LEARNING POINTS

- Systematic reviews are 'studies of studies' that follow a defined structure to identify, evaluate and summarise all available evidence addressing a particular research question
- Key characteristics of a systematic review include a set of objectives with pre-defined inclusion criteria, explicit and reproducible methodology, comprehensive searches that aim to identify all relevant studies, assessment of the quality of included studies, and a standardised presentation and synthesis of the characteristics and findings of the included studies
- Meta-analysis is a statistical analysis that aims to produce a single summary estimate, with associated confidence interval, based on a weighted average of the effect size estimates from individual studies
- Heterogeneity is variability between the true effects in the different studies

Acknowledgements

We thank Chris Metcalfe and Matthias Egger for sharing lecture materials that contributed to this chapter.

 REFERENCE

Lawlor DA, Hopker SW (2001) The effectiveness of exercise as an intervention in the management of depression: systematic review and meta-regression analysis of randomised controlled trials. *BMJ* **322**(7289): 763–67.

 RECOMMENDED READING

CASP Systematic Reviews Appraisal Tool (2011) http://www.sph.nhs.uk/sph-files/casp-appraisal-tools/S.Reviews%20Appraisal%20Tool.pdf/view [cited 2011 Dec. 30];

Centre for Reviews and Dissemination (2009) *Systematic Reviews: CRD's Guidance for Undertaking Reviews in Health Care.* York: CRD, University of York.

Higgins JPT, Altman DG, Gotzsche PC, Juni P, Moher D, Oxman AD, *et al.* (2011) The Cochrane Collaboration's tool for assessing risk of bias in randomised trials. *BMJ* **343**: d5928.

Higgins JPT, Green S (2011) *Cochrane Handbook for Systematic Reviews of Interventions. Version 5.1.0.* The Cochrane Collaboration.

Higgins JPT, Thompson SG, Deeks JJ, Altman DG (2003) Measuring inconsistency in meta-analyses. *BMJ* **327**(7414): 557–60.

Moher D, Liberati A, Tetzlaff J, Altman DG (2009) Preferred reporting items for systematic reviews and meta-analyses: the PRISMA statement. *Ann Intern Med* **151**(4): 264–9, W64.

Sterne JA, Sutton AJ, Ioannidis JP, Terrin N, Jones DR, Lau J, *et al.* (2011) Recommendations for examining and interpreting funnel plot asymmetry in meta-analyses of randomised controlled trials. *BMJ* **343**: d4002.

13

Health economics

William Hollingworth and Sian Noble
University of Bristol

Learning objectives

In this chapter you will learn:

- ✓ to explain basic concepts of economics and how they relate to health;
- ✓ to distinguish the main types of economic evaluation;
- ✓ to understand the key steps in costing health care;
- ✓ to understand the Quality Adjusted Life Year (QALY) and its limitations;
- ✓ to interpret the results of an economic evaluation.

What is economic evaluation?

Economic evaluation is the comparison of the *costs and outcomes of two or more alternative courses of action.* If you bought this book, you have already conducted an informal economic evaluation. This involved comparing the cost of this book and the expected benefits of the information it contains against the cost and expected benefits of alternative books on the topic. In health, economic evaluation commonly compares the cost and outcomes of different methods of prevention, diagnosis or treatment.

The economic context of health care decisions

Higher income countries spend up to 16% of their wealth on health care. In the UK and Nordic countries the public purse pays for more than 80% of health expenditures, whereas in the United States and Switzerland the figure is closer to 50% (Figure 13.1). Funds are raised through general taxation or compulsory contributions by employers or individuals and are then used to pay for the care of vulnerable subgroups (e.g. the elderly and poor) or all citizens. For many of us, health care is free or heavily subsidised at the time of use. We never know its cost, and we do not consider whether it is public money well spent.

Epidemiology, Evidence-based Medicine and Public Health Lecture Notes, Sixth Edition. Yoav Ben-Shlomo, Sara T. Brookes and Matthew Hickman.
© 2013 Y. Ben-Shlomo, S. T. Brookes and M. Hickman. Published 2013 by John Wiley & Sons, Ltd.

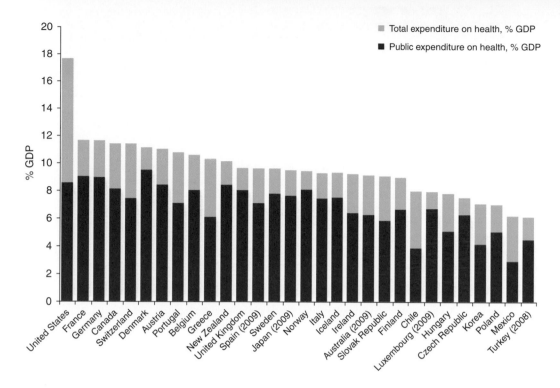

Figure 13.1 Total expenditure on health and public expenditure on health as % gross domestic product (GDP) in OECD countries in 2010. (When 2010 data were unavailable, previous years data were used as indicated in parentheses.) *Source:* Based on data from OECD (2012) *Total expenditure on health*, Health: Key Tables from OECD, No. 1. http://dx.doi.org/10.1787/hlthxp-total-table-2012-1-en and OECD (2012) *Public expenditure on health*, Health: Key Tables from OECD, No. 3. http://dx.doi.org/10.1787/hlthxp-pub-table-2012-1-en.

Health care use is often initiated by a patient deciding to see a doctor. In a system with 'free' care, this decision can be based on medical and not financial considerations. This creates more equitable access; however it may lead to overuse of health services for trivial reasons, sometimes referred to as **moral hazard**. During the medical consultation, treatment decisions are often taken by the doctor with some patient input. Decisions should be based on sound evidence about treatment effectiveness for the patient (**evidence-based medicine**) and affordability for the population. In practice they may also be adversely influenced by incomplete evidence, commercial marketing, and even financial incentives if doctors are paid per procedure (sometimes referred to as **supplier induced demand**). By providing high-quality evidence on the costs and outcomes of alternative ways of providing health care, economic evaluation aims to improve the health of the population for any fixed level of public expenditure.

The design of an economic evaluation

Key elements of study design discussed in previous chapters also apply to economic studies. For example, a specification of the **P**atient group, **I**ntervention, **C**omparator(s) and **O**utcome (**PICO** – see Chapter 8) is essential. In economic evaluation the outcome of interest is frequently expressed as a ratio, such as the additional cost per life year gained.

An economic evaluation conducted alongside a randomised controlled trial (RCT) would, typically, provide stronger evidence than an evaluation based on a cohort study. Regrettably, many RCTs do not include an economic evaluation, although regulators are increasingly demanding proof of efficiency before approval of new drugs and devices. In the absence of relevant information from RCTs, policy-makers rely on

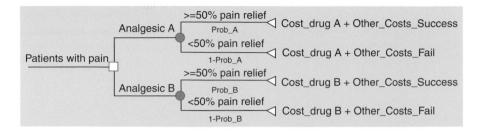

Figure 13.2 A simple decision analysis model to compare the cost effectiveness of two analgesics.

   The probability of successful pain relief with drug A (Prob_A) and drug B (Prob_B) can be estimated from RCTs or the best available observational data. If economic data from an RCT are unavailable, the costs of prescribing drugs A and B (Cost_drugA and Cost_drugB) and the other costs of treating patients with successful (Other_Costs_Success) and unsuccessful (Other_Costs_Fail) pain relief can be estimated from observational studies. These six parameters allow estimation of the additional cost per patient with substantial pain relief of drug A versus drug B.

   For example if: Prob_A = 0.75; Prob_B = 0.50; Cost_drugA = £100; Cost_drugB = £50; Other_Costs_Success = £20 and Other_Costs_Fail = £40, then the cost effectiveness of drug A versus drug B is:

$$[(£100 + (0.75)*£20 + (1 - 0.75)*£40) - (£50 + (0.50)*£20 + (1 - 0.50)*£40)]/(0.75 - 0.50)$$

This equates to £180 for every additional patient with substantial pain relief from drug A.

economic evidence generated by decision analysis models. These models define the possible clinical pathways resulting from alternative interventions (Figure 13.2) and then use literature reviews to draw together the best available evidence on the probability of each pathway, the expected costs and impact on patient health. Clearly these models are only as valid as the studies upon which they are based.

Efficiency is in the eye of the beholder

It is essential to consider the boundaries of the economic evaluation. A programme to prevent obesity in children is unlikely to appear cost-effective during the first few years, but may prove a wise investment over subsequent decades as the cohort develops fewer weight-related diseases. Therefore, for chronic diseases the appropriate time horizon for the economic evaluation is often the lifetime of the patient group. This has important implications for expensive new treatments where effectiveness can be proven relatively quickly by an RCT, but efficiency may not become apparent until long after the end of the RCT follow-up.

   A natural starting point for an integrated health system is to ask whether the money it spends on

a health technology is justified by the improvement it achieves in patient health. However, this health-system perspective may inadvertently lead to blinkered decision making, whereby costs are shifted onto other elements of society. For example centralisation of health care into larger clinics or hospitals might save the health system money at the expense of patients, carers and society through greater travel costs and more time off work. Given this, a strong argument can be made that, in making public spending decisions, we should take an all-encompassing (societal) viewpoint.

   In everyday life, we are accustomed to thinking about costs in terms of monetary values. However money is just an imperfect indicator of the value of the resources used. For example, a doctor-led clinic-based routine follow-up of women with breast cancer could be replaced with a nurse-led telephone based approach. The financial cost of the doctor-led clinics may be no higher than the nurse-led telephone follow-up if the clinics are of short duration and conducted by low-salaried junior doctors. However, the true **opportunity cost** of the doctor led clinics may be much higher if these routine follow-up visits are preventing other women with incident breast cancer receiving prompt treatment at the clinic. The concept of opportunity cost acknowledges that the true cost of using a scarce resource in one way is its unavailability to provide alternative services.

How much does it cost?

The costing process involves identification of resource items affected by the intervention, measurement of patient use of these items and valuation to assign costs to resources used. Identification is governed by the chosen perspective of the analysis. From a health system perspective, an evaluation of a new drug for multiple sclerosis would go no further than tracking patient use of community, primary and secondary care health services. A broader societal perspective would require additional information on lost productivity due to ill health, care provided by friends and family and social services, and patient expenses related to the illness (e.g. travel to hospital, purchase of mobility equipment).

The introduction of electronic records has greatly increased the potential to use routinely collected data to measure resources (e.g. tests, prescriptions, procedures) used in hospitals and primary care. However, there are drawbacks. Records are often fragmented across different health system sectors and difficult to access. Records are usually established for clinical and/or payment purposes rather than research and therefore may not contain sufficient information for accurate costing. Therefore, patient self-report in the form of questionnaires or diaries is often used, but may be affected by **loss to follow-up and recall bias**. The degree of detail required for costing will vary. A study evaluating electronic prescribing would require direct observation of the prescription process. In other studies such minute detail on the duration of a clinic visit would be unnecessary.

Many health systems publish the unit costs of health care, for example the average cost of a MRI scan of the spine, which can be used to value the resources used by patients. However, in an RCT comparing rapid versus conventional MRI of the spine an average cost would not be sufficient and a unit cost must be calculated from scratch. This would include allocating the purchase cost of the imaging equipment across its lifetime (annuitisation) and apportioning salaries, maintenance, estate and other costs to every minute of machine use. It is particularly difficult to generalise the valuation of resource use between nations. General practitioners in the United States, United Kingdom and the Netherlands are paid up to twice as much as their counterparts in Belgium and Sweden, even after adjusting for the cost of living.

Is it worth it?

The typical goal of an intervention is to use resources to optimise health measured by clinical outcomes such as mortality or bone density, or patient-reported outcomes such as pain or quality of life (known as **technical efficiency**). If one outcome is of overriding importance then a **Cost Effectiveness Analysis (CEA)** (Table 13.1) could be used to summarise whether any additional costs of the intervention are justified by gains in health. For example an evaluation of acupuncture versus conventional care for patients with pain could calculate the extra cost per additional patient who has a 50% reduction in pain score at 3 months. If more than one aspect of health, for instance pain *and* function, are considered important outcomes of treatment, analysts can choose to simply tabulate the costs and all outcomes in a **Cost Consequences Study (CCS)**. In a CCS, the reader is left

Table 13.1 Types of economic evaluation.

	What outcome(s) are used	How are results presented[a]
Cost-effectiveness analysis	A primary physical measure e.g. 50% reduction in pain score	Extra cost per extra unit of unit of primary outcome measure
Cost consequences study	More than one important outcome measure e.g. 50% reduction in pain score, 50% increase in mobility score and patient satisfaction score	Costs and outcomes are presented in tabular form with no aggregation
Cost benefit analysis	Money	Benefit–cost ratio of intervention.
Cost utility analysis	QALYs	Extra cost per QALY gained

[a]if no intervention is dominant.

to weigh up the potentially conflicting evidence on disparate cost and outcomes to reach a conclusion about the most efficient method of care.

Less frequently, analysts use **Cost Benefit Analysis (CBA)** to place a monetary value on treatment programmes. This is simplest in areas where citizens are familiar with paying for care. For example, people who might benefit from a new type of In Vitro Fertilisation (IVF) could be asked how much they would be willing to pay (WTP) for a cycle of this therapy, based on evidence that it increases the chances of birth from 20% to 30%. If the WTP of those who might benefit is greater than the additional costs of this new type of IVF, then this provides evidence that it is an efficient use of health care resources.

Policy-makers aim to create a health care system that is both **technically and allocatively efficient**. This means that money spent on each sector of care (e.g. oncology, orthopaedics or mental health) would not result in more health benefits if reallocated elsewhere in the health system. These allocative comparisons would be aided by a universal outcome measure. This measure needs to be flexible enough to be applicable in trials with outcomes as diverse as mortality, depression, and vision. **Quality Adjusted Life Years (QALYs)** used in **Cost-Utility Analysis (CUA)** aim to provide such a universal measure (see Table 13.1 which compares the 4 different types of analysis)

What is a QALY?

QALYs measure health outcomes by weighting years of life by a factor (Q) that represents the patient's health-related quality of life. Q is anchored at 1 (perfect health) and 0 (a health state considered to be as bad as death) and is estimated for all health states between these extremes and a small number of health states that might be considered worse than death. A QALY is simply the number of years that a patient spends in each health state multiplied by the quality of life weight, Q, of that state. For example, a patient who spends 2 years in an imperfect health state, where $Q = 0.75$, would achieve 1.5 QALYs (0.75×2). Q is generally estimated indirectly via a questionnaire such as the *EQ-5D*. The questionnaire asks the patient to categorise current health in various dimensions – for example, mobility, pain, and mental health. Every possible combination of questionnaire response is given a quality weight, Q. These weights are derived from surveys of the public's valuations for the health states described by the questionnaire.

There are concerns that in the attempt to measure and value a very broad range of dimensions of health, QALY questionnaires such as the EQ-5D have sacrificed responsiveness to small but important changes within an individual dimension. Additionally, there is disagreement about the appropriate group to use in the valuation survey. Should it be the general population who can take a dispassionate, but perhaps ill-informed, approach to valuing ill health? Or should it be patient groups who have experienced the health state? Perhaps the most persistent question about QALYs is whether they result in fair interpersonal comparisons of treatment effectiveness. The CUA methodology typically does not differentiate between a QALY resulting from treatment of a congenital condition in a child and a QALY resulting from palliative care in an elderly patient with a terminal illness. It is debatable whether this neutral stance reflects public opinion. For these and other reasons, QALYs remain controversial; in the UK they currently play an important role in national health care decision making, whereas in Germany their role is less prominent.

What are the results of an economic evaluation?

In essence, there are only four possible results from an economic evaluation of a new intervention versus current care (**Cost Effectiveness Plane (CEP)**; (Figure 13.3)). Many new drugs are in the North East (NE) quadrant; they are more expensive, but more effective than existing treatment options. But that need not be the case. 'Breakthrough' drugs (e.g. Penicillin) can be both effective and cost saving (i.e. dominant in the South East quadrant) if the initial cost of the drug is recouped through future health care avoided. When the most effective intervention is simply not affordable, policy makers may opt for an intervention in the South West quadrant which is slightly less effective but will not bankrupt the health system. Sadly, the history of medicine also has a number of examples of new technologies (e.g. Thalidomide for morning sickness) that fall into the North West quadrant, more costly and eventually seen to

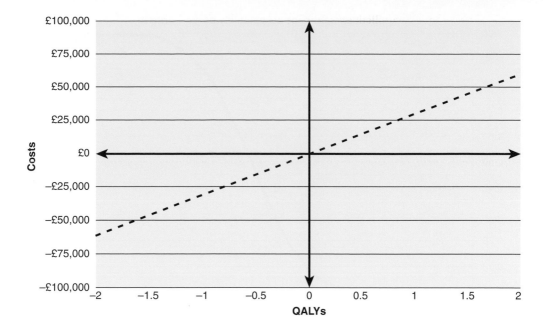

Figure 13.3 Cost effectiveness plane.

be harmful (i.e. dominated). Most controversy and headlines in high-income countries concern interventions in the NE quadrant. Can public funds afford to pay for all health care that is effective, no matter how expensive or marginally effective it is? Assuming that the answer is no, then one solution for differentiating between more efficient and less efficient innovations would be to define a cost-effectiveness threshold. For example, the UK Government has indicated that it is unwilling to fund interventions that yield less than one QALY per £30,000 spent (i.e. anything above and to the left of the dashed line in Figure 13.3).

The key finding of an economic evaluation is often summarised in an **Incremental Cost Effectiveness Ratio (ICER)**. This is simply the difference in cost between the intervention and the comparator $(C_i - C_c)$ divided by the difference in effectiveness $(E_i - E_c)$. A worked example, based on a UK evaluation of a new drug for advanced liver cancer, is provided in Table 13.2. In that example, the drug was effective, but the large additional cost resulted in a high ICER suggesting that it might not be an efficient use of public money.

In countries such as the UK where there is a relatively established threshold, the ICER is commonly converted into a **Net Monetary Benefit (NMB)** statistic (Table 13.2). The NMB is attractive because it simplifies interpretation, a new treatment with a negative NMB is not cost-effective, and enables straightforward calculation of confidence intervals.

Table 13.2 Worked example of calculating the ICER and NMB.

Intervention	Total QALYs	Total Costs
New drug	1.08	£28,359
Best supportive care	0.72	£9,739
ICER	(£28,359 − £9,739) / (1.08 − 0.72) = **£51,722**	
NMB$_{(30,000)}$	(1.08 − 0.72) * £30,000 − (£28,359 − £9,739) = **−£7,820**	

ICER=Incremental cost-effectiveness ratio
NMB$_{(30,000)}$ = net monetary benefit statistic (at a £30,000 threshold)

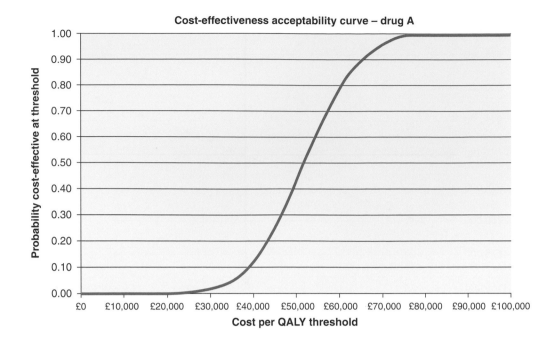

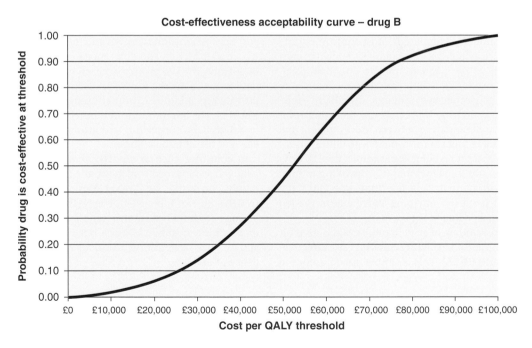

Figure 13.4 Cost effectiveness acceptability curves.
Note: The probability that a drug is cost-effective can be estimated by plotting a line up from a chosen threshold on the horizontal axis (e.g. £30,000 per QALY) to the curve and then across to read off the probability from the vertical axis. An approximate lower (and upper) 95% confidence limit can be estimated by plotting a line across from 0.025 (0.975) on the vertical axis to the curve and then down to read off the cost per QALY limit from the horizontal axis.

Interpreting the result

The **cost effectiveness acceptability curve (CEAC)** (Figure 13.4) is becoming a popular way of presenting the degree of certainty about the result of an economic evaluation. These graphs can be interpreted by scanning across the horizontal axis to a conventional cost-effectiveness threshold (£30,000 per QALY in the UK) and reading off the associated probability of cost-effectiveness from the vertical axis. In Figure 13.4, both drugs A and B are probably not cost-effective at the recommended threshold (p<0.50). However while drug A is almost certainly not cost-effective (approximate 95% confidence interval of £31,000 to £72,000 per QALY), the case is far from proven for drug B (approximate 95% confidence interval of £12,000 to £91,000 per QALY). A larger RCT with longer follow-up might provide a more definitive answer.

Uncertainty can also be addressed through **sensitivity analysis** where key assumptions of the analysis, for example the drug or device cost, are varied to determine the robustness of conclusions.

What happens next?

Even if the benefits of an intervention have been clearly shown to justify the costs these results form just one part of the decision-making process. Political objectives such as promotion of equality and budgetary considerations (i.e. what will we stop doing in order to afford this new treatment?) will also be taken into account before the intervention is recommended.

Summary

Economic evaluation is a key component of evidence-based medicine. It represents a shift in thinking away from 'what is the most effective way of improving this patient's health?' and towards 'what is the most efficient way of using a healthcare budget to optimise the health and wellbeing of the population?'

 KEY LEARNING POINTS

- Economic evaluations allow one to make rationale choices between treatments
- Costs and benefits are commonly calculated from a health system or societal perspective

---

- Costing requires identification, measurement and valuation of resources
- There are four main types of economic evaluation: cost-effectiveness, cost-consequence, cost-benefit and cost-utility analysis
- QALYs combine health-related quality of life and survival, enabling comparison of treatments across different domains of health care with a common metric
- An economic evaluation may indicate that a new intervention is dominant (effective and cost-saving), dominated (ineffective and costly) or effective but more expensive
- The trade off between the costs and effectiveness of therapies can be summarised by the Incremental Cost Effectiveness Ratio and Net Monetary Benefit statistic
- Statistical uncertainty can be quantified using a confidence interval or Cost Effectiveness Acceptability Curve
- Sensitivity analyses are usually undertaken to see if the conclusions are robust to various assumptions

 FURTHER READING

Drummond MF, Sculpher MJ, Torrance GW, O'Brien BJ, Stoddart GL (2005) *Methods for the Economic Evaluation of Health Care Programmes.* Oxford: Oxford University Press.

Drummond MF, Richardson WS, O'Brien BJ, Levine M, Heyland D (1997) Users' guides to the medical literature. XIII. How to use an article on economic analysis of clinical practice. A. Are the results of the study valid? Evidence-Based Medicine Working Group. *JAMA* **277**: 1552–7.

O'Brien BJ, Heyland D, Richardson WS, Levine M, Drummond MF (1997) Users' guides to the medical literature. XIII. How to use an article on economic analysis of clinical practice. B. What are the results and will they help me in caring for my patients? Evidence-Based Medicine Working Group. *JAMA* **277**: 1802–6.

Ramsey S, Willke R, Briggs A, *et al.* (2005) Good research practices for cost-effectiveness analysis alongside clinical trials: the ISPOR RCT-CEA Task Force report. *Value Health* **8**: 521–33.

14

Audit, research ethics and research governance

Joanne Simon and Yoav Ben-Shlomo
University of Bristol

Learning objectives

In this chapter you will learn:

- ✓ how to describe the process around the audit cycle;
- ✓ what the general ethical principles are around research;
- ✓ what is the role of the research ethics committee;
- ✓ what special issues relate to interventional and observational studies;
- ✓ the principles around research with children and incapacitated adults.

How do we know we are doing a good job?

It is common for health care professionals to review the management of patients when something goes very wrong, such as an unexpected death or serious complication post-surgery (**critical incident analysis**). However problems with more minor events, e.g. wound infection rates, or mortality in high-risk patients may not be detected without some sort of formal audit procedure which is intended to detect 'outliers'. These can be both positive (better than expected) or negative (worse than expected) rates of events and the unit of analysis could be at the level of an individual clinician, specialty within a hospital level or at a hospital level. For example the Bristol Royal Infirmary enquiry investigated an excess number of children under the age of one dying from open heart surgery between 1991 and 1995 (between 30 and 35 additional deaths). It concluded

There was no systematic mechanism for monitoring the clinical performance of healthcare professionals or of hospitals. For the future there must be effective systems within hospitals to ensure that clinical performance is monitored. There must also be a system of independent external surveillance to review patterns of performance over time and to identify good and failing performance. (www.bristolinquiry.org.uk/)

Epidemiology, Evidence-based Medicine and Public Health Lecture Notes, Sixth Edition. Yoav Ben-Shlomo, Sara T. Brookes and Matthew Hickman.
© 2013 Y. Ben-Shlomo, S. T. Brookes and M. Hickman. Published 2013 by John Wiley & Sons, Ltd.

The audit cycle

Audit is a form of quality improvement that aims to improve clinical care by critically examining existing practice and identifying any areas for concern. The necessary steps involve:

(1) choosing a topic for the audit;
(2) predefining acceptable standards or using the variation in the distribution of outcomes to identify outliers (see Figure 14.1);
(3) collecting relevant data to address the topic including information on case mix or clinical severity;
(4) analysing the data so that performance is compared to expected outcomes;
(5) implementing any necessary recommendations;
(6) repeating audit after a sufficient time period to enable any improvement to occur.

What's the difference between audit, service evaluation and research?

Unlike research, audit by definition is not designed to obtain new evidence but rather compares actual performance with some agreed level of quality standards. The findings may be unique to the individual hospital or health care system and not generalisable to other situations. Its aim is to improve health care delivery rather than identify new risk factors or new interventions that work. It is concerned with the appropriate implementation of evidence or consensus based guidelines rather than their development. It usually uses existing data rather than collecting new data though the process of extracting that data may be similar to that used in research. **Service evaluation** can be considered even one stage earlier than audit as its primary purpose is simply to measure what and how services are actually delivered without reference to any specific quality standard as in audit. Both audit and research, however, may have ethical implications (see below) though usually audit and service evaluation do not require formal ethical review by a research ethics committee. Appendix 14.1 highlights the differences between research, audit and service evaluation.

Ethical issues

Research ethics can be defined as the sustained analysis of motives of, procedures for and social effects of biomedical research (Murphy, 2004,

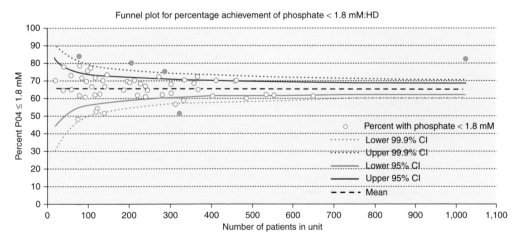

Figure 14.1 Cross-sectional **statistical process control** chart showing the control of phosphate level in patients on renal replacement therapy across different renal units in the United Kingdom. The x-axis indicates whether the unit is large or small and the graph shows different confidence intervals so one can infer the probability that the result may have occurred by chance. There are four high performing units and one low performing unit outside the 99.9% confidence limits.
Source: taken from Hodsman A, Ben-Shlomo Y, Roderick P *et al.* (2011) The 'centre effect' in nephrology: what do differences between nephrology centres tell us about clinical performance in patient management? *Nephron Clin Pract* **119**: c10–c17. Reproduced with permission from S. Karger AG Basel.

p. 1). Any clinical, biomedical, epidemiological or social-science research which involves direct contact with NHS patients or healthy participants should be undertaken in accordance with commonly agreed standards of good ethical practice. The *Declaration of Helsinki*, first written in 1963 by the World Medical Association, lays down a set of ethical principles for medical research. The fundamental and widely accepted ethical principles can be broadly classified as:

- Beneficence (to do good)
- Nonmaleficence (first, do no harm)
- Autonomy (individual's right to choose)
- Justice (fairness and equality)
- Truthfulness (informed consent, confidentiality)

Historical events, such as the Nuremberg Trials (Nazi doctors experimented on prisoners under the pretext of medical research) and the Tuskegee syphilis study (where African-American men with syphilis were never asked for consent and had penicillin knowingly withheld after its introduction so that doctors could study the natural history of the disease), led to the need for a statement of ethical issues in research, such as the Declaration of Helsinki, and for arrangements for the ethical review of proposed research in order to protect the research participants and promote high-quality research.

For research involving patients of the United Kingdom National Health Service (NHS), their tissue or their data, ethical review and favourable ethical opinion is sought prospectively from an NHS Research Ethics Committee. Research undertaken by academic staff or students involving participants outside of the NHS should be reviewed by ethical committees within the host Higher Education Institution. Ethical review must occur before any research related activity takes place. Other developed countries have different but equivalent bodies such as Institutional Review Boards (IRBs) in the United States or Independent Ethics Committees. Ethics committees must not only consider key ethical aspects of the research but also its validity; poor quality research can be unethical because it may have no benefit in terms of new knowledge whilst have some risk for the participants. It may also put future participants at harm if the research is misleading (for example the scare concerning MMR vaccination and risk of autism leading to a decline in population vaccination rates)

Ethical issues in Randomised Controlled Trials (RCTs)

All research studies raise ethical issues, such as **participant confidentiality**. However RCTs involve more difficult issues than observational studies, because they mean that the choice of treatment is not made by patients and clinicians but is instead devolved to a process of random allocation. This means that a patient in an RCT may receive a new untested treatment, or not be able to choose a new active treatment if allocated to the placebo group.

Before one can undertake an RCT, the health professionals treating the patients must be uncertain about whether the treatments being evaluated are better, worse or the same as any existing treatment or a placebo. This is called **clinical equipoise**. If there is existing evidence that a new treatment is superior then clinicians should not participate. However, in reality, most clinicians will have some preference or 'hunch' that one treatment is better than another, but they will need to suspend these views to conduct an RCT to provide clear evidence. Often, RCT results are different from clinicians' hunches. For example a recent large RCT of a drug that inhibits the cholesteryl ester transfer protein (CETP) and raises HDL-cholesterol, associated with a reduced risk of heart disease, actually found an increased risk of cardiovascular events. Despite improving HDL-cholesterol, it was unclear why patients on active treatment had a higher mortality rate though the drug did unexpectedly raise the participants' blood pressure (Barter *et al.*, 2007).

As described in more detail below patients must give **informed consent** to participate in an RCT and must understand that the treatment they receive will be determined by chance through randomisation. If one of the treatments is a placebo group then the patients must know this. They should not be coerced to take part or given financial incentive other than any expenses that arise from participation. Even if they consent to participate, they are entitled to withdraw from the study at any time and this should in no way compromise their future treatment. For informed consent to be ethically valid the investigator must disclose all risks and benefits and the participant must be competent to understand this. Independent research ethics committee must review and approve studies before they are undertaken.

One special aspect of RCTs is the use of 'sham' procedures to maintain blinding. In a drug trial it is usually straightforward to create an identical looking placebo so that participants cannot tell whether they are taking the active or placebo medication. This is more complex for nonmedical interventions, especially surgical interventions. In this case a sham procedure may be used though this may have risk in itself. For example, a RCT of foetal nigral transplantation for Parkinson's disease randomised patients to the insertion of aborted material using stereotactic surgery. The placebo group underwent the same procedure and had partial burr holes made in the skull but no needle or foetal material was inserted (Olanow *et al.*, 2003).

Ethical issues in observational studies

Observational studies are usually less problematic and of lower risk as the researchers simply measure characteristics of the participants using questionnaires, tissue, imaging or physiological measures. One issue that may arise in such studies is opportunistic identification of clinical abnormalities and it is good practice to have an explicit protocol for how these will be handled as well as obtaining consent from the participants as to whether they would wish to have this information feedback to them and/or their general practitioners. For example many epidemiological studies will measure blood pressure and there are clear evidence-based guidelines on what constitutes a level worthy of treatment if it is sustained over several readings or over a 24-hour period. However, studies of MRI brain imaging in the elderly will find a high prevalence of asymptomatic brain infarcts (around 18% in subjects between 75 and 97 years in the Rotterdam study). In this case it is less clear that feeding back abnormal results is helpful as it may cause participant anxiety without necessarily any improvement in health care (Vernooij *et al.*, 2007).

Informed consent

Informed consent is at the heart of ethical research. Most studies involving individuals must have appropriate arrangements for obtaining consent from potential research participants. Informed consent must be:

- voluntary and freely given;
- fully informed;
- recorded in writing or some other means if there are literacy issues.

Potential participants should be given a written information sheet and informed consent form, which has received approval from a relevant research ethics committee. The written information sheet should contain the following elements: why they have been selected, what is the purpose of the research, what will happen to them if they agree, any risks or benefits, how their information will be kept confidential, what if something goes wrong, how to find out further information.

Obtaining informed consent should be seen as a process of communication and discussion between researcher and participant. The researcher has a duty to ensure the participant truly understands what is being asked of them, and that they are willing to voluntarily give full, informed consent. Researchers should be very careful not to coerce the participant or to emphasise the potential benefits, nor attempt to minimise the risks or disadvantages of participation. Coercion may be implicit rather than explicit if the recruiting clinician has a long standing relationship with the patient who may find it hard to refuse the invitation. Participants have the right to ask questions of the researcher, and be given reasonable time to consider their decision to participate before confirming their willingness to participate both verbally and in writing. All participants must have given informed consent before any aspect of the research starts.

Vulnerable groups (children and incapacitated adults)

Children

Informed consent must be obtained from the child's parent (or legal guardian) as appropriate. When parental consent is obtained, the *assent* (voluntary agreement) of the child should also be sought by researchers, as appropriate to the child's age and level of understanding. A full explanation of the research must be given to the parent (or legal guardian) of the child, in accordance with the principles described earlier, including the provision of written information and opportunity for questions and time for consideration. The parent (or legal guardian) may then give informed consent for the child to participate in the study.

The child should also be given information about the research. This will be age-appropriate and offered according to the child's level of understanding. Often the use of visual aids or cartoons can explain basic information for young children. Verbal assent should be sought from the child, and recorded in the research notes, as well as the child's medical record (for clinical trials). Older children may wish to sign a consent form. For children over the age of 16 this would constitute legally valid consent.

Written information provided to children should be written in age-appropriate language that the child could understand. Different versions of the research information should therefore be produced for different age ranges e.g. under 5s, 6–12 year olds, 13–15 year olds and over 16.

Incapacitated adults

Incapacitated adults do not have mental capacity to make decisions for themselves. This may be because of unconsciousness, mental illness, or other causes, to the extent that the person does not have sufficient understanding or ability to make or communicate responsible decisions. Special arrangements exist to ensure the interests of incapacitated adults recruited into research studies are protected. For investigational medicinal product (drug) trials, or trials of medical devices in England, Wales and Northern Ireland the provisions for inclusion of incapacitated adults are laid down in the Medicines for Human Use (Clinical Trials) Regulations 2004 and as amended. In Scotland, these regulations and also the Adults with Incapacity (Scotland) Act 2004 (regulations 4 to 16 and Parts 3 and 5 of Schedule 1) will also apply. Such requirements are considered suitable for other types of clinical research.

When considering a patient who is unable to consent for themselves for suitability for a trial, the decision on whether to consent to, or refuse, participation in a trial will be taken by a *legal representative* who is independent of the research team and should act on the basis of the person's presumed wishes. The type and hierarchy of legal representative who should be approached to give informed consent on behalf of an incapacitated adult prior to inclusion of the subject in the trial is given in Table 14.1 (note that arrangements for Scotland are slightly different).

Table 14.1 Type and hierarchy of legal representative who can give informed consent on behalf of an incapacitated adult prior to inclusion of the subject in the trial.

England, Wales and Northern Ireland	Scotland
1. Personal legal representative	*1. Personal legal representative*
A person not connected with the conduct of the trial who is:	1A. Any guardian or welfare attorney who has power to consent to the adult's participation in research.
(a) suitable to act as the legal representative by virtue of their relationship with the adult, *and*	1B. If there is no such person, the adult's nearest relative as defined in section 87(1) of the Adults with Incapacity (Scotland) Act 2000.
(b) available and willing to do so.	
2. Professional legal representative	*2. Professional legal representative*
A person not connected with the conduct of the trial who is:	A person not connected with the conduct of the trial who is:
(a) the doctor primarily responsible for the adult's medical treatment, or	(a) the doctor primarily responsible for the adult's medical treatment, or
(b) a person nominated by the relevant health care provider (e.g. an acute NHS Trust or Health Board).	(b) a person nominated by the relevant health care provider.
A professional legal representative may be approached if no suitable personal legal representative is available.	A professional legal representative may be approached if it is not reasonably practicable to contact either 1A or 1B before the decision to enter the adult into the trial is made. Informed consent must be given before the subject is entered into the trial.

The appropriate legal representative should be provided with an approved Legal Representative Information Sheet and Legal Representative Informed Consent Form to document the consent process.

The consent given by the legal representative remains valid in law even if the patient recovers capacity. However, at this point, the patient should be informed about the trial and asked to decide whether or not they should continue in the trial, and consent to continue should be sought.

Research governance

Research governance can be defined as the broad range of regulations, principles and standards of good practice that exist to achieve, and continuously improve, research quality across all aspects of health care in the UK and worldwide. In the UK, the Department of Health published the first Research Governance Framework for Health and Social Care in 2001, and this was updated in 2005 and sets out to:

* safeguard participants in research;
* protect researchers/investigators (by providing a clear framework to work within);
* enhance ethical and scientific quality;
* minimise risk;
* monitor practice and performance;
* promote good practice and ensure lessons are learned.

Research governance includes research that is concerned with the protection and promotion of public health, undertaken in or by the Department of Health, its non-Departmental Public Bodies and the NHS, or within social care agencies. It includes clinical and nonclinical research; and any research undertaken by industry, charities, research councils and universities within the health and social care systems. Everyone who undertakes healthcare research (research involving individuals, their tissue or their data) therefore has responsibilities for research governance. This includes lead researchers, research nurses, students undertaking research, as well as NHS organisations where research takes place and universities who may employ or supervise researchers or act as sponsor organisations.

Research governance should be considered at all stages of the research, from the initial development and design of the research project, through it's set-up, conduct, analysis and reporting. Researchers need to ensure that:

* day to day responsibility for elements of each research project is clearly stated;
* research follows the agreed protocol;
* research participants receive the appropriate care while participating in the research;
* data protection, integrity and confidentiality of all records is intact;
* reporting adverse incidents or suspected misconduct is undertaken.

Research governance approval is required from any NHS Trust before the research can take place on their premises, or access patients, their tissue or their data. All research documents such as research protocol, participant information sheets and informed consent forms, details of NHS Research Ethics Committee approval, researcher CV are submitted for governance checks. Current systems for multi-centre research review the research governance compliance at a nominated lead NHS Trust, and local information only is submitted to the local NHS Trusts. The Integrated Research Application System (www.myresearchproject.org.uk) is used for submission of research information to NHS Research Ethics Committees as well as NHS research governance approval.

 KEY LEARNING POINTS

* Audit is a process to ensure that delivery of health care meets accepted standards of care and can identify both exemplars of very good or very poor practice

* To complete the audit cycle, one must demonstrate that any identified deficiencies have been acted upon and there has been improvement

* All research has ethical implications but these tend to be more serious with RCTs than observational studies especially around the issue of clinical equipoise. RCTs may also use sham procedures to maintain blinding

* In general terms, it is essential to avoid any unnecessary harm to participants, ensure they

are fully informed prior to consent and maintain participant confidentiality

- Studies of children need to seek child assent as well as parental consent
- Special rules apply to research with incapacitated adults where is needs to be shown that the research could not be done in any other way and is in the participants' best interest
- Research ethics committees must approve research studies before they commence and there are often governance procedures that ensure that the research is undertaken to the highest level.

 ## REFERENCES

Barter PJ, Caulfield M, Eriksson M, *et al.* (2007) Effects of Torcetrapib in patients at high risk for coronary events. *NEJM* **357**: 2109–22.

Hodsman A, Ben-Shlomo Y, Roderick P, *et al.* (2011) The 'centre effect' in nephrology: what do differences between nephrology centres tell us about clinical performance in patient management? *Nephron Clin Pract* **119**: c10–c17.

Olanow CW, Goetz CG, Kordower JH, *et al.* (2003) A double-blind controlled trial of bilateral fetal nigral transplantation in Parkinson's disease. *Ann Neurol* **54**: 403–14.

Vernooij MW, Ikram MA, Tanghe HL, *et al.* (2007) Incidental findings on brain MRI in the general population. *N Engl J Med* **357**: 1821–8.

 ## FURTHER READING

Bristol Royal Infirmary Inquiry (2001) *Learning from Bristol: the report of the public inquiry into children's heart surgery at the Bristol Royal Infirmary 1984–1995.* Norwich: Stationery Office, (CM 5207.) Available at www.bristol-inquiry.org.uk/

Campbell A, Jones G, Gillett G (2001) *Medical Ethics*, 3rd edn. Oxford: Oxford University Press.

Hope T, Savulescu J, Hendrick J (2008) *Medical Ethics and Law. The Core Curriculum*, 2nd revised edn. London: Churchill Livingstone.

Murphy, Timothy (2004) *Case Studies in Biomedical Research Ethics.* Cambridge, MA: MIT Press.

UK National Research Ethics Service website: http://www.nres.npsa.nhs.uk/

Appendix 14.1 Differentiating research, service evaluation and clinical audit

Research	Service Evaluation*	Clinical Audit
The attempt to derive generalisable new knowledge including studies that aim to generate hypotheses as well as studies that aim to test them.	Designed and conducted solely to define or judge current care.	Designed and conducted to produce information to inform delivery of best care.
Quantitative research – designed to test a hypothesis. Qualitative research – identifies/ explores themes following established methodology.	Designed to answer: 'What standard does this service achieve?'	Designed to answer: 'Does this service reach a predetermined standard?'
Addresses clearly defined questions, aims and objectives	Measures current service without reference to a standard.	Measures against a standard.
Quantitative research – may involve evaluating or comparing interventions, particularly new ones. Qualitative research – usually involves studying how interventions and relationships are experienced.	Involves an intervention in use only. The choice of treatment is that of the clinician and patient according to guidance, professional standards and/or patient preference.	Involves an intervention in use only. The choice of treatment is that of the clinician and patient according to guidance, professional standards and/or patient preference.
Usually involves collecting data that are additional to those for routine care but may include data collected routinely. May involve treatments, samples or investigations additional to routine care.	Usually involves analysis of existing data but may include administration of interview or questionnaire.	Usually involves analysis of existing data but may include administration of simple interview or questionnaire.
Quantitative research – study design may involve allocating patients to intervention groups. Qualitative research – uses a clearly defined sampling framework underpinned by conceptual or theoretical justifications.	No allocation to intervention: the health professional and patient have chosen intervention before service evaluation.	No allocation to intervention: the health professional and patient have chosen intervention before audit.
May involve randomisation.	No randomisation.	No randomisation.
Normally requires REC review. Refer to www.nres.npsa.nhs.uk/applications/apply/ for more information	Does not require REC review.	Does not require REC review.

*Service development and quality improvement may fall into this category
Source: adapted from Defining Research: NRES guidance to help you decide if your project requires review by a Research Ethics Committee, NHS National Patient Safety Agency 2010.

Self-assessment questions – Part 2: Evidence-based medicine

Q1 Do tired doctors make more medical errors? (modified from Landrigan *et al., N Engl J Med* 2004)

Newly qualified doctors (PRHOs) typically work the greatest number of hours per week which may mean that they are especially prone to fatigue related errors. Whilst there is evidence that sleep deprivation impairs neurobehavioural performance, it is still unclear whether there is an increased risk of medical errors.

The Intern Sleep and Patient Safety Study was conducted in the medical intensive care unit and coronary care unit of a large academic hospital in Boston. PRHOs between July 2002 and June 2003 were allocated to work either the traditional schedule (work week average of 77 to 81 hours with up to 34 continuous hours of scheduled work, when clinic occurred after they were on call) or the intervention schedule (maximal scheduled hours 60–63 per week, with consecutive hours of work limited to approximately 16 hours). The allocation was done by the research team using random numbers and none of the team had any prior knowledge of the PRHOs' past academic record or clinical performance. During any week, all PRHOs on each unit were working the same schedule. The aim of the intervention schedule was to improve opportunities for sleep while minimising errors. The primary outcome of the study was the number of serious medical errors in which PRHOs were directly involved, this was recorded through direct observation by physicians. Blinding of these physician observers was not possible as they had to undertake the same work patterns.

During the study there were 634 admissions in total. The patients' and PRHOs' characteristics were very similar within the two schedules. All the PRHOs who were randomised completed the study except for one doctor allocated to the traditional schedule who dropped out due to ill-health. Table QB.1 presents the rates of serious errors and preventable adverse events per 1000 patient-days within each schedule.

(a) What is the null hypothesis?

(b) Does the table provide any evidence of an association between the type of schedule and the rate of 'serious medical errors'? Comment on the rate ratio, confidence interval, and P value.

(c) What type of errors does the intervention schedule most effectively reduce? Justify your answer.

(d) Why was it important that the researcher who decided whether a PRHO was allocated to either the intervention or traditional schedule had no knowledge about the PRHO? What do we call the design procedure employed in this type of study to prevent this potential bias? If this does not occur how could the results have been biased.

(e) What is meant by 'blinding' and did it occur in this study? If a study is unblinded what might occur? How could this have affected the results in this study?

(f) What other type of bias may effect this type of study design? Did it occur in this specific study?

Epidemiology, Evidence-based Medicine and Public Health Lecture Notes, Sixth Edition. Yoav Ben-Shlomo, Sara T. Brookes and Matthew Hickman.
© 2013 Y. Ben-Shlomo, S. T. Brookes and M. Hickman. Published 2013 by John Wiley & Sons, Ltd.

Table QB.1 Incidence of serious medical errors.

	Rate per 1000 patient-days				
	Intervention schedule	Traditional schedule	Rate ratio*	95% confidence interval	P value
Serious medical errors	100.1	136.0	0.74	0.57 to 0.95	0.016
Medication	82.5	99.7	0.83	0.61 to 1.17	0.19
Procedural	6.6	8.5	0.78	0.24 to 2.29	0.64
Diagnostic	3.3	18.6	0.18	0.03 to 0.59	<0.001
Other	7.7	9.3	0.83	0.28 to 2.29	0.71
Preventable adverse events#	16.5	20.9	0.79	0.39 to 1.54	0.47

*Rate ratio can be interpreted similarly to the risk ratio
#Injury due to a non-intercepted serious error in medical management

(g) In addition to the potential biases mentioned in questions d–f, what other explanations should be considered before concluding that the intervention schedule reduces the rate of serious errors? How likely are each of these?

(h) Assuming the association between work schedule and serious errors is true, why is it important to look at the association between work schedule and preventable adverse events before any policy changes are made. What else should also be considered?

(i) Does the intervention schedule lead to fewer preventable adverse events? Please comment on the rate ratio, confidence interval and P value? How precise is the estimate of the rate ratio?

(j) How generalisable are the findings? Would you suggest implementation of the intervention schedule into the UK?

Q2 Blinding in RCTs

For each of the following trial designs, state whether it is possible to blind patients and/or researchers to the allocation of treatments

(a) A drug trial of a new antidepressant compared to placebo where the outcome measure is a patient rated depression scale

(b) Group versus individual speech therapy sessions for patients who have a language difficulty (dysphasia) after a stroke where the outcome measure is a recorded conversation reading a specific piece of text

(c) A hypertensive trial where patients are given a drug (beta-blocker) that also slows down heart rate or an identical looking placebo and a nurse measures the blood pressure.

(d) A RCT of two different joint prostheses for osteoarthritis of the hip with the outcome measure being hip flexion without pain done by the researcher and a patient administered quality of life score.

(e) A trial of acupuncture for arthritic pain using a patient completed pain index and participants who have never previously had acupuncture.

Q3 Economic evaluation

The economic evaluation was conducted as part of a randomised controlled trial which examined the effectiveness, acceptability and accessibility of a general practitioner with special interest (GPSI) dermatology service compared with routine hospital outpatient care. Patients who were referred to a hospital outpatient dermatology clinic and were deemed suitable to be managed by a general practitioner with special interest were randomised to either usual care (i.e. hospital outpatient care) or the GPSI service.

Resources were measured for the patients for nine months following randomisation. Most of the NHS resources were measured through computerised systems. Resources used by patients and their companions, and information on time off work (lost production) were measured through patient self completed postal questionnaires.

Two types of evaluation using differing perspectives were conducted.

(I) A primary outcome measure, the dermatology life quality index score, and costs were evaluated from an NHS perspective.

(II) This outcome measure and others (an access score, patient satisfaction with the consultation, satisfaction with facilities, attendance rates, and waiting times) and costs were evaluated from several perspectives (NHS, patient and companion, societal lost production).

A sensitivity analysis was conducted which extended the collection of NHS resources for an additional 3 months (12 months in total). (Based on Coast J, Noble S, Noble A, Horrocks S, Asim O, Peters TJ, Salisbury C (2005) *BMJ* **331**(7530): 1444–8.)

(a) Identify the types of resource use that you would collect if the evaluation was from
   i. an NHS/health service provider perspective
   ii. societal perspective
(b) What are the potential problems with using self-completed questionnaires to measure patient costs and time off work?
(c) A **cost-effectiveness analysis** could be used for the first type of evaluation. What is the **PICO** for this analysis?
(d) What type of economic evaluation might you use for the second type of evaluation?
(e) The **cost-effectiveness analysis** will give evidence as to which is the most **technically efficient** provision of care. If this evaluation was to aid the creation of an allocatively efficient health care system what outcome measure(s) should be used.
(f) Comparing the new GPSI service with routine outpatient care, the results from the first type of evaluation were in the North East quadrant of the **cost-effectiveness plane**. What does this mean?
(g) How should uncertainty in relation to the **cost-effectiveness analysis** be represented?
(h) Why do you think the **sensitivity analysis** was conducted?

Q4 Diagnostic tests
(a) The abstract of a recent publication has reported the following performance measures for a new diagnostic test: sensitivity 50%, specificity 98%, positive predictive value 86%, negative predictive value 89%.
   i. What percentage of patients with the disease are correctly identified by the test?
   ii. Given a positive test result, what is the risk of having the disease?
   iii. What is the false positive rate of this test?
   iv. What percentage of patients with a negative test will still have the disease?
   v. Is this test more useful for ruling out or ruling in the diagnosis?
(b) When assessing a new diagnostic test:
   i. It should have a high specificity (>90%) if it is important not to miss new cases of disease. True or false?
   ii. If it is more expensive than existing tests it should not be introduced. True or false?
   iii. If subsequent investigation of people who test positive is invasive and risky, then the test should have a high positive predictive value. True or false?
   iv. Cohort studies are the best study design to evaluate whether a new diagnostic test improves health. True or false?
   v. The best diagnostic test has 100% sensitivity and 100% specificity. True or false?

Q5 Prognosis

State which of the following questions are true about prognosis (T) and which are not (F):
(a) A 2-year-old girl has glue ear. Is she likely to have long-term hearing impairment?
(b) A 60-year-old man has just been diagnosed with lung cancer. What is his chance of surviving 10 years?
(c) A 9-year-old boy has symptoms of dystonia (neurological movement disorder). What is the most likely cause?
(d) An injecting drug user (female, 30 years old) has just been diagnosed with hepatitis C. How likely is she to develop liver cancer?

(e) A nursery-age child is diagnosed with measles. Is he likely to pass this on to unvaccinated family members through household contact?

Q6 Systematic reviews

The figure shows the results from a Cochrane systematic review of randomised controlled trials of exercise-based rehabilitation for people with coronary heart disease. The majority of patients randomised had suffered an acute myocardial infarction and were middle-aged men. The following questions refer to this systematic review.

Which of the following statements are true/false?
(a) The results are presented as a field plot
(b) Whether treatment increased or decreased mortality is shown in the figure
(c) The pooled effect shows that exercise-based cardiac rehabilitation is better than usual care
(d) The trials with the longest bars are the biggest
(e) The size of the square for each trial represents the precision of the estimate

Review: Exercise-based rehabilitation for coronary heart disease
Comparison: 01 Exercise only versus usual care
Outcome: 01 Total Mortality

Study	Treatment n/N	Control n/N	Relative risk (fixed) 95% CI	Weight (%)	Relative risk (fixed) 95% CI
Anderson 81	4/46	3/42		2.5	1.22 [0.29, 5.12]
Behtall 90	16/113	12/116		9.6	1.37 [0.68, 2.76]
Carson 82	12/151	21/152		16.9	0.58 [0.29, 1.13]
Erdman 86	4/40	0/40		0.4	9.00 [0.50, 161.87]
Holmback 94	1/34	1/35		0.8	1.03 [0.07, 15.81]
Kentala 72	5/152	8/146		6.6	0.60 [0.20, 1.79]
NEHDP	15/323	24/328		19.3	0.63 [0.34, 1.19]
Siv arajan 82	3/88	2/84		1.7	1.43 [0.25, 8.36]
Speccia 96	5/125	13/131		10.3	0.40 [0.15, 1.10]
Stern 83	0/42	1/29		1.4	0.23 [0.01, 5.52]
Vecchio 81	0/25	2/25		2.0	0.20 [0.01, 3.97]
Wilhemson 75	28/158	35/157		28.4	0.79 [0.51, 1.24]
Total (95% CI)	93/1297	122/1285		100.0	0.76 [0.59, 0.98]

Test for heterogeneity chi-square = 10.50 df = 11 p = 0.4858
Test for overall effect = −2.08 p = 0.04

−1   −2   1   5   10
Favours treatment   Favours control

Part 3

Public health

15

Public health

Matthew Hickman, Ruth Kipping and David Gunnell
University of Bristol

Learning objectives

In this chapter you will learn:

- ✓ to define public health and distinguish between public health and individual health care;
- ✓ to identify how public health is measured or diagnosed;
- ✓ to identify types of public health intervention.

Introduction

Public health has been defined as: 'the science and art of preventing disease, prolonging life, and promoting health through organised efforts of society'. Public health focuses on improving the health of *entire populations* rather than on individual patients. The population is the patient. Tools for improving population health range from the development of new clinical services for treating disease, screening programmes to detect disease at an early (treatable) stage, immunisation to prevent the transmission of infectious diseases, to legislation to prohibit actions or behaviours, or health improvement in schools and workplaces. Public health aims to encompass the whole clinical iceberg (see Figure 15.1).

Public health seeks to target all ill health comprising the population that are asymptomatic or prodromal (unaware of illness), the population that have not yet presented to medical services as well as population being managed by health care services.

Public health practice

Public health is an interdisciplinary practice – with public health specialists operating locally, nationally and internationally; within healthcare services, local authorities, the voluntary sector and other government bodies – and drawing on a multitude of skills. As we write this chapter UK public health along with the NHS is being reorganised. This is not new – and however public health is organised the type of problems specialists tackle and the approach they take will be similar. What is common and critical is the population approach, i.e. that health needs are identified and assessed and interventions delivered and evaluated at a population level.

Epidemiology, Evidence-based Medicine and Public Health Lecture Notes, Sixth Edition. Yoav Ben-Shlomo, Sara T. Brookes and Matthew Hickman.
© 2013 Y. Ben-Shlomo, S. T. Brookes and M. Hickman. Published 2013 by John Wiley & Sons, Ltd.

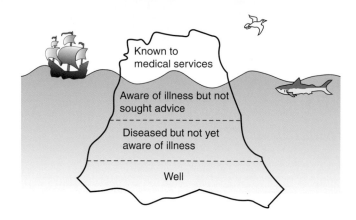

Figure 15.1 Clinical iceberg.

The three domains of public health in the UK are:

Health improvement	Improving services	Health protection
Inequalities	Clinical effectiveness	Infectious diseases
Education	Efficiency	Chemicals and poisons
Housing	Service planning	Radiation
Employment	Audit and evaluation	Emergency response
Family/community	Clinical governance	Environmental health hazards
Lifestyles	Equity	
Surveillance and monitoring of specific diseases and risk factors		

Many of these are covered elsewhere in the book – including infectious disease epidemiology and **health protection**; and **evidence based medicine** which underpins improving services. The issues in health improvement emphasise that public health aims to reduce inequalities as well as improve population health and that public health interventions can operate at multiple levels. As well as the domains above, public health is concerned with **Health Impact Assessment (HIA)** – UK and international examples of which are collated at the HIA Gateway. HIA is defined by WHO as 'A combination of procedures, methods and tools by which a policy, programme or project may be judged as to its potential effects on the health of a population, and the distribution of those effects within the population'.

The United States Communicable Disease Control has identified ten public health achievements of the twentieth century (Figure 15.2).

It is estimated that the average lifespan in the US increased by >30 years during the twentieth century and that 25 years (~3/4) of the gain is attributable to public health. Similar gains have occurred in other industrial/developed countries. The contribution of public health interventions include: eradication of smallpox, elimination of polio, and control of many other infections through 'vaccination'; reductions in motor vehicle accidents due to improvements in driving and 'motor-vehicle safety'; reductions in environmental exposure and occupational injury through ensuring 'safer work places'; improved sanitation, availability of clean water, and antimicrobials leading to better 'control of infectious diseases'; reductions in risk behaviours, such as smoking, and control of blood pressure and early detection have contributed to a decline in 'deaths from coronary heart disease and stroke'; better hygiene and nutrition of mothers and babies has contributed to reductions in neonatal and maternal mortality; and the many anti-smoking campaigns and policies have led to changes in public perceptions of the dangers and acceptability of smoking by the public and substantial reductions in smoking and environmental exposure to tobacco in the population. Morbidity and socioeconomic circumstances also have improved through 'safer and healthier foods' reducing frequency of diseases associated with nutritional deficiency (such as rickets and pellagra); family planning/contraceptive services reducing family size and transmission of sexually transmitted infections; and fluoridation has made substantial reductions in tooth decay and loss.

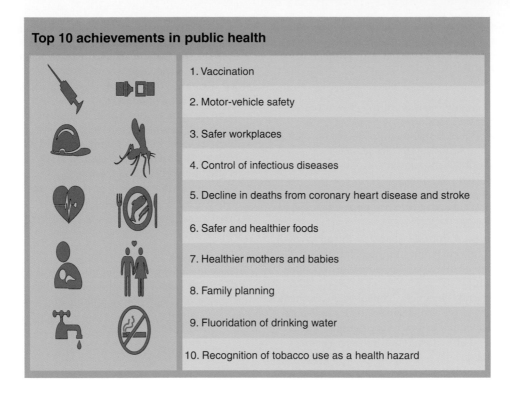

Top 10 achievements in public health

1. Vaccination

2. Motor-vehicle safety

3. Safer workplaces

4. Control of infectious diseases

5. Decline in deaths from coronary heart disease and stroke

6. Safer and healthier foods

7. Healthier mothers and babies

8. Family planning

9. Fluoridation of drinking water

10. Recognition of tobacco use as a health hazard

Figure 15.2 The twentieth century's ten great public health achievements (in developed countries). *Source*: http://www.cdc.gov.

These represent a range of different interventions:

- *primary prevention*: such as vaccination and health promotion campaigns; legislation and enforcement to promote safer driving, and safer work places;
- *environmental and social changes*: including improved nutrition and availability of clean water and fluoridated water;
- *medical advances*: such as hygiene during child birth and other surgical interventions; and more aggressive identification and treatment of early signs of heart disease.

The health problems affecting low and middle income countries differ from those of industrialised nations – and some of the public health achievements of the twentieth century identified above are as yet unresolved in developing countries. For example, there were approximately 6.5 million deaths in children under five in African and Southeast Asian countries in 2008 (Black *et al.*, 2010). The top six causes were: pneumonia (18%); diarrhoea (15%); neonatal birth complications (12%); neonatal asphyxia (9%) or sepsis (6%) and malaria (8%). Key interventions to prevent these deaths include: clean/sterile delivery, nutrition and nutritional deficiencies (e.g. vitamin A and zinc), antibiotics, water sanitation, vaccination (Hib and measles), oral rehydration, and mosquito (insecticide treated) nets. Key public health interventions in developed and developing countries can be medical, educational, social or legal.

Public health diagnosis

The steps to improving public health are analogous to clinical medicine but with slightly different tools. We need to 'diagnose' the problem. The tools at our disposal are information on the population, routine data on mortality and morbidity, hospitalisation, public health surveillance data, population health surveys and other epidemiological studies. Some of the key sources used in the UK are listed below. These allow us to measure rates of disease in the population, and consider variations in health and disease in different populations and over time.

(1) 10 yearly census (http://www.ons.gov.uk/census/index.html);
(2) mortality statistics (http://www.ons.gov.uk/about/who-we-are/our-services/unpublished-data/vital-events-data/mortality-records);
(3) cancer registration data (http://www.statistics.gov.uk/CCI/SearchRes.asp?Term=cancer);
(4) hospital episode statistics (http://www.dh.gov.uk/en/Publicationsandstatistics/Statistics/HospitalEpisodeStatistics/index.htm);
(5) general practice consultation statistics (http://www.ic.nhs.uk/statistics-and-data-collections/primary-care/general-practice/trends-in-consultation-rates-in-general-practice–1995-2009; http://www.gprd.com/home/default.asp; http://www.qresearch.org/SitePages/Home.aspx; http://www.thin-uk.com/);
(6) notification data: infectious disease (e.g. meningitis, mumps), congenital malformations, maternal deaths;
(7) laboratory reporting statistics (e.g. sentinel surveillance and other routine information on laboratory tests and diagnoses);
(8) morbidity surveys: National Psychiatric Morbidity Survey; Health Survey for England (to give prevalence of e.g. CVD, asthma);
(9) lifestyle surveys: General Health Survey, Health Survey for England (prevalence of smoking, obesity. alcohol, exercise etc.);
(10) qualitative and quantitative research studies.
(11) national confidential enquiries – e.g. maternal mortality, peri-operative deaths and suicide and homicide by people in contact with mental health services.

In England analysis of these data sources are routinely undertaken at a local level and published as a **Joint Strategic Needs Assessment**, to inform commissioning of NHS and local authority services, and in an annual independent report of the Director of Public Health. Importantly these tools also allow public health specialists to address specific questions such as:

- Is the CHD death rate in a local population higher than the regional or national average, and are the rates re-vascularisation higher or lower than expected?
- Do increases in cannabis exposure cause increases in schizophrenia?
- Is breast cancer survival in Britain improving compared to other European countries?
- What causes Sudden Infant Death Syndrome (cot death) and how can we prevent it?
- Is childhood obesity increasing?
- Has Chlamydia screening reduced the incidence of pelvic inflammatory disease?
- What strategies could be used to prevent suicide?

and many more.

These questions can be reformulated as a PICO as discussed earlier – the difference is that we are measuring the intervention and the outcome at a population level.

Public health interventions

After making our diagnosis we need to prescribe an intervention or select a management that can address the health problem. This will involve a critical appraisal of the evidence on effectiveness of alternative interventions in the same way as evidence-based medicine is recommended for clinical practice. For example, from 1995 to 2005 the proportion of children (aged 2–15) classified as obese increased from 11% to 18% (establishing the need for public health action). A **Cochrane review** of primary prevention studies suggested that the majority did not demonstrate strong evidence and that many studies were limited in design, duration or analysis; but that perhaps comprehensive strategies which address diet and physical activity, change the environment, and involve psychosocial support have the best change of preventing obesity (Summerbell, 2005). Strategies adopted by local governments and health trusts, therefore, have tended to be multifaceted.

Unlike clinical medicine the implementation or delivery of the intervention may require the development of health strategies, mobilisation of resources and introduction of new services and persuasion of other government partners to adapt or change their policies (as highlighted below).

Improving population health can involve restricting individual freedom. Since public health interventions and strategies operate at a population level; they may create a tension between individual choices and the public health. For example, local residents launched a legal challenge through a judicial review of the decision in South England by South Central Strategic Health Authority to add fluoride to the local water supply.

Cigarette smoking, heavy drinking and obesity are related to multiple causes of death and cause substantial premature mortality in UK. For instance:

- Smoking is related to over 40 causes of death and morbidity, and causes approximately 100,000 deaths per year are due to smoking including a third of persistent smokers.
- Alcohol abuse and misuse is associated with over 50 causes of death and morbidity, with estimates of direct and indirect causes of mortality annually ranging from 20 000 to 70 000 deaths per year; population levels of drinking in the UK have increased in the last 20 years consistent with increases in the number of people dying from liver disease (one of the few major causes of death which is increasing and the mean age of diagnosis and death is decreasing).
- By 2008 approximately 1 in 4 men and women were obese, a twofold and 150% increase respectively. Obesity is associated with Type 2 diabetes, osteoarthritis, coronary heart disease and some cancers, and will add substantially to the risk of death and disability if present with smoking and alcohol misuse.

Interventions to reduce these behaviours have adopted a range of methods and styles. The Nuffield School on Bioethics classified a **Public Health Intervention Ladder** in the degree of social control on individual choice (see Table 15.1).

Table 15.1 Public Health Intervention Ladder

Eliminate choice: Introduce laws that entirely eliminate choice	Seatbelt legislation, drink drive laws, bans on alcohol sales in those under 18
Restrict choice. Introduce laws that restrict the options available to people	Banning smoking in public places; banning transfatty acids as an ingredient of processed food in restaurants*; banning 'happy hours' and reducing drinking hours*
Guide choice through disincentives. Introduce financial or other disincentives to influence people's behaviour	Increasing taxes on cigarettes; introducing a minimum price per unit of alcohol*
Guide choices through incentives. Introduce financial or other incentives to influence people's behaviours	Offering tax-breaks on buying bicycles for travelling to work; subsidising gym membership; contingency management (interventions in which substance misusing people receive tangible, positive reinforcers for objective evidence of behaviour change) as part of the treatment of people with alcohol, smoking, or weight problems
Guide choices through changing the default policy.	Changing the standard side dish in school meals from chips to a healthier alternative; changing nature of drinking environments so that alcohol served with food*)
Enable choice. Help individuals to change their behaviours	Providing free 'smoking cessation' programmes; exercise prescription; provide brief interventions for alcohol, or smoking in general practice, A&E and other health and social settings
Provide information. Inform and educate the public	Campaigns to encourage people to walk more or eat five portions of fruit and vegetables a day; food labelling to identify health and unhealthy foods*; smoking warnings on cigarette packs; information on recommended drinking levels and units of alcohol
Do nothing or simply monitor the current situation	Several of the suggestions above * have yet to be introduced; monitor trends in alcohol harm, such as emergency and inpatient admissions and assaults http://www.nwph.net/alcohol)

Note: Several of the interventions suggested marked as (*) have yet to be introduced;

Public health action

We examine two further examples of public health analysis and intervention: on prevention of suicide and sudden infant death syndrome (SIDS).

Suicide Prevention

Suicide is an important cause of premature mortality, especially among young people, and is the most severe outcome of mental illness. For example, each year during the 1990s in the UK there were approximately:

- 4,500 deaths from suicide;
- >200,000 hospital attendances for self-harm;
- 1 million individuals experience suicidal thoughts;
- 2 million people prescribed an antidepressant;

- 5 million adults with neurotic symptoms;
- 150 million working days lost through mental illness;

Suicide is a complex public health problem, (as shown in Figure 15.3).

There are multiple potential influences and causes of suicide. Another way of looking at suicide and injury prevention is to construct a **Haddon Matrix** (Haddon, 1999) which describes risk and protective factors in terms of the person, agent or event, and environment and whether they occur before, during or after the injury. We will focus on one potential source of prevention – the method of suicide – and show how the 'restriction' or 'elimination' of choice' can reduce the overall number of suicides. The figures show that for men and women the rate of suicide by domestic gas fell as coal gas which had high carbon monoxide (CO) content and was highly toxic was

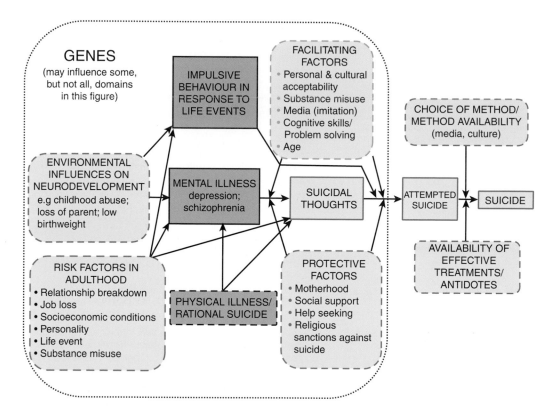

Figure 15.3 Studying suicide from the lifecourse perspective.
Source: After Gunnell D, Lewis G (2005) Studying suicide from the lifecourse perspective: implications for prevention. *Br J Psychiatry* **187**: 206–8. With permission from The Royal College of Psychiatrists.

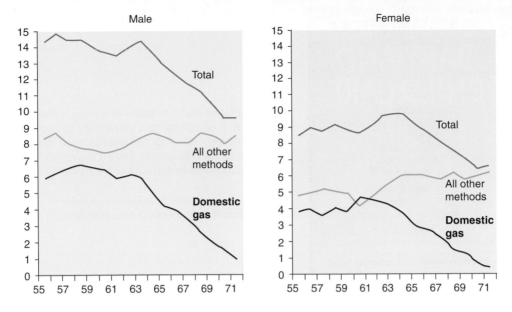

Figure 15.4 Suicide deaths (rates per 100,000) by mode (domestic gas vs. other methods) in men and women, 1955–1971.
Source: after Kreitman N (1976) The coal gas story: United Kingdom suicide rates, 1960–71 *Brit J Prev Soc Med* **30:** 86–93, with permission from BMJ Publishing Group Ltd.

gradually replaced by natural gas (low CO), until by 1970s there was no domestic supply based on coal gas and no suicides from this method. What is remarkable – and critical to suicide prevention – is that the reduction in deaths from domestic gas have not been replaced by other methods. In the 1950s and early 1960s coal gas was the commonest method of suicide; its withdrawal and eventual removal led to approximately 9,000 fewer suicides (Figure 15.4).

This observation has led to interest in controlling other methods of suicide. For example, the introduction of legislation restricting the quantity of paracetamol that could be bought over the counter is associated with a reduction in suicide deaths due to paracetamol as well as declines in liver transplants. More recent bans on coproxamol also are estimated to have prevented around 150–250 poisoning deaths per year in the UK. These interventions and evaluations of impact are derived from the examination of routine data sets and an assessment of the natural history and causal influences on disease. Worldwide the commonest method of suicide is pesticide self-poisoning – accounting for over 250,000 deaths per year – bans on the most toxic pesticides may have a profound impact on the incidence of suicide worldwide.

SIDS prevention

Sudden Infant Death Syndrome (SIDS) or 'cot death' was responsible for approximately 900 deaths per year (1 in 500 children in the first year of life) in UK in the 1970s/1980s, with marked seasonal variation peaking in winter months. Some researchers thought it was possible that infants sleeping position (prone – lying on stomach vs. supine – lying on back) may influence risk. Advice on the sleeping position of babies was largely unchanged since the 1940s when the most popular child-rearing book suggested that babies should be encouraged to sleep on their stomach, i.e. a prone sleeping position – as illustrated in Figure 15.5.

A case control study examining potential causes of SIDS with 72 cases and 144 controls found the following (Fleming *et al.*, 1990, p. 85):

- Odds Ratio (OR) of prone sleeping: 8.8 (95% CI 7.0–11.0; p < 0.001);

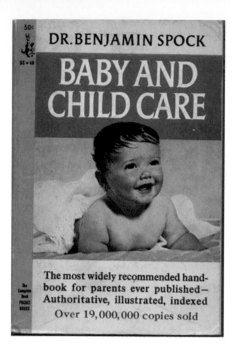

"...There are two disadvantages to a baby's sleeping on his back. If he vomits, he's more likely to choke on the vomitus. Also, he tends to keep his head turned toward the same side-usually toward the center of the room. This may flatten that side of his head..."

"...I think it is preferable to accustom a baby to sleeping on his stomach from the start if he is willing..."

Figure 15.5 Example of advice on baby sleeping position from 1940s onwards.

- OR per extra duvet/blanket tog (measure of heat insulation) above 8: 1.14 (1.03–1.28);
- OR associated with exposure to all night heating: 2.7 (1.4–5.2).

Because SIDS are rare events the OR is equivalent to the Risk Ratio – and shows how much more likely SIDS is if a baby is exposed to the risk (e.g. that prone sleeping is over 8 times more likely to lead SIDS than sleeping on back). This led to an intervention – to 'provide information' including a publicity campaign (see Figure 15.6) – that sought to counteract previous advice and encourage parents to place baby on their back (and emphasise that healthy babies are unlikely to choke when on their backs); as well as advice to prevent the baby overheating.

The success of the campaign in changing practice can be seen in the national mortality statistics. After the campaign SIDS more than halved from an average of 900 during 1980s down to 450 per year by 1992.

Recently it was suggested that sufficient evidence had accumulated by 1970 to recommend placing infants to sleep on their back (as shown in a cumulative meta-analysis by Gilbert (2005), though of course the techniques of systematic reviews, meta-analysis and evidence-based medicine were not in practice then.

Summary

In summary, public health is concerned with the health of communities and populations. In public health, diagnoses are made through assessment of routine mortality and morbidity statistics, health and lifestyle surveys. Public health interventions may involve healthcare or other services that can influence personal, societal and environmental influences on health and risk – their impact also is measured at the population level.

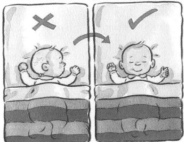

The safest way for your baby to sleep is on the back.

Babies who sleep on their backs are safer and healthier. If babies vomit, they are more likely to choke on their front. If your baby has rolled onto his tummy, turn him onto his back and tuck him in, but don't feel you have to keep getting up all night to check.

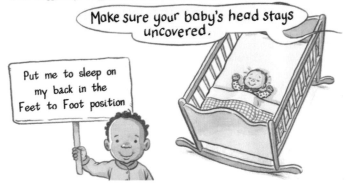

At some point babies will learn to roll onto their front. When your baby can roll from back to front and back again, on his own, then leave him to find his own position. At the start of any sleep time, put him on his back. Babies settle more easily on their backs if they have been placed to sleep that way from the very beginning. If your baby won't settle, keep trying.

It can be dangerous if your baby's head gets covered when she sleeps. Place her with her feet to the foot of the cot, with the bedclothes firmly tucked in and no higher than the shoulders, so she can't wriggle down under the covers. If she wriggles up and gets uncovered – don't worry.

Make sure your baby's head stays uncovered.

Put me to sleep on my back in the Feet to Foot position

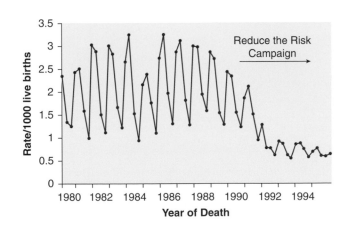

Figure 15.6 Campaign literature on baby sleeping position and time trends in SIDS deaths by year (before and after the 'Back to Sleep' campaign in the 1990s).

KEY LEARNING POINTS

- Public health focuses on improving the health of entire populations rather than on individual patients
- The three domains of public health in the UK are: health improvement, improving services and health protection
- Public health interventions can be medical, educational, social or legal – and can encompass a range of ways of encouraging healthy behaviour or reducing unhealthy choices
- Routine health and census data and epidemiological studies provide tools for assessing health of the population

tions from 1940 to 2002. *Int J Epidemiol* **34**: 874–87.

Gunnell D, Lewis G (2005) Studying suicide from the lifecourse perspective: implications for prevention. *Br J Psychiatry* **187**: 206–8.

Haddon W (1999) The changing approach to the epidemiology, prevention, and amelioration of trauma: the transition to approaches etiologically rather than descriptively based. Injury Classic. *Inj Prev* **5**: 231–5.

Kreitman N (1976) The coal gas story: United Kingdom suicide rates, 1960–71. *Brit J Prev Soc Med* **30**: 86–93.

Summerbell C, Waters E, Edmunds L, *et al.* (2005) Interventions for preventing obesity in children. *Cochrane Database of Systematic Reviews* Issue 3.

 ## REFERENCES

Black RE, Cousens S, Johnson HL, *et al.* (2010) Global, regional, and national causes of child mortality in 2008: a systematic analysis. *The Lancet* **375**: 1969–87.

Fleming P *et al.* (1990) Interaction between bedding and sleeping position in the sudden infant death syndrome: a population based case-control study. *BMJ* **301**: 85.

Gilbert R, Salanti G, Harden M, See S (2002) Infant sleeping position and the sudden infant death syndrome: systematic review of observational studies and historical review of recommenda-

 ## FURTHER READING AND RESOURCES

Health Protection Agency: www.hpa.org.uk

Faculty of Public Health: www.fph.org.uk

Association of Schools of Public Health: http://www.whatispublichealth.org/what/index.html

CDC MMWR: http://www.whatispublichealth.org/impact/index.html

http://www.dh.gov.uk/en/Publichealth/Obesity/index.htm

http://www.nuffieldbioethics.org/public-health/public-health-policy-process-and-practice

16

Screening

Angela E. Raffle
University of Bristol

Learning objectives

In this chapter you will learn:

- ✓ the principles behind screening for disease;
- ✓ the notion that screening is a programme and not a test;
- ✓ screening can cause harm as well as benefit;
- ✓ the need for controlled trials to evaluate screening;
- ✓ the key biases that need to be considered in interpreting data;
- ✓ the need for balanced information to inform the public about screening.

History of screening

The first UK **screening** programmes were for **communicable diseases**, for example 'mass miniature radiography' for detecting tuberculosis. The aim was mainly to prevent disease transmission. Direct benefit to the screened individual was secondary. The TB screening programme stopped once prevalence became low.

The first UK noncommunicable disease screening was cervical cytology testing introduced in the 1960s. Back then there was little recognition of the complexity of delivering a comprehensive screening programme, and for the first two decades of its existence the cervical screening programme was highly controversial, made little or no impact on deaths from cervical cancer, and led to considerable overtreatment of inconsequential symptomless tissue change.

The lessons from this experience were taken to heart and led to the establishment in the 1990s of the UK National Screening Committee (NSC). The NSC aim is to ensure that sound evidence underpins all screening policy, and that all screening programmes are delivered according to rigorous quality standards. Criteria, modified from the 1968 World Health Organisation's **Wilson's Criteria**, are used by the NSC to help assess which potential screening programmes could be worthwhile (see Appendix 16.1 for the detailed list).

To evaluate the pros and cons of a screening programme, one must understand:

- what screening is;
- what screening does;
- why good-quality research is essential before introducing screening;
- what a practising doctor needs to know for advising his or her patients.

Epidemiology, Evidence-based Medicine and Public Health Lecture Notes, Sixth Edition. Yoav Ben-Shlomo, Sara T. Brookes and Matthew Hickman. © 2013 Y. Ben-Shlomo, S. T. Brookes and M. Hickman. Published 2013 by John Wiley & Sons, Ltd.

What is screening?

In a nutshell, screening means tests done on healthy people to reduce their risk of a nasty health outcome in the future.

A more careful version of this explanation is that screening means:

- tests or inquiries;
- it is performed on people who do not have (are asymptomatic) or have not recognised the signs or symptoms of the condition being tested for;
- it is carried out where the stated or implied purpose is to reduce risk for such individuals of future ill health in relation to the condition being tested for; or
- it is carried out to give information about risk that is deemed valuable for such individuals even though risk cannot be altered.

Screening is thus a form of **secondary prevention** when disease is detected early in its natural history thereby allowing intervention, in theory, to improve prognosis.

Screening is a programme not just a test. The test alone cannot achieve any improvement in outcome, so screening comprises a sequence of events. It must be delivered as a well-organised programme of interrelated activities. It encompasses all necessary steps from identifying the eligible population through to delivering interventions and supporting individuals who suffer adverse effects.

The initial screen is usually followed by further tests for the positives. The screening test is a bit like a sieve that divides a higher risk group and a lower risk group. It does not give certainty. Usually, the people with a positive screening test then need to go on to have more tests. This can be described as the diagnostic phase, or as the 'sorting' phase.

Across the globe there is huge variation in policymaking and delivery. From place to place and over time, examples exist of screening programmes that vary widely in terms of:

- how soundly they are based on evidence;
- how well they are delivered (see Figure 16.1).

What this means is that whilst some screening is evidence-based and high-quality, and leads to more public good than harm at affordable cost, this is not universally the case. Some screening is not based on sound evidence, and some is delivered haphazardly so cannot achieve its potential benefits. This kind of screening does more public harm than good, and is not best value use of resources. It may nevertheless be commercially profitable and highly popular with consumers.

Screening for inherited disorders needs just the same rigour as other screening. Some screening involves testing for inherited or heritable disorders, in people without signs or symptoms and without genetic susceptibility. Such testing can yield information that affects other family members, who did not themselves have a test or give consent to the information being uncovered. Other than this special feature, the same screening principles apply.

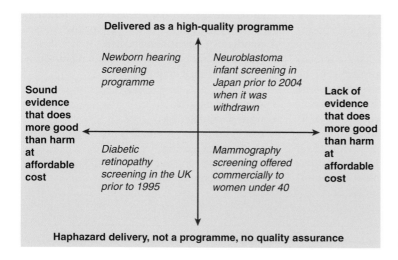

Figure 16.1 Variation in evidence-based policy-making and service delivery for screening.

What screening does

Screening causes harm as well as benefit. Offering screening to a population leads to diverse consequences. Some individuals may benefit, and some are harmed.

The consequences can be shown using a flowchart. Figure 16.2 shows the screening process and the main outcomes, using bowel cancer as an illustration. Those helped are the people who are identified as cases, receive intervention and have longer life expectancy as a result. Those with an adverse or equivocal outcome are those who have intervention for a condition that would not have become manifest during their natural lifespan, those who suffer complications, those with false alarms, and those who are falsely reassured,

Overdetection is a major downside of many screening programmes yet it is invisible to the public. Many people believe the main harm of screening is the anxiety it causes, although participants tend to say that this is a price worth paying given the benefits. Of greater concern in public health terms is the over-diagnosis and over-treatment inherent in many screening programmes. Breast screening for example leads to some women having breast removal, radiotherapy and chemotherapy for tissue change that would never have caused a problem. It is of course impossible to distinguish the woman who has had life-saving treatment, from the woman who has had unnecessary treatment. This means that paradoxically the popularity of the programme is enhanced by over diagnosis because everyone who is treated tends to the belief that for them it has been life saving.

Screening may change the perception of disease. Once it is suggested that a disease could be screened for, this tends to create an impression that every case could be prevented if only 'more was done'. This can alter the experience for patients and relatives, who may find it harder to accept the condition and may feel convinced that if somebody had found it sooner then the illness could have been avoided. For this reason it is important to explain screening as a means of reducing risk, rather than a means of 'prevention'. To the lay public prevention tends to mean total prevention.

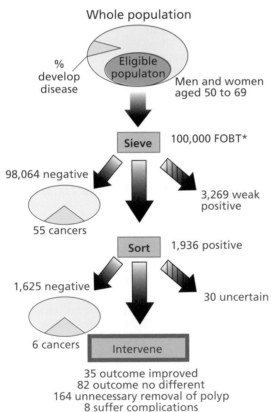

Figure 16.2 The numbers in the flow diagram for bowel cancer screening (Information used in 1998 for planning the UK bowel screening pilots).
*FOBT – faecal occult blood test screen for bowel cancer.
Source: AE Raffle and JAM Gray (2007) Screening Evidence and Practice. Oxford: Oxford University Press.

Why controlled trials are necessary

Health outcomes in observational studies are likely to be very good even if screening makes no difference. If all you do is measure health outcomes in screened individuals then you will quickly become convinced that screening reduces risk for all kinds of conditions. This is because of three key biases. To control for these biases we need well conducted randomised controlled trials. The three key biases are:

- *healthy screenee effect* – the people who come for screening tend to be healthier than those who do not, therefore outcome in screened individuals tends to be better than in the background population;

- *length time effect* – screening is best at picking up long-lasting non-progressive or slowly-progressive pathological conditions, and tends to miss the poor prognosis rapidly-progressing cases; outcome is therefore automatically better in screen-detected cases compared with clinically detected cases even if screening makes no difference to outcome;
- *lead time effect* – survival time for people with screen-detected disease appears longer because you start the clock sooner.

Neuroblastoma screening provides a case study of why controlled trials of screening are important. Marketing and promotion in the 1980s of screening for neuroblastoma, an infant tumour, prompted a review of evidence by a panel of experts who met in Chicago. Despite the fact that observational studies showed excellent survival in screen-detected cases the experts concluded that these cases could in fact be biologically different from the serious cases that the screening was aiming to help. The panel recommended no adoption of screening, and that **randomised controlled trials (RCTs)** were needed. Two major RCTs were then conducted. These revealed that deaths were higher in screened infants than in controls, because of overtreatment and consequent deaths from the complications of treatment. Once this evidence was clear, then Japan, which had pioneered neuroblastoma screening, ceased their national programme.

    Test performance is important, and there is always a trade-off between finding as many cases as possible, and avoiding too many false alarms and overtreatment. In screening, as with other kinds of testing, it is crucial to define what you mean by a 'case' and to assess how well the test or tests can separate cases from noncases. The standard measures of **sensitivity**, **specificity**, **positive predictive value** and **likelihood ratios** are used (see Chapter 9). The choice of cut-offs for defining what constitutes a positive result is a balancing act between avoiding too many missed cases (sensitivity) versus avoiding too many false alarms (specificity) and the potential for overtreatment. Inevitably, the case-definition for what is being found through screening, for example aortic aneurysm greater than 5.5 cms, is not synonymous with the condition you are hoping to avert, that is, an aneurysm

that will fatally rupture. This is why overtreatment happens even though the cases are 'true positives'.

Advice to provide a good service to patients

Make sure you know how to find key information. Up to date details of the national screening programmes in the UK are all available online and they are constantly changing as quality improves and new evidence emerges. The different kinds of screening are:

- *antenatal and newborn* – which are linked because staff caring for newborn babies are often key to taking actions that flow from the results of antenatal findings;
- *childhood* – for example vision screening, growth screening;
- *adult* – for example abdominal aortic aneurysm screening, bowel cancer screening, diabetic retinopathy screening.

Be clear on the basics. When helping a patient who is deciding whether to be screened make sure you know:

- what exactly is the programme aiming to reduce the risk of?
- who is eligible?
- what does the screen (sieving phase) involve?
- what does the sort involve in terms of further tests?
- what is the intervention?

Develop your skills in helping patients choose in accordance with their values. Your job is to help your patient to understand the good and the bad about screening, to help them weigh up what matters to them, and to support them through the process if they choose to be screened. You also need to respect their decision if they choose not to be screened.

    Keep your knowledge up to date. If your job involves being responsible for delivering any part of a screening service then make sure you find out what training is available, and that you keep up to date and follow any quality checks and failsafe procedures.

Be aware that information in the mass media may not be balanced. Information that your patients receive via newspapers, magazines and direct mailed adverts, may be slanted towards 'selling' screening. 'News stories' are often little more than adverts, having come directly from public relations experts working for companies providing screening. Often journalists will have received payment or favours to encourage them to write positively about private screening clinics. You need to help your patients to make sense of this information. They may be unaware of the commercial motivation for offering screening. They may not realise they are only being offered a test and not a proper programme, and that evidence may be lacking.

Regulation of the content of screening advertising is being developed. Concerns have been raised by the British Medical Association and by the Royal Colleges about the need to protect consumers from highly misleading advertising claims about screening. When selling a mortgage, or stocks and shares, the seller is legally bound to explain the risks for example of house repossession, or that shares can lose value. In stark contrast to this, when selling health screening, there is free reign to use all the skilful techniques of advertising, to play on fears, to keep silent on hazards and lack of proven benefit, to imply that this is a 'once-only offer', and to quote testimonials from fictitious grateful customers, carefully chosen to appeal to those most likely to be influenced — 'thank you from me, my husband, and my golden retriever'. The BMA Board of Science is pushing for changes that will ensure consumers have a right to know:

- all the consequences based on the best available evidence, not just from the test but also from subsequent steps;
- that any benefit can only come about if the test is part of a high-quality programme, and how any other steps in the programme will be provided;
- the financial gain for the person offering the test;
- exactly what they will be charged and what this does and does not cover;

- the desirability of seeking independent advice from a qualified medical practitioner who has no financial interest in the matter.

 KEY LEARNING POINTS

- Initially screening was used for infectious disease but it is now advocated for chronic diseases like cancer
- Screening is done on healthy (or asymptomatic) people to improve their long term health outcomes
- It requires a programme of interrelated activities
- The screening test acts as a sieve for sorting out who may require further testing
- Overdetection and overtreatment due to false positive tests are a major downside
- Observational studies will overestimate the benefits of screening due to healthy screenee effect, length time and lead time biases
- Well-conducted trials are required to provide a sound evidence base for screening
- The public need to be aware of both the potential positive and negative consequences of being screened

 FURTHER READING AND RESOURCES

Raffle A (2010) Guest Editorial: Advertising private tests for well people. *Clinical Evidence* 2 June.

Raffle A (2011) Health Knowledge Interactive Learning Module on Screening http://www.healthknowledge.org.uk/interactive-learning/screening (last accessed 22 March 2011).

Raffle A, Gray JAM (2007) Screening; Evidence and Practice. Oxford: Oxford University Press, 2007. (Details of the neuroblastoma case study are on pp. 89–92.)

UK Screening Portal, web resources for the UK National Screening Programmes. http://www.screening.nhs.uk/ (last accessed 22 March 2011).

Appendix 16.1: UK National Screening Committee criteria

(Taken from http://www.screening.nhs.uk/criteria)

The Condition

(1) The condition should be an important health problem.

(2) The epidemiology and natural history of the condition, including development from latent to declared disease, should be adequately understood and there should be a detectable risk factor, disease marker, latent period or early symptomatic stage.

(3) All the cost-effective primary prevention interventions should have been implemented as far as practicable.

(4) If the carriers of a mutation are identified as a result of screening the natural history of people with this status should be understood, including the psychological implications.

The Test

(5) There should be a simple, safe, precise and validated screening test.

(6) The distribution of test values in the target population should be known and a suitable cut-off level defined and agreed.

(7) The test should be acceptable to the population.

(8) There should be an agreed policy on the further diagnostic investigation of individuals with a positive test result and on the choices available to those individuals.

(9) If the test is for mutations the criteria used to select the subset of mutations to be covered by screening, if all possible mutations are not being tested, should be clearly set out.

The Treatment

(10) There should be an effective treatment or intervention for patients identified through early detection, with evidence of early treatment leading to better outcomes than late treatment.

(11) There should be agreed evidence based policies covering which individuals should be offered treatment and the appropriate treatment to be offered.

(12) Clinical management of the condition and patient outcomes should be optimised in all

health care providers prior to participation in a screening programme.

The Screening Programme

(13) There should be evidence from high quality Randomised Controlled Trials that the screening programme is effective in reducing mortality or morbidity. Where screening is aimed solely at providing information to allow the person being screened to make an 'informed choice' (e.g. Down's syndrome, cystic fibrosis carrier screening), there must be evidence from high quality trials that the test accurately measures risk. The information that is provided about the test and its outcome must be of value and readily understood by the individual being screened.

(14) There should be evidence that the complete screening programme (test, diagnostic procedures, treatment/intervention) is clinically, socially and ethically acceptable to health professionals and the public.

(15) The benefit from the screening programme should outweigh the physical and psychological harm (caused by the test, diagnostic procedures and treatment).

(16) The opportunity cost of the screening programme (including testing, diagnosis and treatment, administration, training and quality assurance) should be economically balanced in relation to expenditure on medical care as a whole (i.e. value for money). Assessment against this criteria should have regard to evidence from cost benefit and/or cost effectiveness analyses and have regard to the effective use of available resource.

(17) All other options for managing the condition should have been considered (e.g. improving treatment, providing other services), to ensure that no more cost effective intervention could be introduced or current interventions increased within the resources available.

(18) There should be a plan for managing and monitoring the screening programme and an agreed set of quality assurance standards.

(19) Adequate staffing and facilities for testing, diagnosis, treatment and programme management should be available prior to the commencement of the screening programme.

(20) Evidence-based information, explaining the consequences of testing, investigation and

treatment, should be made available to potential participants to assist them in making an informed choice.

(21) Public pressure for widening the eligibility criteria for reducing the screening interval, and for increasing the sensitivity of the testing process, should be anticipated. Decisions about these parameters should be scientifically justifiable to the public.

(22) If screening is for a mutation the programme should be acceptable to people identified as carriers and to other family members.

17

Infectious disease epidemiology and surveillance

Caroline Trotter,[1] Isabel Oliver[2] and Matthew Hickman[1]
[1]University of Bristol
[2]South West Health Protection Agency

Learning objectives

In this chapter you will learn:

✓ key concepts and terminology in infectious disease epidemiology;

✓ principles of and methods for infectious disease surveillance and outbreak management.

Introduction

An **infectious disease** is an illness resulting from the transmission of a pathogenic biological agent – including some viruses, bacteria, fungi, protozoa, parasites and prions – to a susceptible host. A **communicable disease** is an infectious disease that can be transmitted directly or indirectly from person to person. The 'germ theory' of disease, attributing the presence of disease to specific micro-organisms, was firmly established in the late 19th century by the work of Louis Pasteur and Robert Koch. Earlier studies by John Snow and William Budd, who are often considered among the forefathers of modern epidemiology, had demonstrated the contagiousness of cholera and typhoid through contaminated water, although not the specific agents responsible. This knowledge provided the scientific basis for infectious disease control, which is among the key public health successes of the twentieth century: including, as highlighted in Chapter 15, improvements in hygiene, the advent of effective antibiotic therapy and successful vaccination programmes.

Despite these advances, the **burden of infectious disease** remains high, particularly in low-income countries and we face new challenges from emerging infections and organisms resistant to antimicrobials. Globally, an estimated 68% of the 8.8 million deaths in children under 5 years are due to infectious diseases, with the most common causes being pneumonia (18%), diarrhoea (15%) and malaria (8%) (Black, 2010). In England, the mortality associated with infectious disease is much lower (although, still an estimated 10% of deaths overall have an underlying infectious

---

Epidemiology, Evidence-based Medicine and Public Health Lecture Notes, Sixth Edition. Yoav Ben-Shlomo, Sara T. Brookes and Matthew Hickman.
© 2013 Y. Ben-Shlomo, S. T. Brookes and M. Hickman. Published 2013 by John Wiley & Sons, Ltd.

cause) but the financial burden remains high at around £6 billion per annum, with respiratory infections, infectious intestinal disease, health-care acquired infections and HIV/AIDS contributing the greatest cost.

There are many reasons why infections continue to take their toll. In the poorest countries inadequate health care and sanitation play a large role, and effective interventions may not be available, deliverable or affordable for those most in need. Globally, new infectious agents continue to emerge; three examples among a long list in recent decades include the recognition of HIV/AIDS in the 1980s, the emergence of variant CJD in humans arising from the BSE epidemic in cattle in the 1990s, and an epidemic of Severe Acute Respiratory Syndrome due to the SARS-coronavirus in the 2000s. Other communicable diseases have been able to re-emerge due to pathogen evolution (drug resistance) or changes in the host population (e.g. tuberculosis facilitated by HIV). This means that despite improvements in understanding, treatment and prevention, the threat from infectious diseases remains.

What are the characteristics of infectious disease epidemiology?

During the course of this book you have learnt about different study designs, epidemiological and statistical methods. These can just as well be applied to infectious diseases as noninfectious diseases. However, there are some special features of infectious diseases that do not apply to noncommunicable diseases. Communicable diseases can generally be transmitted from person to person, so the incidence of new infections depends on the prevalence of infection (or rather infectious individuals) in the population. Critically treatment or prevention of infection in one person can avert infections in other people. Other important characteristics of infectious disease which distinguish it from noninfectious or chronic disease include:

- **immunity** – following infection or vaccination individuals may become immune (resistant) to future infections. Some pathogens are strongly immunogenic (e.g. measles infection provokes

long-lasting immunity that protects against future infection), others are weakly immunogenic (e.g. gonorrhoea) and therefore people may become infected again;
- **carrier state** – an individual may be infected and able to infect others without displaying any symptoms of disease;
- *urgency* – there is sometime a need to act quickly to respond to an outbreak.

Other key features of infectious agents

Once a person is exposed to an infectious agent, they may resist infection if they are immune or may become infected. The figure shows dynamics of infection/disease and infectiousness. If they are infected, there is often an **incubation period** between the time of infection and the time when symptoms develop. This is usually followed by a period of clinical illness with symptoms dependent on the infection although, for some organisms it is possible to have asymptomatic infection (also known as a carrier state). Following infection there is a **latent period** during which the person infected is not infectious (not able to transmit the disease to others). Following this period, and, depending on the organism, the person may become infectious before, during and / or after the period of clinical symptoms which can pose challenges to the control of disease (Figure 17.1).

Transmission

Infectious diseases can be transmitted by various, and sometimes multiple, means (see below for some examples). Understanding how infections are transmitted is central to developing appropriate and effective control measures (see Table 17.1).

A useful measure of transmissibility (the intrinsic potential for an infectious agent to spread) is the **basic reproduction number**. Also known as **R0**, this can be defined as the average number of secondary cases produced by one primary case in a wholly susceptible population. The estimated R0 for influenza is around 2–3, whereas measles has an R0 of around 12–18. Other things being equal, the larger the value of R0, the more difficult the infection is to control. Often, some proportion of the population is not susceptible to the infection because they are immune, so that the

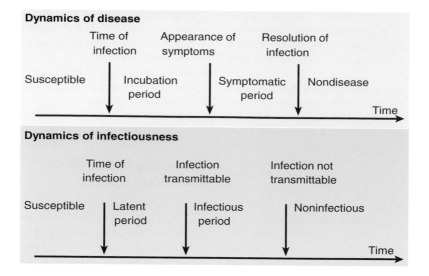

Figure 17.1 Dynamics of disease and infectiousness.

number of cases infected by a primary case is less than R0. The actual average number of secondary cases produced by an infectious primary case is known as the **effective reproduction number (R)**.

Occurrence of infectious diseases

If the effective reproduction number, R, is less than one (i.e. each case gives rise to fewer than one secondary case) then the infection cannot persist in the population and will eventually die out. We can reduce R by reducing the number of susceptible people in the population, for example through vaccination. R0 can be used to estimate the proportion of the population that needs to be vaccinated to prevent sustained spread of the infection; this is given by $1 - 1/R0$ and is known as

the **herd immunity threshold**. If the vaccination coverage consistently exceeds this threshold then the disease will eventually die out. **Herd immunity** therefore refers to the proportion of a host population which is immune to an infection, but also relates to the concept that the presence of immune individuals protects those who are not themselves immune.

If R is greater than 1 then the incidence of the disease is increasing in the population giving rise to an **epidemic**. An epidemic occurs when the incidence of disease, in a given population and during a given period, substantially exceeds the expected incidence. **Outbreak** is often used interchangeably with epidemic, but is sometimes used more specifically to refer to an epidemic in a geographically or demographically localised population. A **pandemic** is a worldwide epidemic – as

Table 17.1 Modes of transmission and examples.

Mode of transmission	Example
Direct physical contact / transfer of body fluids – touching an infected person, including sexual intercourse	Staphylococcus, gonococcus, HIV, hepatitis B, ebola
Inhalation of droplets containing the infectious agent (aerosol)	Tuberculosis, measles, influenza
Vertical transmission (mother to foetus)	Hepatitis B, HIV, syphilis, rubella
Parenteral – bloodborne through needlestick/injection or transfusion	HIV, hepatitis B, hepatitis C
Ingestion of food or water that is contaminated	Salmonella, campylobacter, cholera, vCJD, hepatitis A
Vector borne – through animal carrier/zoonosis	Malaria (mosquito), Lyme disease (deer ticks)

recently occurred in relation to swine flu. An **endemic** infection is one that occurs regularly in a given population and can be maintained in that population without external influence (i.e. R is around 1). For example, in the UK chickenpox is endemic, malaria is not.

Control of infectious diseases

Interrupting transmission is a key aim of infectious disease control. More specifically, *control* can be defined as a reduction in the incidence, prevalence, morbidity or mortality of an infectious disease to a locally acceptable level. **Elimination** refers to a reduction to zero of the incidence of disease or infection in a defined geographical area. **Eradication** is the permanent reduction to zero of the worldwide incidence of infection (Dowdle, 1998).

To date smallpox is the only infectious disease of humans that has been eradicated (as certified by WHO in 1979), with poliovirus currently being targeted as the second. **Vaccines** have been highly successful in combating formerly common childhood diseases such as measles and pertussis (whooping cough). Successful immunisation programmes rely upon the availability of safe and effective **vaccines**, targeted at the age groups at highest risk. High uptake ensures that individuals are protected, but because of herd immunity, it is not necessary to immunise 100% of the population.

The current national routine childhood immunisation schedule in the UK includes vaccines that protect against the following infections:

2 months:
- diphtheria, tetanus, pertussis, polio and Haemophilus influenzae type b (Hib, a bacterial infection that can cause severe pneumonia or meningitis in young children) given as a 5-in-1 single injection known as DTaP/IPV/Hib
- pneumococcal infection

3 months:
- 5-in-1, second dose (DTaP/IPV/Hib)
- meningitis C

4 months:
- 5-in-1, third dose (DTaP/IPV/Hib)

- pneumococcal infection, second dose
- meningitis C, second dose

between 12 and 13 months:
- meningitis C, third dose
- Hib, fourth dose (Hib/MenC given as a single jab)
- MMR (measles, mumps and rubella), given as a single jab
- pneumococcal infection, third dose

3 years and 4 months, or soon after:
- MMR second jab
- diphtheria, tetanus, pertussis and polio (DtaP/IPV), given as a 4-in-1 pre-school booster

around 12–13 years:
- cervical cancer (HPV) vaccine, which protects against cervical cancer (girls only): three jabs given within six months

around 13–18 years:
- diphtheria, tetanus and polio booster (Td/IPV), given as a single jab

In addition, the elderly and those at high risk are offered seasonal influenza vaccine each year.

There are many infections for which vaccines are not currently available so disease control measures must therefore rely on other ways of interrupting transmission. Returning to R0, the factors influencing the basic reproduction number and potential control measures targeting these factors are shown in Table 17.2, illustrated using the example of sexually transmitted infections.

Surveillance of infectious diseases

Public health surveillance refers to the ongoing, systematic collection, analysis and interpretation of data essential to the planning, implementation, and evaluation of public health practice, closely integrated with the timely dissemination of these data to those responsible for prevention and control. Put more simply, surveillance provides information for public health action.

Clearly it is not possible or desirable to monitor all infections, but some infectious diseases

Table 17.2 Factors influencing basic reproduction number for an STI and potential control measures targeting these factors.

Factors influencing R0	Potential control measures
$R_0 =$ probability of effective contact	Condoms, acyclovir (treatment for herpes simplex virus), anti-retroviral therapy
x number of contacts	Education, negotiating skills
x duration of infectiousness	case ascertainment (screening, partner notification), treatment, compliance, accessibility of services

are deemed important enough to be included in national and international surveillance systems. The criteria that are applied to determine this 'importance' include:

- Is it an important public health problem, for example because of high mortality/morbidity or significant epidemic potential?
- Is the disease amenable to public health action?
- Is it feasible to undertake surveillance – is the relevant information available?

We undertake surveillance to monitor trends including the identification of outbreaks, to guide immediate public health action such as outbreak control, to guide the planning, implementation, and evaluation of programmes to prevent and control disease and to evaluate public health policy.

In the UK statutory notifications are a key source of surveillance information. Clinicians have a legal requirement under public health legislation to notify, on suspicion, each case of a notifiable disease. The current list of notifiable infectious diseases in the UK is given In Box 17.1.

Other key sources of surveillance information include laboratory reports, voluntary reports from clinicians, hospital activity data, general practice consultations and vaccination coverage data, as well as epidemiological studies. Enhanced surveillance systems are sometimes established for diseases of particular public health importance. These systems collect a more detailed set of information on each case in order to characterise better the distribution or infection or behavioural risk or in response to a new or emerging problem to improve our understanding of it or to monitor a new vaccination programme. For example, enhanced surveillance has been established for syphilis,

hepatitis B, TB, and severe group A streptococcal disease.

Outbreak investigation

An outbreak is the occurrence of more cases of a specific infection than expected in a particular time and place and/or among a specific group of people. Outbreak investigations in order to identify the source of infection, the mode and/or vehicle of transmission and inform further control measures are usually conducted in the context of a multidisciplinary outbreak control team. The aims of any outbreak investigation are to implement control measures as soon as possible to prevent further cases and to improve our knowledge to prevent future outbreaks. The earlier the response, the greater the opportunity for prevention.

- *Confirmation:* the first step in an outbreak investigation is to establish the existence of an outbreak, that there are indeed more cases of a particular infection than we would expect. This may require analysis of surveillance data. An excess of cases may not necessarily indicate that there is an outbreak, for example, there may have been changes in local surveillance or improvements in diagnosis. Laboratory confirmation of some cases is required to verify the diagnosis.
- *Control:* once the outbreak is confirmed it is essential to implement any immediate control measures such as hygiene measures, exclusion of cases from certain settings, if appropriate, (for example, infected food handlers from work), provision of information to the population at risk or prophylaxis with antimicrobials, vaccine or immunoglobulin.
- *Cases:* A key task is to identify the cases. A **case definition**, a standard set of criteria to decide

Box 17.1 Diseases notifiable (to Local Authority Proper Officers) under the Health Protection (Notification) Regulations 2010.

- Acute encephalitis
- Acute meningitis
- Acute poliomyelitis
- Acute infectious hepatitis
- Anthrax
- Botulism
- Brucellosis
- Cholera
- Diphtheria
- Enteric fever (typhoid or paratyphoid fever)
- Food poisoning
- Haemolytic uraemic syndrome (HUS)
- Infectious bloody diarrhoea
- Invasive group A streptococcal disease and scarlet fever
- Legionnaires' Disease
- Leprosy
- Malaria
- Measles
- Meningococcal septicaemia
- Mumps
- Plague
- Rabies
- Rubella
- SARS
- Smallpox
- Tetanus
- Tuberculosis
- Typhus
- Viral haemorrhagic fever (VHF)
- Whooping cough
- Yellow fever

of describing the outbreak in terms of person, time and place (descriptive epidemiology). Outbreaks are traditionally characterised by time, by drawing a graph of the number of cases by their date of onset. This is referred to as an **epidemic curve**. The epidemic curve provides a great deal of information and can show how the outbreak is spread through the population, at what point we are in the epidemic and its overall pattern. If the disease and its incubation period are known the epidemic curve can point at possible times when persons were exposed. Characterising the outbreak by person (age, sex, …) can help identify which people are at risk. Characterising the outbreak by place provides information on the geographic extent of a problem and may also show patterns that provide clues to the identity and origins of the problem. Descriptive epidemiology helps us identify the population at risk and develop hypothesis such as the source of the outbreak or the mode of transmission. Any hypothesis developed through descriptive epidemiology should then be tested using analytical studies such as case-control or cohort studies to confirm an association between the risk factor and disease (covered in earlier chapters).

Figure 17.2 shows an example of an epidemic curve from a famous (in terms of epidemiology history) cholera outbreak in Golden Square, Broad Street, London, 1854. The pump handle was removed when the epidemic was waning and appears to have had no effect, although it has been suggested that the closure of the pump may have prevented recurrence of the epidemic (Smith, 2002).

Environmental investigations are generally undertaken in conjunction with epidemiological investigations. These may include visits and inspections to locations of interest such as schools or farms to identify possible risks or sources and environmental and/or food sampling followed by investigations in the laboratory. Local authorities and other regulators have legal powers to control environmental sources of infection. Control measures should be implemented as soon as possible as new information becomes available. Once the investigation has concluded and the end of the outbreak has been declared it is important that the findings are written up as an outbreak report and communicated to help prevent future outbreaks and inform public health action.

whether a person should be classified as having the disease under study and being part of the outbreak, is required to help us identify the cases. The case definition usually includes clinical information, demographic characteristics and information about location and time.
- *Characterise*: Once the cases have been identified, demographic, clinical and risk-factor information is obtained from them with the aim

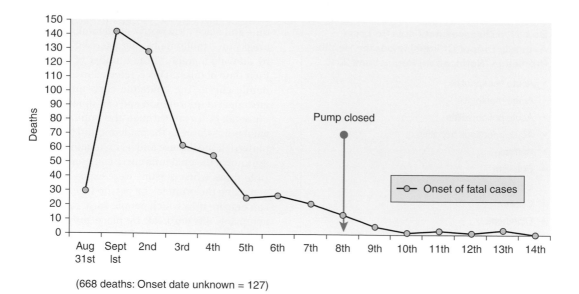

(668 deaths: Onset date unknown = 127)

Figure 17.2 Epidemic curve of cholera outbreak in Golden Square, Broad Street, London, 1854.
Source: Smith (2002).

 KEY LEARNING POINTS

- As communicable diseases generally are transmitted from person to person, the incidence of new infections depends on the prevalence or number of infectious individuals in the population; and treatment or prevention of infection in one person can avert infections in other people

- Understanding how infections are transmitted is central to developing appropriate and effective control measures

- R0 or the basic reproduction number is the average number of secondary cases produced by one primary case in a wholly susceptible population. R0 varies for different infections. The larger the value of R0, the more difficult the infection is to control

- R or the effective reproduction number is the actual average number of secondary cases produced by an infectious primary case. If R < 1 then the infection cannot persist in the population and will eventually die out. We can reduce R by reducing the number of susceptible people in the population, for example through vaccination or other control measures

- The herd immunity threshold is a measure of the proportion of the population that needs to be immune (e.g. through vaccination) to prevent sustained spread of the infection (1 − 1/R0). Herd immunity refers to the concept that the presence of immune individuals protects those who are not themselves immune

- Public health surveillance is the ongoing, systematic collection, analysis and interpretation of data essential to the planning, implementation, and evaluation of public health practice, that is, information for public health action

- An outbreak is the occurrence of more cases of a specific infection than expected in a particular time and place and/or among a specific group of people. The aims of any outbreak investigation are to implement control measures as soon as possible to prevent further cases and to improve our knowledge to prevent future outbreaks

 REFERENCES

Black RE, Cousens S, Johnson HL, *et al.* (2010) Global, regional, and national causes of child mortality in 2008: a systematic analysis. *The Lancet* **375**: 1969–87.

Davey Smith G (2002) Commentary: Behind the Broad Street pump: aetiology, epidemiology and prevention of cholera in mid-19th century Britain *Int. J. Epidemiol* **31**: 920–32.

Dowdle WR (1998) The principles of disease elimination and eradication. *Bull World Health Organ* **76** (Suppl 2): 22–5.

 ## FURTHER READING

Giesecke J (2001) *Modern Infectious Disease Epidemiology*. London: Arnold Publishers Group.

Hawker J, Begg N, Blair I, Reintjes R and Weinberg J (2005) *Communicable Disease Control Handbook*. Oxford: Blackwell Science.

Health Protection Agency (2005) *Health Protection in the 21st Century: Understanding the Burden of Disease; Preparing for the Future*, www.hpa.org.uk

Heymann DL (2004), *Control of Communicable Diseases Manual*, 18th edn. Washington DC, USA: American Public Health Association.

M'iKanatha N (ed.) (2007) *Infectious Disease Surveillance*. Oxford: Blackwell.

World Heath Organisation, www.who.int

18

Inequalities in health

Bruna Galobardes, Mona Jeffreys and George Davey Smith
University of Bristol

Learning objectives

In this chapter you will learn:

✓ what inequalities in health are and why they are amenable to change;

✓ different axes of inequalities in health, how to measure them and their cumulative effect on health;

✓ understand different life course patterns of health inequalities and what they tell us about the disease;

✓ understand and interpret relative and absolute health inequalities;

✓ understand possible mechanisms to minimise health inequalities and the role that doctors can play in achieving this.

Definitions: what are health inequalities?

Health inequalities are variations in health between population groups resulting from a variety of societal and economic processes that are unequally distributed within or between populations.

Health inequalities do not arise because of mere physiological ('normal') differences between population subgroups. For example, we will not characterise as inequality the higher incidence of breast cancer in women compared to men because it is explained by inherent biological characteristics (e.g. volume of breast tissue and hormonal levels). However, if a higher breast cancer incidence were to be partly determined by reduced access and/or standard of care among women compared to men, this would then constitute a gender inequality.

The World Health Organisation (WHO) distinguishes between health inequalities and **health inequities**, defining health inequalities as all types of variations in health (e.g. a different prevalence of dementia by age group would be referred to as a health inequality) and health inequities as those variations that are 'attributable to the external environment and conditions mainly outside the control of the individuals concerned' (WHO, 2011). However, before the WHO made this distinction, the term health inequalities was already well established and has continued to be used in the UK and elsewhere (in research as well as in government) to refer exclusively to those variations in health that are avoidable and 'unfair' as described in the first paragraph. Thus, following this tradition, this is how the term health inequalities is used in this chapter.

Epidemiology, Evidence-based Medicine and Public Health Lecture Notes, Sixth Edition. Yoav Ben-Shlomo, Sara T. Brookes and Matthew Hickman.
© 2013 Y. Ben-Shlomo, S. T. Brookes and M. Hickman. Published 2013 by John Wiley & Sons, Ltd.

There are great variations in the magnitude and direction of health inequalities across populations and over time, indicating that health inequalities are modifiable and the likely result of changes in specific exposures. A recent review on the decline of cardiovascular disease in high income countries highlighted however, that the role of the social determinants in explaining this decrease is often context-dependent (Harper *et al.*, 2011). The socioeconomic patterning of adiposity also illustrates this. Obesity is currently more prevalent among poor people in high income countries but among rich people in low income countries (McLaren, 2007; Subramanian *et al.*, 2011). The socioeconomic patterning of adiposity within a country has changed in successive cohorts. The higher prevalence of adiposity we observe in today's poorer children in rich income countries like the UK did not exist in cohorts born earlier in the century. These changes over time and across countries are due to environmental, and therefore modifiable, factors. These factors relate to an individual's choices of diet and physical activity, as well as to the societal determinants of equal access to and affordability of healthy diet and opportunities for physical activity that are differently distributed across socioeconomic groups.

Axes of inequalities, how to measure them and current patterns

Societies develop and maintain systems of social stratification along multiple dimensions. We present here four different but interrelated axes of inequalities: socioeconomic position including social class; geography; gender and ethnicity or race.

Socioeconomic inequalities in health

Socioeconomic position (SEP) refers to the social and economic factors that influence what positions individuals or groups hold within the structure of a society (Lynch and Kaplan, 2000). A variety of other terms, such as **social class** or **socioeconomic status**, are often used interchangeably although they have different theoretical bases

and, therefore, interpretations. There is no single best indicator of SEP suitable for all study aims and applicable at all time points in all settings. Each indicator measures different, although related, aspects of socioeconomic stratification. SEP measures are based on individual characteristics such as educational level, occupation (NS-SEC and previously the Registrar General Social Class in the UK), household condition or amenities and income. However, especially when using routine datasets, an area-based or ecological measure is derived, based on census-derived variables (e.g. percentage of unemployed and low income) to produce a deprivation indicator, for example the **Index of Multiple Deprivation** (Communities and Local Government, 2008; Scottish Government, 2012; Welsh Government, 2011) which can then be used to characterise small geographical areas where individuals live. This is often done in **ecological studies** (see Chapter 5).

The magnitude of inequality for a given outcome can be expressed in terms of the relative index of inequality (RII) or, for absolute differences, the slope index inequality (SII). These indices summarise the inequalities that arise throughout the whole population and not just the extreme groups. They are useful when comparing inequalities across countries or over time as they also take into account changes in the size of the socioeconomic groups, such as the decrease over time of people working in manual occupations. It is important to note that the unit over which the RII and SII are calculated may vary. As some of the examples in this chapter illustrate it can be an area (comparing the hypothetically best-off with the worst-off areas as in Figure 18.1) or an individual (comparing the hypothetical person with the lowest occupational level with the person with the highest occupational level as in Figure 18.2).

Figure 18.1 shows the RII of premature mortality from 1921 to 2007 in Britain using the Breadline Britain Index, a measure of poverty (Thomas *et al.*, 2010). The RII is interpreted as the relative rate of mortality for the hypothetically worst-off compared with the hypothetically best-off areas (in this case parliamentary constituencies), assuming a linear relationship between poverty and mortality risk. From an initial almost 2.5 times higher risk of premature mortality in the worst–off area, the differentials diminished until the early 1970s, showing that health inequalities can be diminished, but have been increasing in recent decades, reaching a peak at 2.8. It is important to note though that

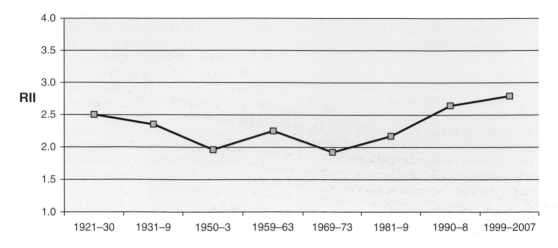

Figure 18.1 Relative Index of Inequality (RII) of premature mortality (0–64 years) from 1921 to 2007 in Britain. *Source*: Adapted from Thomas *et al*. (2010).

this recent increasing trend in inequalities is in relative terms and has occurred in the presence of an increasing life expectancy across all population groups. Thus, the increase in relative inequalities currently arises because of a faster improvement in health in best-off areas compared to the improvement in the worst-off areas (see Section on p. 166 Relative versus absolute health inequalities).

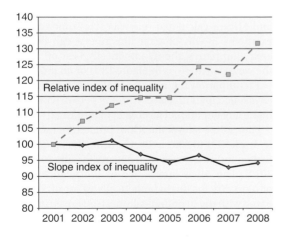

Figure 18.2 Absolute (slope index of inequality) and relative (relative index of inequality) inequalities in mortality rates of NS-SEC classes (socioeconomic groups based on occupation) by year (2001 as reference year=100), in men aged 25–64 in the UK.
Source: Adapted from Langford and Johnson (2010).

Geographical inequalities

Geographical inequalities in health have been extensively described between and within countries. The recent WHO Commission on Social Determinants of Health highlighted the extent of variation in health inequalities across the globe (WHO, 2008). Figure 18.3 shows the variation between countries in infant mortality from just over 20/1,000 live births in Colombia to just over 120 in Mozambique. The lowest mortality rate of 2/1,000 live births is in Iceland (not in the graph). In addition, the figure shows dramatic inequalities within countries as the differences in survival between offspring of educated and non-educated mothers.

Inequalities in health persist also between rich nations. The variation in cancer survival rates across 21 European countries shows that survival is lower in UK than the European average (Figure 18.4) (Eurocare, 2012). This has been the driver of several initiatives in the UK to ensure earlier diagnosis of cancer, such as the National Awareness and Early Diagnosis Initiative for cancer. Finally, similar large variations have been described within rich countries. Figure 18.5A shows that within a small area of London important differences in life expectancy remain. Travelling east from Westminster the life expectancy of a man decreases nearly one year at each stop of the London Underground, resulting in a six year difference from a men leaving in Canning Town. These differences are even larger in Glasgow (Figure 18.5B).

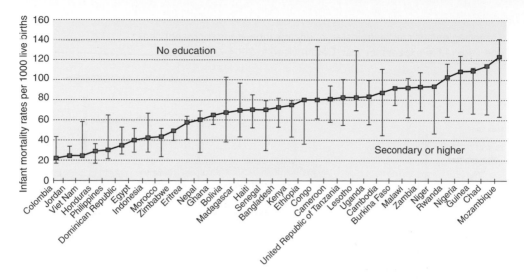

Data from the Demographic and Health Surveys (DHS, nd) derived from STATcomplier, The continuous dark the represents average infant mortality rates for countries; the end-points of the bars indicate the infant mortality rates for mothers with no education and for mothers with secondary or higher education.

Figure 18.3 Infant mortality rates between countries and within country by mother's educational group.
Source: Reproduced from WHO Commission on the Social Determinants of Health (2008).

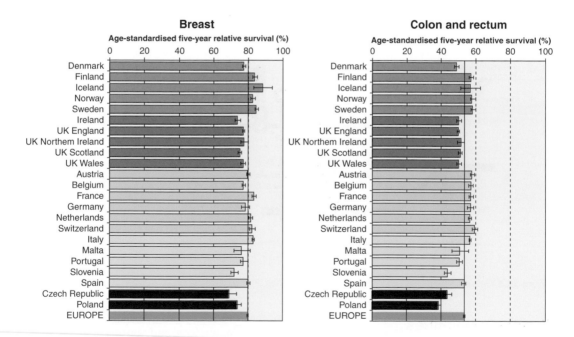

Figure 18.4 Age-standardised five-year relative survival of breast and colon and rectum cancers in 21 European countries.
Source: Reproduced from EUROCARE-4 Database on Cancer Survival in Europe (2012).

(A)

Travelling east from Westminster; every two tube stops represent over one year of life expectancy lost. Data revised to 2004–08

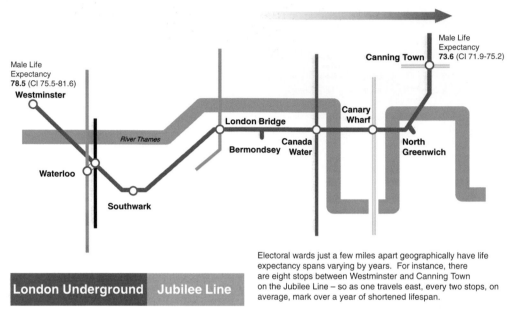

Male Life
Expectancy
73.6 (CI 71.9-75.2)

Canning Town

Male Life
Expectancy
78.5 (CI 75.5-81.6)
Westminster

**Canary
Wharf**

London Bridge

River Thames

**Canada
Water**

Bermondsey

**North
Greenwich**

Waterloo

Southwark

Electoral wards just a few miles apart geographically have life expectancy spans varying by years. For instance, there are eight stops between Westminster and Canning Town on the Jubilee Line – so as one travels east, every two stops, on average, mark over a year of shortened lifespan.

London Underground **Jubilee Line**

Source: Analysis by London Health Observatory of ONS and GLA data for 2004-08. Department of Health.

(B)

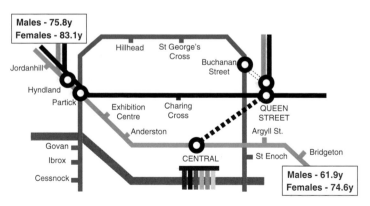

Males - 75.8y
Females - 83.1y

Hillhead   St George's
Cross
Buchanan
Street

Jordanhill

Hyndland
Partick

Exhibition   Charing
Centre   Cross

**QUEEN
STREET**

Anderston

Argyll St.

Govan

Ibrox

CENTRAL

St Enoch

Bridgeton

Cessnock

Males - 61.9y
Females - 74.6y

Life expectancy data refers to 2001-5 and was extracted from the GCPH community health and well-being profiles. Adapted from the SPT travel map by Gerry McCartney.

Figure 18.5 Geographical differences in life expectancy in London (A) and Glasgow (B).

Gender inequalities

Gender inequalities are those variations that cannot be explained by inherent physiological differences between sexes. Gender inequalities persist across most societies and arise through a variety of mechanisms involving unequal access to and control over material and non-material resources, access to education, work and political power, unfair divisions of work, leisure and control over one's life and health (Shaw *et al.*, 2004). Women constitute 64% of the illiterate adults, tend to have

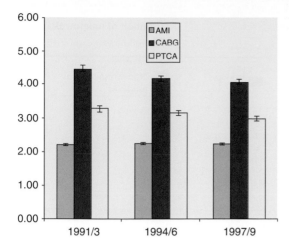

Figure 18.6 Male:female ratio (age-standardised) for acute myocardial infarction (AMI), and revascularisation procedures (CABG or PTCA), with 95% confidence intervals for ages 40 + years, in England between 1991 and 1999. *Source:* Reproduced from Shaw *et al.* (2004).

less well paid and secure jobs, and for equivalent employment receive 20 to 30% lower income than men.

Even in societies where gender inequalities are less prominent, differentials in pay, political power and access to and quality of health care exist. Figure 18.6 shows that in England women receive less revascularisation, a surgical procedure that provides new or additional blood supply to an organ, compared to men over and above differences in need (Shaw *et al.*, 2004). While men are twice as likely to be admitted to hospital with an acute myocardial infarction, the differentials in terms of health care they receive (revascularisation) are much larger. Although the severity, co-morbidity and presentation of myocardial infarction are likely to be different between men and women it seems unlikely these factors can explain a 3- to 4.5-fold higher revascularisation rates in men given that differentials in myocardial infarction diagnosis is only 2-fold.

Race and ethnicity

Race and ethnicity are two related, but differing concepts (Bhopal, 2004). Race was defined on the basis of visible physical characteristics, and is primarily a biological rather than social construct. Ethnicity, on the other hand, is primarily a social construct. One's ethnicity is a mix of culture and heritage, which may include ancestry, religion, language etc. These terms are often used synonymously, and the measurement of ethnicity often incorporates some measures of race.

The use of racial/ethnic groups, both in terms of how they are defined and analysed, is in constant flux. Until recently, it was common for researchers or health care providers to assign race/ethnicity to study participants; increasingly, it is more common to use self-identification. Clearly the options of race/ethnic groups that research participants are given with which to identify will affect the data that are collected. For example, ethnicity was first asked as a direct question in the UK census in 1991, although country of birth had been used for many decades prior to this. In the 2001 census, the question was expanded to allow identification with pre-defined mixed race/ethnicity categories. The questions used are likely to be further refined for the 2011 census. Although this refinement is in some ways useful, the lack of comparability over time in the populations enumerated causes problems for monitoring the health of population subgroups.

The measurement of ethnic inequalities in health in the UK has been further hampered by the lack of ethnicity information in routinely collected data sources, although this is improving. For example, a recent report documented cancer incidence and survival statistics by ethnicity (National Cancer Intelligence Network, 2009). To overcome the relatively high level of missing ethnicity data, three approaches were used, to create plausible ranges of relative risks of cancer associated with the minority ethnic groups (Asian, Black, Chinese and Mixed) compared to the White group. Results for prostate cancer from this report are shown in Figure 18.7, showing the marked increase in risk in Black compared to White men. Furthermore, once diagnosed, Black men in the United States have a poorer prognosis than White men (Evans *et al.*, 2008) though data in the UK suggests that this may not be the case highlighting the potential importance of a national health service in reducing inequalities in prognosis.

It is important to note that these different dimensions of inequalities are *not mutually exclusive* and research shows that the resulting inequality for overlapping groups is not simply additive. The health of a woman of manual social class, belonging to an ethnic minority, living in a poor area may be much worse than what would be

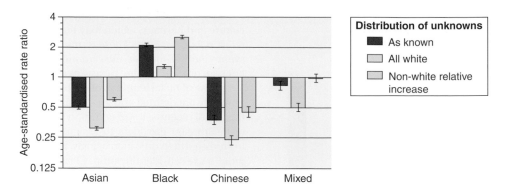

Figure 18.7 Rate ratio of prostate cancer in selected ethnic groups, compared to White men in England, 2002–2006. *Source*: Reproduced from National Cancer Intelligence Network report (2009).

expected by simply adding the effects due of each dimension of inequality.

Relative versus absolute health inequalities

Relative indicators measure inequality in terms of the ratio between the least advantaged and the most advantaged groups whereas the absolute indicators measure inequality in terms of the difference in health outcomes between groups (see also Chapter 2). Thus, absolute levels of health between groups (by SEP, gender, ethnicity, etc.) are important in determining the absolute levels of inequality. To illustrate this, Figure 18.2 (above) shows the increase of the relative index of inequality between 2001 and 2008 between occupational groups in the UK (Langford and Johnson, 2010). This relative increase in inequalities has occurred at a time when mortality rates have steadily decreased in all occupational groups. Absolute inequalities (as measured by the slope index of inequality) show a general decrease between 2001 and 2008 with the fastest decreases occurring between 2004 and 2007 and a recent increase in 2008.

Considering absolute and relative risks is also relevant to understand the contribution that different risks factors can have in reducing health inequalities of an outcome if these risk factors were to be eliminated (or lowered) from the population. Despite research suggesting that novel factors

were needed to explain the mechanisms that generate health inequalities in cardiovascular disease, a recent study showed that targeting traditional CHD risk factors was the most successful approach to eliminating inequalities in CHD in absolute terms (Kivimaki *et al.*, 2008). If the best practice interventions relating to four traditional CHD risk factors (lowering blood pressure, cholesterol and glucose and eliminating smoking) were successfully implemented across all socioeconomic groups this would eliminate most of the socioeconomic gradient in CHD mortality in absolute terms. Interestingly, this research showed how cholesterol, a risk factor not socially patterned in relative terms (there was little or no association between cholesterol levels and employment grade), resulted in the second most important contribution after smoking, in terms of reducing inequalities in absolute terms (contributed proportionally more to diminish CHD from the lower SEP groups as it is more prevalent in these). This work is based on an assumption that remains a real challenge, and that is how to implement these interventions (e.g. smoking cessation) with equal success across socioeconomic groups.

Life course inequalities

Life course epidemiology investigates the long-term effects on health and chronic disease risk of physical and social hazards during gestation, childhood, adolescence, young adulthood and later adult life and it is particularly relevant to understanding how socioeconomic circumstances influence health (Kuh and Ben-Shlomo, 2004). It explicitly incorporates time of exposure and can be conceptualised at individual level, across generations, and through population disease trends. There is sufficient evidence showing that socioeconomic inequalities in health accumulate throughout the life course. Establishing whether the social distribution of a disease occurs at different time periods using indicators that reflect accumulation of life course social disadvantage; or, examining whether one particular measure of SEP relates more closely to an outcome, can point to the temporal nature of exposures related to this health outcome. For example, poor socioeconomic circumstances during childhood are particularly important in determining higher risk of stomach cancer mortality, pointing to early life exposure to Helicobacter pylori as the most relevant time of exposure in determining disease risk in adulthood. On the other hand, childhood SEP, together with socioeconomic conditions in adult life, both contributed to determining mortality from CHD, lung cancer and respiratory-related deaths. The relative contribution of child versus adult SEP varied by country, as well as reflecting different life-course cumulative exposure to smoking and other risk factors in different countries (Harper *et al.*, 2011). Furthermore, childhood socioeconomic circumstances affected not only survival but also the exposures that determined an increase risk of incident CHD.

Current research shows that the most likely model explaining life-course SEP effects on CHD is the cumulative effects model where additive effects of SEP throughout childhood and adulthood increase the risk of adult CHD. Accumulation of risks throughout life can be due to clustered and temporally linked exposures. For example, children from lower socioeconomic backgrounds are more likely to be of low birth-weight, have poorer diets, be more exposed to passive smoking and to infectious agents and have fewer educational opportunities. Exposures may also form chains of risk, where coming from a family background of low SEP leads to low educational attainment which in turn will increase the probability of working in an occupation with a high risk of toxic exposures and of having low income.

Despite many challenges, the **life course framework** is perhaps the best way to address the central research questions with respect to health inequalities – to describe and monitor, and to contribute to understanding **aetiology**.

Reducing the health inequalities gap

The great variation on health inequalities across populations and time indicates that these are avoidable. Whether the wider determinants (e.g. redistribution of wealth, achieving full employment, eradicating child poverty, smoking bans, etc.) or the more proximal factors (e.g. smoking cessation, health promotion for disadvantaged groups, etc.) of health inequalities are targeted depends on the political and policy choices that different countries make (see Chapter 16).

Tackling the wider determinants of health inequalities has the potential to eliminate inequality at its roots, but requires political enforcement and determination as these policies are rarely popular (see Chapter 20). Given that many subgroups of the population do not reach sufficient income for what has been estimated is needed for a healthy living means that undoubtedly these groups will remain with worse levels of health (Morris *et al.*, 2000). Less controversial approaches focus on tackling the proximal risk factors generating health inequalities, for example smoking cessation, healthy diet or increasing physical activity, either at a wider populational level or by selectively targeting subgroups of the population that need them most.

Doctors have an impact on health inequalities (Royal College of Physicians, 2010). Tackling the wider determinants of health among the most disadvantaged patients includes understanding and successfully targeting the determinants of health behaviours (e.g. understanding and dealing with the relatively greater behavioural change that to stop smoking represents for a person of poorer socioeconomic background whose parents, friends and work colleagues smoke) but also promoting culture change and advocacy to target the wider determinants of inequalities. In addition, the medical profession can inadvertently generate or perpetuate health inequalities. When a new intervention is implemented, for example breast cancer screening, the population subgroups who avail themselves of this tend to be the richer and/or more educated. Thus it is these subgroups with already better health outcomes (e.g. lower breast cancer mortality rate) who tend to benefit most from the intervention, creating, or widening, an existing health inequality. In an effort to avoid this, a **Health Inequality Impact Assessment** should be a key stage prior to the implementation of any new intervention, so that an assessment exercise is carried out that considers how certain groups may be differentially affected by a policy or intervention.

 KEY LEARNING POINTS

- There are extensive variations, mostly in the magnitude but also in the direction, of health inequalities suggesting that inequalities are avoidable
- Whilst traditionally epidemiologists have described these inequalities, it is essential to understand why they arise
- A life-course approach provides a helpful model to understand how exposures can either accumulate or act in particular sensitive periods of life to determine future disease risk.
- Tackling health inequalities requires intervening in both the wider and more proximal determinants of these inequalities.
- Doctors have a role in helping individuals modify behaviours, ensuring equal access to health care and acting as advocates to influence political action

 REFERENCES

Bhopal R (2004) Glossary of terms relating to ethnicity and race: for reflection and debate. *J Epidemiol Community Health* **58**(6): 441–5.

Communities and Local Government, (2008) http://www.communities.gov.uk/publications/communities/indiciesdeprivation07, accessed. 2011;

Eurocare (2012) http://www.eurocare.it/Results/tabid/79/Default.aspx (accessed. 2012)

Evans S, Metcalfe C, Ibrahim F, *et al.* (2008) Investigating Black-White differences in prostate cancer prognosis: A systematic review and meta-analysis. *Int J Cancer* **123**(2): 430–5.

Harper S, Lynch J, Davey Smith G (2011) Social determinants and the decline of cardiovascular diseases: understanding the links. *Annu Rev Public Health* **32**: 36–9.

Kivimaki M, Shipley MJ, Ferrie JE, *et al.* (2008) Best-practice interventions to reduce socioeconomic inequalities of coronary heart disease mortality in UK: a prospective occupational cohort study. *Lancet.* **372**(9650): 1648–54.

Kuh D, Ben-Shlomo Y (2004) *A Life Course Approach to Chronic Disease Epidemiology.* 2nd edn. Oxford: Oxford University Press.

Langford A, Johnson B (2010) Trends in social inequalities in male mortality, 2001-08. Intercensal estimates for England and Wales. *Health Stat Q.* **47**: 5–32.

Lynch J, Kaplan G (2000) Socioeconomic position. In: Berkman LF, Kawachi I (eds). *Social Epidemiology.* 1st edn. Oxford: Oxford University Press, pp. 13–35.

McLaren L (2007) Socioeconomic status and obesity. *Epidemiol Rev.* **29**(1): 29–48.

Morris JN, Donkin AJ, Wonderling D, *et al.* (2000) A minimum income for healthy living. *J Epidemiol Community Health* **54**(12): 885–9.

National Cancer Intelligence Network (2009) *Cancer Incidence and Survival by Major Ethnic Group, England, 2002–2006.* London: Cancer Research UK.

Royal College of Physicians (2010) *How Doctors Can Close the Gap. Tackling the Social Determinants of Health through Culture Change, Advocacy and Education.* London: RCP Policy Statement.

Scottish Government (2012) http://www.scotland.gov.uk/Topics/Statistics/SIMD/ (accessed March 2012).

Shaw M, Maxwell R, Rees K, *et al.* (2004) Gender and age inequity in the provision of coronary revascularisation in England in the 1990s: is it getting better? *Social Science & Medicine.* **59**(12): 2499–2507.

Subramanian SV, Perkins JM, Ozaltin E, *et al.* Weight of nations: a socioeconomic analysis of women in low- to middle-income countries. *The American Journal of Clinical Nutrition.* **93**(2): 413–21.

Thomas B, Dorling D, Smith GD (2010) Inequalities in premature mortality in Britain: observational study from 1921 to 2007. *BMJ.* **341**(): c3639.

Welsh Government (2011) http://wales.gov.uk/topics/statistics/theme/wimd/?lang=en (accessed March 2012) .

WHO (2008) Commission on Social Determinants of Health. Closing the gap in a generation: health equity through action on the social determinants of health. Final Report of the Commission on Social Determinants of Health. 2008; Geneva: World Health Organisation.

WHO (2011) http://www.who.int/hia/about/glos/en/index1.html (accessed. 2011).

 FURTHER READING

'Fair Society Healthy Lives' (The Marmot Review) http://www.instituteofhealthequity.org/projects/fair-society-healthy-lives-the-marmot-review

19

Health improvement

Bruce Bolam
Victorian Health Promotion Foundation

Learning objectives

In this chapter you will learn to:

✓ define health improvement, the determinants of health and the ethics of prevention;

✓ explain high-risk and population approaches to prevention;

✓ outline the roles of behaviour change, empowerment and social change in health improvement;

✓ outline key messages and actions for health improvement in medical practice.

What is health improvement and disease prevention?

Health is a state of complete physical, mental and social well-being and not merely the absence of disease or infirmity.

(World Health Organisation, 1946)

Health improvement is about preventing disease and death, and improving quality of life and well-being. Interventions can be implemented at different stages of the natural history of disease (see Table 19.1) and at individual, community and population levels to:

• Add years to life by reducing avoidable death;
• Add health to life by reducing disability and disease;
• Add life to years by enhancing quality of life.

Health promotion is the process of enabling people to increase control over, and to improve, their health.

(World Health Organisation, 1986)

Alongside this definition, the Ottowa charter for Health Promotion recommended:

• building *healthy public policy* – through legislation, fiscal measures, taxation and organisational change in all government policies;
• creating *supportive environments* – through physical and social living and working conditions that are safe and sustainable;
• strengthening *community action* – through empowerment and community development;
• developing *personal skills* – through provision of information, health education to support the personal and social development of individuals;
• *reorienting health services* – to broaden from curative medicine to the prevention of disease.

Epidemiology, Evidence-based Medicine and Public Health Lecture Notes, Sixth Edition. Yoav Ben-Shlomo, Sara T. Brookes and Matthew Hickman.
© 2013 Y. Ben-Shlomo, S. T. Brookes and M. Hickman. Published 2013 by John Wiley & Sons, Ltd.

Table 19.1 Different levels of prevention strategies.

Level	Aim	Example	Service context
Primary prevention	To avoid disease starting – reducing the incidence of disease by controlling the risk factors for morbidity and mortality	Immunisation	Public health
Secondary prevention	To detect disease early – reducing the prevalence of disease by shortening its duration through early identification and prompt intervention	Cancer screening	GP and hospital services
Tertiary prevention	To limit the damage caused by disease – reducing the progress and severity of established disease	Stroke rehabilitation	Rehabilitation and palliative services

The ethics of health improvement

In 2007, the Nuffield Council on Bioethics proposed a stewardship model of public health that maintains ethically acceptable goals for preventative interventions including:

- promoting the health of children and other vulnerable people;
- helping people to overcome addictions and other unhealthy behaviours;
- ensuring that it is easy for people to lead a healthy life, for example by providing convenient and safe opportunities for exercise.

These goals must be tempered by recognition that preventative programmes should:

- not attempt to coerce adults to lead healthy lives;
- minimise interventions that are introduced without individual consent of those affected, or without a just mandate, such as democratic decision-making;
- seek to minimise interventions that are perceived as unduly intrusive and in conflict with important personal values.

To outweigh the adverse impact of state intervention on individual liberty, the justification for action must be stronger each step up the **public health intervention ladder** (see Box 19.1 and Table 15.1).

Box 19.1 Nuffield Council on Bioethics ladder of public health intervention.

Eliminate choice – for example through compulsory isolation of patients with infectious diseases

Restrict choice – for example removing unhealthy ingredients from foods, or removing unhealthy foods from restaurants

Guide choice through disincentives – for example through taxes on cigarettes, or by discouraging the use of cars in inner cities through charging schemes or limitations of parking spaces

Guide choices through incentives – for example offering tax-breaks for the purchase of bicycles that are used as a means of travelling to work

Guide choices through changing the default policy – for example, in a restaurant, instead of providing chips as a standard side dish, menus could be changed to provide a more healthy option as standard

Enable choice – for example by offering participation smoking cessation services, building cycle lanes, or providing free fruit in schools

Provide information – for example as part of campaigns to encourage people to walk more or eat five portions of fruit and vegetables per day

Do nothing or simply monitor the current situation

The determinants of health

Increasing the control people have over their health necessitates action to tackle the determinants of health. In 1974, the Lalonde report for the Canadian government argued that the health of individuals and society was determined by four major factors, or fields:

The main determinants of health

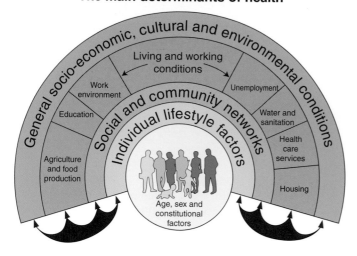

Figure 19.1 Whitehead and Dahlgren model of health determinants. *Source*: Dahlgren G, Whitehead M (1991) *Policies and Strategies to Promote Social Equity in Health.* Institute for Future Studies, Stockholm (Mimeo).

- genetics and biology;
- behaviour or lifestyle;
- physical and social environments;
- the organisation of health services.

These fields are further illustrated by Whitehead and Dahlgren's model of the social **determinants of health**:

The uneven distribution of the determinants of health across society leads to wide variation in the control individuals have over their health and this results in inequalities in health between groups.

The 2008 report of the WHO Commission on the Social Determinants of Health maintained that social inequalities in health come about through differential exposure to risk factors for, vulnerability to and consequences of disease. For example, economic recession commonly leads to higher levels of unemployment among manual and unskilled workers. Unemployment in turn leads to loss of self-esteem and social isolation, thus increasing vulnerability to depression. An unemployed, depressed person has less economic and social resources to cope with the consequences of this and other illnesses, leading to worse long-term prognosis and lower likelihood of returning to work.

The Commission recommended three principal actions to tackle the social determinants of health:

- Improve the conditions of daily life – the circumstances in which people are born, grow, live, work, and age.

- Tackle the inequitable distribution of power, money, and resources – the structural drivers of the conditions of daily life.
- Measure and understand the problem and assess the impact of action – using epidemiology to understand the problems and evaluate interventions.

Upstream determinants of health such as housing and economic conditions shape the distribution of downstream disease risk factors in the population. Health improvement policy typically addresses common 'SNAP' behavioural risk factors for disease in the population or individual: smoking; nutrition; alcohol, and physical activity. Clinical risk factor management in turn often targets reductions in biological risk markers linked to these behaviours.

High-risk and population approaches to prevention

There is a continuous distribution of many disease risk-factors in populations and therefore preventative interventions to reduce risk can be implemented across a whole population or targeted towards individuals or groups at particularly high risk. Geoffrey Rose observed that the relative merits of population and high risk strategies depends in large part upon the relationship between the exposure, such as serum cholesterol, blood pressure, alcohol or salt intake, and the outcome, such as coronary heart disease (CHD), stroke or chronic liver disease (Rose, 1981).

Where exposure to significant risk is limited to a small proportion of the population, a high-risk strategy will benefit the majority of individuals at risk and make a significant contribution to reduction in the total burden of disease. A high-risk approach has the advantages of a high benefit-to-risk ratio and clear patient and clinician motivation. Any individual at high risk of disease will benefit from targeted risk factor reduction in the clinical setting, regardless of the distribution of risk in the wider population.

In many circumstances, however, high-risk groups constitute a minority of the population and larger absolute improvements in population health can be made by reducing risk across the whole population. When an exposure is normally distributed in the population and the risk of disease by exposure approximately linear, then the majority of disease will occur among the 'normal' part of the population. This gives rise to the observation that 'a large number of people at small risk may give rise to a larger number of cases of disease than the small number of cases who are at high risk'. In this context, a population approach will have the greatest impact on the total burden of disease as it reduces disease incidence in both high risk and 'normal' population sub-groups (see Figure 19.2).

For example, Figure 19.3 shows the relationship between serum cholesterol (blue bars) and risk of CHD (red line) and the proportion of CHD deaths by serum cholesterol (% above bars). Thus, elevated or high serum cholesterol, over 6.5 or 8 mmol/l respectively, is associated with a greater than tenfold risk of CHD. The 10% of the population with elevated or high serum cholesterol

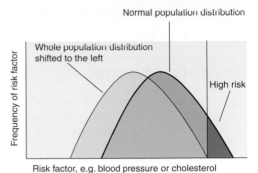

Figure 19.2 The population approach to disease prevention. Shifting whole population distribution to the left offers a small benefit to a lot of people.

accounts for 30 per cent of all CHD deaths. Counter intuitively, 70% of all CHD deaths occur among the remainder of the population with 'normal' serum cholesterol.

Similarly, about 30% of bone fractures occur in the 10% of the population with low bone density. Interventions targeting this high-risk group will fail to prevent the 70% of fractures that occur in the rest of population.

A population approach is simpler as it does not require identification of high-risk groups. But there is relatively little advantage conferred to the majority of low-risk persons. For example, many hundreds of people must not smoke in workplaces to prevent one death attributable to environmental tobacco smoke. This dilemma is known as the **prevention paradox**: that a population benefit is achieved by changes in a large number of people who may not individually benefit. In addition, the high-risk group will often remain high-risk subsequent to population level intervention and

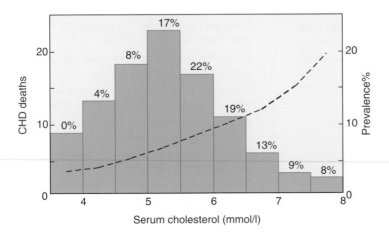

Figure 19.3 Distribution of CHD deaths across population. *Source*: Adapted from Rose G (1981) Strategy of prevention: lessons from cardiovascular disease. *BMJ* **282**: 1847–51.

therefore social inequalities in disease outcomes will persist.

Behaviour change

The determinants of behaviour are complex, being influenced by inherited, learnt and contextual factors over the life-course of the individual. The provision of scientifically accurate, accessible information is a necessary but insufficient condition for individual behaviour change. For example, advice to drink alcohol in moderation can be undermined by social norms and marketing that promote drinking; wide availability of cheap alcohol; physical and psychosocial enjoyment derived from alcohol consumption, and a lifetime of established drinking habits. Thus, an approach to health improvement based solely on public or patient education will rarely succeed. Guidance on behaviour change from the National Institute for Health and Clinical Excellence (NICE) recommends that clinicians working with individuals should select interventions that motivate and support people to:

- understand the short, medium and longer-term consequences of their health-related behaviours, for themselves and others;
- feel positive about the benefits of health-enhancing behaviours and changing their behaviour;
- plan their changes in terms of easy steps over time;
- recognise how their social contexts and relationships may affect their behaviour, and identify and plan for situations that might undermine the changes they are trying to make;
- plan explicit 'if–then' coping strategies to prevent relapse;
- make a personal commitment to adopt health-enhancing behaviours by setting and recording goals to undertake clearly defined behaviours, in particular contexts, over a specified time;
- share their behaviour change goals with others.

Brief interventions for behaviour change

Brief interventions involve opportunistic advice, discussion, negotiation or encouragement provided by clinicians to support patient behaviour change. There is good evidence that brief interventions to reduce alcohol misuse, promote smoking cessation and increase physical activity are highly **cost-effective**. Although an individual brief intervention will rarely lead to observed behaviour change, the cumulative effect of multiple interactions of this type over the course of a lifetime or illness, tailored to the individual patient and supported by specialists when necessary, can result in positive outcomes. The erroneous assumption that clinical advice on lifestyle never results in behaviour change is one of the principal barriers to uptake of these highly cost-effective interventions.

Brief interventions commonly involve assessment of current behaviour and risk, the use of motivational interviewing techniques to encourage change, and planning action tailored to the individual. For example, NICE guidance on smoking cessation recommends the following.

- Clinicians should ask people who smoke how interested they are in quitting.
- If they want to stop, they should refer them to an intensive support service such as NHS Stop Smoking Services.
- If they are unwilling or unable to accept a referral, offer a stop smoking aid such as pharmacotherapy.
- Set up monitoring systems so they and other health professionals can know whether or not their patients smoke.

Other approaches, such as *FRAMES* (Box 19.2) use **motivational interviewing** techniques.

Box 19.2 FRAMES – an approach to motivational interviewing.

- **Feedback** – give an objective assessment of the risks associated with current behaviour
- **Responsibility** – encourage the patient to see them self as responsible for change
- **Advice-giving** – provide non-judgemental, evidence-based recommendations for change
- **Menu** – provide a variety of self-directed and treatment options for change
- **Empathy** – show sympathy for the feelings and experiences of the patient
- **Self-efficacy** – encourage the patient's belief in them self to make change

The role of empowerment and social change

Empowerment means increasing the opportunities, resources and beliefs that individuals or communities have to control their life circumstances. An empowerment approach is taken in health improvement to enable individuals or groups to achieve better outcomes for themselves in the long term. Interventions of this type are often focused at a given community:

- Community of place – for example neighbourhood, city or nation
- Community of interest – for example occupational group or football club
- Community of identity – for example peer group, sexual orientation or gender

Community-level interventions may also focus on specific setting such as schools or hospitals. Often, action to tackle the determinants of health will be needed and this can include a political dimension. For example, tax-breaks on the purchase of bicycles for NHS staff and provision of bike locks and showers at healthcare facilities will encourage those who live close by to cycle to work. Changes in transport policy will be needed to prioritise walking, cycling and public transport over car use as the principal means of transport to healthcare sites from further afield.

Through advocacy and leadership on specific social issues, clinicians and others have helped pave the way for legislative or policy change that help bring about structural change in society and establish new population norms of behaviour. Change on this scale requires high-level political commitment and the integration of national policies and legislation impacting the issue of concern.

Tobacco control – an example of integrated health improvement

Tobacco control aims to reduce the harm arising from tobacco use. Richard Doll's prospective **cohort study** of smoking among British doctors in the 1950s provided the first authoritative evidence of the long-term effects of smoking on morbidity and mortality, and the dose-response relationship between exposure in number of cigarettes smoked and disease outcomes. Since that time researchers, clinicians, legislators and many other advocates have steadily worked to document and develop interventions to reduce the harms of smoking. Much of this change has been incremental and highly political, going against many vested commercial and other interests in society.

The 2005 WHO Framework Convention on Tobacco Control embodies an evidence-based set of legislative and other measures to control the global epidemic of tobacco smoking to which 168 countries have committed. This is supported by the MPOWER framework, a succinct expression of the six most important, evidence-based measures to control tobacco use at a population level.

- **M**onitor tobacco use and prevention policies
- **P**rotect people from second-hand tobacco smoke
- **O**ffer help to quit tobacco use
- **W**arn about the dangers of tobacco
- **E**nforce bans on tobacco advertising, improvement and sponsorship
- **R**aise taxes on tobacco

Progress in tobacco control is reflected in the reductions in smoking prevalence observed in many high-income countries over the past sixty years, down from highs of around 50% of adults smoking in the postwar period to around 20% today. Unfortunately, this downward trend in rich countries has been counterbalanced by a steady upward trend in tobacco production and consumption in low-income countries, and this represents a key challenge for tobacco control and global health advocates.

Health improvement in medical practice

All medical practitioners have a crucial role to play in health improvement:

- at an individual level, by encouraging and enabling healthy living and self-care behaviours for patients, staff and themselves;

- at a service level, by leading the development of quality healthcare that promotes the health of staff and patients;
- at a community level, by advocating for interventions that address the determinants of health.

The prominence medical practitioners have in promoting awareness of and debate about health cannot be underestimated. This status makes medical practitioners important role-models and leaders for health in the wider community, for good or ill. Every medical practitioner has an ethical responsibility to actively promote evidence-based messages and practices for the prevention of disease and improvement of health in their immediate sphere of professional influence.

Many specialities have specific health improvement remits, for example the prevention and treatment of blood-borne viruses and sexually-transmissible diseases in genitourinary medicine. The two specialities that have the largest proportion of their work focused towards health improvement and primary prevention are general practice and public health medicine.

The Royal College of General Practitioners curriculum statement five on promoting health and preventing disease focuses on promoting health behaviours and supporting patients to care for themselves safely and effectively, but also recognises the importance of developing practice-level approaches to tackling social inequalities in the health of the registered population. (http://www.gmc-uk.org/5_Healthy_people_01.pdf_30450948.pdf)

The Faculty of Public Health recognises health improvement as one of the three pillars of preventative practice, the others being health service development and health protection. Public health specialists work to promote health by influencing the lifestyle and socio-economic, environmental and educational determinants of individual, community and population health. (http://www.fph.org.uk/)

 KEY LEARNING POINTS

- Health improvement is the process of enabling people to increase control over and improve their health
- Preventative interventions can be focused at individual, community and population levels and at primary, secondary and tertiary stages in the natural history of disease
- An ethical balance must be struck between individual liberty and the benefits of action to prevent disease and prolong life
- Preventative interventions that target those at high risk of disease are common in medical practice and have significant benefits for the individual, although they typically make relatively little contribution to the overall health of the population
- Preventative interventions at a population level make the most contribution to reduction of incident cases when excess risk is widely distributed in the population, as a large number of people at low risk of disease will give rise to more cases than a small number of people at high risk, but suffer from the prevention paradox
- Motivational interviewing and brief interventions to bring about behaviour change are evidence-based clinical skills that medical practitioners can use
- Community empowerment and social change is necessary to tackle the determinants of ill health and inequality
- All medical practitioners have important roles to play in promoting health at individual, service and community levels

 REFERENCES

Dahlgren G, Whitehead M (1991) *Policies and Strategies to Promote Social Equity in Health*. Institute for Future Studies, Stockholm (Mimeo).

Rose G (1981) Strategy of prevention: lessons from cardiovascular disease. *BMJ* **282**: 1847–1851.

20

Evaluating public health and complex interventions

Yoav Ben-Shlomo and Rona Campbell
University of Bristol

Learning objectives

In this chapter you will learn:

- ✓ to understand the varied methods used to evaluate public health or complex interventions;
- ✓ to describe the features of a cluster randomised controlled trial and when it may be appropriate to use this design;
- ✓ how we can we use time trend or before/after designs;
- ✓ what the role is of natural experiments;
- ✓ how ecological data within and between areas can be of value.

What is a complex intervention?

The methods used to evaluate health service interventions have been covered in Chapter 11. Our gold standard is the parallel group **randomised controlled trial** (**RCT**) which, if undertaken well, provides very strong evidence as to whether an intervention is causally related to improved health outcomes or not. These are ideally suited to studies of drugs where it is usually possible to blind the subjects and researchers to which intervention has been given. As methods of conducting trials have developed and expanded so have the types of interventions that such trials are used to evaluate – from a single drug to a single nonpharmacological intervention, such as surgery, to a **complex intervention** such as a stroke unit or a smoking cessation programme.

A complex health care intervention is defined as one that consists of several separate components, each of which is considered essential to the functioning of the intervention as a whole. A smoking cessation programme, for example, might consist of written information, media coverage, physician advice and cognitive behaviour therapy. Unfortunately there are several reasons why it is often very difficult or simply not feasible to conduct a parallel RCT to public health interventions or complex health service research questions. Instead we use different sorts of designs some of which are still randomised (cluster randomised trials) and some that are based on special types of observational studies.

Epidemiology, Evidence-based Medicine and Public Health Lecture Notes, Sixth Edition. Yoav Ben-Shlomo, Sara T. Brookes and Matthew Hickman.
© 2013 Y. Ben-Shlomo, S. T. Brookes and M. Hickman. Published 2013 by John Wiley & Sons, Ltd.

Cluster randomised controlled trials

A **cluster randomised trial** differs from conventional RCTs in that a cluster rather than an individual is the unit of randomisation. Examples of clusters include (a) hospitals, (b) general practices, (c) geographical areas (d) schools, (e) prisons, (f) workplaces etc. In each cluster all potential subjects receive the same intervention rather than being randomised to different treatment options.

Why do we randomise by cluster?

The usual reason is that it is not practical to randomise by individual. Public health interventions are generally delivered at a group rather than individual level so it is sensible to evaluate them at this level. For example, a work-based health promotion campaign would be unpopular if only some of the workers were offered the intervention since those not receiving it may feel hard done by. On the other hand it would be fine to randomise workplaces to either all workers receiving the intervention or no workers receiving it. One of the main issues is **contamination**, which is when the intervention also gets delivered to some of the control group. For example, if we tried to randomise individuals to a media campaign that uses local newspapers, it would be difficult to prevent the control group being contaminated by the intervention. In this instance, different geographical areas could be randomised to either receive the media campaign or not.

As noted in Chapter 14, it is usual to seek informed consent prior to randomisation in a parallel group design RCT. This approach is referred to as opt in consent. In a cluster RCT consent to participate has first to be sought at the group level. Randomisation of the clusters follows and consent from the individual is often obtained using opt-out consent an approach which usually involves individuals returning a form if they do not want to receive the allocated intervention or to have their outcome data used in the analysis. Opt out consent is used in population health improvement research because obtaining individual written consent may limit recruitment and introduce bias which may seriously undermine the validity of the research. It is argued that in minimally invasive epidemiological research, individual consent should be waived where (a) the benefits to society are potentially high, (b) the risk to individuals low, and (c) the effort and cost of obtaining individual consent may be prohibitive. Because groups rather than individuals are randomised, cluster trials also require additional design and analysis considerations and the advantages and disadvantages of this approach are explained further in Table 20.1.

Example: Peer led intervention for smoking prevention in teenagers: the ASSIST cluster RCT
Health education lessons in schools have not been shown to be very effective in reducing teenage smoking. However, young people may be more influenced by their peers than teachers. The ASSIST trial studied the smoking behaviour of 10,730 young people aged 12–13 years in 59 schools in England and Wales. Schools were randomised within strata (based on size of school, level of entitlement to free school meals etc.) so that 29 schools received usual health education and 30 schools received the intervention. The intervention required students to identify influential peers in their year group who then went on a 2-day participatory learning course outside school which covered the harms of smoking as well as listening and supportive skills. Peer supporters were then encouraged to discuss smoking during informal conversations with their friends. After two years follow-up, the odds ratio of smoking in the intervention compared to control schools was 0.78 (95% CI 0.64 to 0.96) demonstrating a 22% relative reduction in odds of smoking in the intervention schools (Campbell *et al.*, 2008).

Stepped wedge designs

In some cases it may be hard to recruit clusters if there is a pre-existing belief that the intervention is effective (or a policy decision has been made to implement the intervention even in the absence of evidence) or clusters randomised to the control arm feel little commitment to the study and the necessary data collection given that they will not receive the intervention. In such circumstances, a useful alternative is a **stepped wedge design** whereby all clusters receive the intervention but some receive it immediately whilst others receive it after a delay so there is a period of time when they act as the control arm. (Such a

---

Table 20.1 Advantages and disadvantages of cluster randomisation.

Advantages

(a) Reduces problems of *contamination* so that either practitioners or subjects in the control arm are not inadvertently exposed to the intervention which may result in benefits to those in the control arm indirectly due to the intervention. This will reduce (attenuate) the chance of showing the intervention is beneficial.

(b) May be more cost-effective to deliver intervention at a cluster than individual level.

(c) For public health interventions intended to improve population health, where individual randomisation is not possible, cluster randomisation is the gold standard.

Disadvantages

(a) Larger sample sizes are required as are more sophisticated statistical methods that take into account the clustering effect (e.g. multilevel models). In a two-arm trial one needs at least 8 clusters (4 per arm) as a minimum and the more clusters the better so that any differences between clusters are balanced across the trial arms. Stratified randomisation is one method to help ensure balance so that the clusters are grouped into strata based on a characteristic likely to be related to the outcome being studied e.g. teaching hospital versus district general hospital prior to randomisation in a trial comparing day surgery versus surgery including an inpatient stay.

(b) Recruitment or exclusion bias: individual RCTs first recruit participants and then randomises them avoiding any selection or exclusion bias as the researchers are not aware of which arm the person will be allocated. However in a cluster RCT, if randomisation of the clusters occurs before the participants are recruited then the researchers could influence which participants are included after they know which arm the person has been allocated too which could bias the results.

---

design can also be used in individual level studies.) This often reflects what happens in the 'real world' where a new service cannot be delivered immediately to all areas and has to be introduced to some areas first though often the order is not randomised so that bias may be introduced.

Example: Nutritional supplementation and future cardiovascular risk

There is much scientific interest concerning the role of pre- and postnatal nutrition on later life cardiovascular risk as observational cohort studies have shown that babies born small have more heart disease and diabetes. A national community-based programme to improve the nutrition of children in India was established in the 1980s. This involved providing a cereal based meal with calorie and protein supplementation to pregnant mothers and their children in villages in India. Because the programme had to be implemented in a phased approach, the National Institute of Nutrition in Hyderabad under took a stepped wedge design where 29 villages were selected and 15 were chosen as the intervention and 14 were control villages who all received the intervention after a delay of three years. A follow-up study, conducted when the children were around 16 years of age, showed that children born in the intervention villages were taller, had better measures of insulin metabolism and less stiff arteries though measures of obesity were similar (Kinra *et al.*, 2008).

Why can't we always do RCTs?

Whilst it may be theoretically possible to imagine how one could do a trial for any evaluation, in the real world it is often simply not possible or not ethical to either do an individual or cluster-based RCT. Table 20.2 highlights possible reasons and examples.

Ecological studies

We have previously explained ecological studies in Chapter 5. As well as enabling us to examine aetiological questions (do areas with higher radon levels have a greater risk of lung cancer?) ecological studies can also be used to evaluate policy or area-based interventions. As mentioned previously, the major limitation of this approach is the **ecological fallacy**, i.e. associations that are detected on a group level may not hold on an individual level. Their main advantage is they usually enable fairly rapid evaluation if using routinely collected data such as mortality or administrative data on health care provision. For example, a study from the United States measured age-adjusted rates of suicide mortality across all the states and found

Table 20.2 Reasons why it is difficult or impossible to undertake RCTs.

1. *Experimentation unnecessary* – effects so dramatic that confounding could not explain results, e.g. insulin therapy for insulin dependent diabetes
2. *Rare outcomes* – Either positive or negative outcomes are very rare so very large sample sizes required hence study too expensive e.g. randomising free cycle helmets to children to reduce mortality
3. *Long follow-up* – Effects only seen after a very long follow-up, e.g. risk of leukaemia after metallic break down from hip implants seen after more than 15 years of exposure
4. *Lack of perceived* **equipoise**: Difficult to recruit when people are already convinced that an intervention is beneficial or unlikely to be harmful, for example recruiting children and young people to an RCT of the effectiveness cycling helmets in preventing head injury could be difficult when parents may already be convinced that they are beneficial even if though it is possible that any mechanical advantage is outweighed by a harmful change in risk taking behaviour by the person wearing the helmet or in other vehicle users observing that the cyclist is wearing a helmet
5. *Politics* – Political or legal obstacles, e.g. policy-makers may not wish to know that their policy is not effective or feel that the intervention must be introduced to all at the same time
6. *Contamination* – Control areas may start to take up preventative measures that have been allocated to the intervention areas as a secondary phenomenon
7. *Cost of study* – Both for reasons given above as well as the cost of the intervention, a formal trial may be prohibitively expensive
8. *Readily available intervention* – If, for example, we were interested in the effect of television viewing on obesity it would not be possible to withhold television from some individuals (or clusters)

Source: Modified from Black (1996).

that greater state expenditure on mental health services as well as the number of psychiatrists per 100,000 population predicted lower levels of suicide mortality (Tondo *et al.*, 2006). Despite adjusting for other variables, it is still possible that confounding by other factors remains so that areas that spend more money on mental health services are also areas with better social networks or family support (for which there is probably no routine data) and in fact it is the latter factors rather than the expenditure that is the protective factor.

Natural experiments and before and after studies

A more powerful approach uses, often in hindsight, the good fortune of a **natural experiment**. These are events (sometimes planned but often unplanned) which are usually not in the control of the researchers and which change an exposure in such a way that is unlikely to be related to other confounders – hence in a random way. Ideally the event is sudden with a clear temporal onset. This then allows researchers to study the effect of the experiment where it would either be unethical or impractical to randomise. In some cases the comparison group is another population that have not

received the intervention or in the case where everyone is exposed it is usual to compare outcomes before and after the intervention. These two approaches can be combined. They can be used to study aetiological questions or the impact of some policy.

Example: Smoke free legislation and hospital admissions for acute coronary syndrome
Scotland introduced legislation to ban smoking in public places from the end of March 2006 and in advance of England and Wales. This enabled a comparison both within Scotland, before and after the ban, as well as comparing this with any changes in England. Figure 20.1 shows that for each month admissions reduced after the legislation with an overall 17% reduction (95% confidence interval, 16 to 18%). This compared to a 4% reduction in England during the same period, which is similar to the mean annual decrease of 3% in Scotland observed during the decade before the smoking ban.

Example: Legislation on pesticide sales and suicide mortality
It is quite common to plot longer term time trends or do **time series** analyses with the timing of any major change highlighted. Figure 20.2 shows suicide mortality rates (per 100,000) in Sri Lanka where pesticides are commonly used as a method for overdose. The initial ban of Parathion in 1984 had no effect on the rapidly increasing rates, as

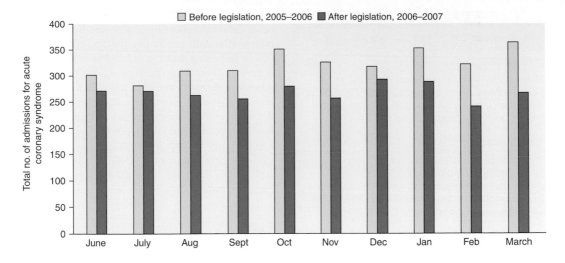

Figure 20.1 Admissions for acute coronary syndrome according to month before and after smoke-free legislation
Source: Pell *et al.*, NEJM (2008).

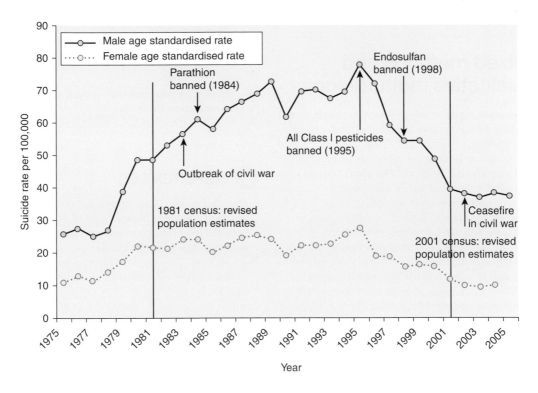

Figure 20.2 Age standardised suicide rates for males and females, Sri Lanka, 1975–2005
Source: Gunnell *et al.*, IJE (2007).

Table 20.3 Advantages and disadvantages of ecological and before and after studies.
Advantages
These studies are much cheaper than conventional RCTs as the intervention happens outside the research setting and often the outcome data come from routine sources such as mortality statistics.
Disadvantages
Without an appropriate comparator population (as in the suicide example) it is always possible that other factors might explain these patterns. However, the rapidity and magnitude of the decline in example above makes this very unlikely.

there were plenty of other agents, but the ban of all Class 1 pesticides in 1995 was followed by a sudden rapid decline for both men and women (see Figure 20.2).

Table 20.3 gives the advantages and disadvantages of ecological and before and after studies.

Mixed methods and qualitative methodology

It is becoming increasingly common that research studies combine both qualitative and quantitative methods within the same project ('mixed methods') as both approaches are often complementary and the results of one approach can feed into and refine the other. As noted in Chapter 11 **qualitative research methods** can be used to observe and inform aspects of randomised trials. These include (a) improving recruitment, (b) how best to measure outcomes of interest, (c) what participants understand when they are invited to take part in a trial and (d) how well an intervention is delivered in a trial (fidelity of implementation). Qualitative and mixed methods can be employed within any of the approaches described above for evaluating complex public health interventions. Qualitative methods are particularly useful when a complex public health intervention is being developed as they can be used to find out whether the intervention is acceptable both to those for whom the intervention is being provided and to those responsible for delivering it and to answer questions about whether or not it is feasible to deliver the intervention. For example, the ASSIST

cluster randomised control trial was preceded by a detailed feasibility study which used both quantitative and qualitative methods. The results of that indicated that it was feasible to implement a peer led smoking prevention intervention in schools and that it would be possible to do a large scale cluster RCT to evaluate the effectiveness of the intervention. Further mixed methods research was then conducted within the trial to access the acceptability of the intervention to the school students (see Audrey *et al.*, 2006 for more details) and school staff and to examine the fidelity of implementation.

 KEY LEARNING POINTS

- It is not always possible to use RCTs for public health interventions and where a trial design is used it is usually a cluster rather than individual level randomised design
- Cluster RCTs are more complex to analyse and require larger sample sizes than individual-based RCTs
- Ecological studies and variations in time trends can be very helpful especially in relation to major policy changes
- Natural experiments can also provide unique insights into causal effects

 REFERENCES

Audrey S, Holliday J, Campbell R (2007) It's good to talk: adolescent perspectives of an informal, peer-led intervention to reduce smoking. *Social Science & Medicine* **63**: 320–34.

Black N (1996) Why we need observational studies to evaluate the effectiveness of health care. *BMJ* **312**: 1215–18.

Campbell R, Starkey F, Holliday J, *et al.* (2008) An informal school-based peer-led intervention for smoking prevention in adolescence (ASSIST): a cluster randomised trial. *The Lancet* **371**: 1595–1602.

Gunnell D, Fernando R, Hewagama M, *et al.* (2007) The impact of pesticide regulations on suicide in Sri Lanka. *International Journal of Epidemiology* **36**: 1242–3.

Kinra S, Rameshwar Sarma KV, Mendu VV, *et al.* (2008) Effect of integration of supplemental nutrition with public health programmes in pregnancy and early childhood on cardiovascular risk in rural Indian adolescents: long term follow-up of Hyderabad nutrition trial. *BMJ* **337**: a605.

Medical Research Council (2011) Using natural experiments to evaluate population health interventions, London: MRC (available from http://www.mrc.ac.uk/Utilities/Documentrecord/index.htm?d=MRC008043)

Pell JP, Haw S, Cobbe S, *et al.* (2008) Smoke-free legislation and hospitalizations for acute coronary syndrome. *N Engl J Med* **359**: 482–91.

Tondo L, Alpert MJ, Baldessarini R (2006) Suicide rates in relation to health care access in the United States: an ecological study. *J Clin Psychiatry* **67**: 517–23.

Victora CG, Habicht JP, Bryce J (2004) Evidence based public health: Moving beyond randomised trials. *Am J Public Health* **94**: 400–5.

21

Health care targets

Maya Gobin and Gabriel Scally
Health Protection Services and University of West of England

Learning objectives

In this chapter you will learn:

- ✓ what are targets within public health policy;
- ✓ the different sorts of targets that can be set;
- ✓ the positive and negative aspects of setting targets;
- ✓ what makes good targets.

Public health policy and target setting

The way in which societies respond to population health problems is generally by agreeing what needs to be done to tackle serious concerns and improve the health of the public. The policies they adopt vary enormously in their sophistication and effect. As the policies adopted, particularly at a national level, have grown both in their span and implications it has been found necessary to back them up with the practical strategies need to support their implementation and, hopefully, success.

The substantial growth in the development of public health policies, whether at a global or national level, has seen increasing attention being paid to the use of targets as a tool in assisting with the implementation of strategies for their achievement. In the United Kingdom (UK) the production of a secession of public health policies, which have expanded into the wider area of cross-sectoral working, has been accompanied by a commensurate growth in the use of targets.

Targets have been a feature of health policy in the UK for a substantial proportion of the history the NHS. In the last ten years, they have been increasingly used as a tool in performance management, not just in health but across the entire public sector. Targets are seen as an integral part of public health planning and programme design. However, setting targets is a complex, imperfect process and there is no inevitably that their use will lead to improvements in outcomes or performance.

What are targets?

There are many definitions of what exactly targets are but the World Health Organisation's (WHO) 1998 definition provides a good basis for exploring their nature.

> '*Health targets* define the concrete steps which may be taken towards the achievement of health goals. Setting targets also provides one approach to the assessment of progress in relation to a defined health policy or programme by defining a benchmark against which progress can be measured.'

Epidemiology, Evidence-based Medicine and Public Health Lecture Notes, Sixth Edition. Yoav Ben-Shlomo, Sara T. Brookes and Matthew Hickman.
© 2013 Y. Ben-Shlomo, S. T. Brookes and M. Hickman. Published 2013 by John Wiley & Sons, Ltd.

Targets specify time bound desired levels of improvement and can be informed, or indeed driven by:

- political policies;
- public priorities or concerns;
- previous performance;
- internal comparison with other units within the organisation;
- external comparison identifying good practice (either in other public organisations or with private sector organisations).

In the health sector high-level targets are considered by many as necessary in order to achieve the goals and objectives set out in health policies and are primarily set for either one or both of the following reasons:

(1) to ensure that activity is directed towards the achievement of health outcomes; and/or
(2) to facilitate the monitoring of progress in order to ensure that health policy goals and objectives are being met.

At a global level, important examples are the **Millennium Development Goals** (see Chapter 22). Targets are also a tool used in managing the performance of individuals, organisations and systems where the targets represent a level of performance/standards that should be achieved. At their best they are used to:

(1) ensuring consistency in the care or service provided; and
(2) challenging the individual, organisation or system to do better.

Targets can be:

- *All-the-time targets* – they are the level of service to be delivered all the time. An example would be 'Never Events'. These are serious failures in patient safety, such as intrathecal injection of vincristin, which the NHS works to try and ensure never occur.
- *Percentage achievement targets* – are commitments to achieve a stated level of performance against a standard. An example of this approach would be a goal of testing 35% of the population aged 16 to 24 years of age for Chlamydia every year.

- *Qualitative targets* – describe the level of service that is expected. An example of this is the 'You're Welcome' quality criteria which set out principles to help health services (including non-NHS provision) become young people friendly.
- *Time-bound target* – is a one-off promise for a certain area. In 2003 the then government set a national target to reduce health inequalities, as measured by infant mortality and life expectancy at birth, by 10% by 2010.

An example of targets used in performance management at a national level in the United Kingdom were Public Service Agreements between the Treasury and other government departments. Each agreement described how targets will be achieved and how performance against these targets would be measured over a three-year period.

Targets can be set in relation to a wide range of elements of policies and programmes. They can relate to inputs, demand, activity, infrastructure, outcomes, outputs and processes. As well as the element to which they are applied, the nature of the target can vary and a major division is into qualitative or quantitative targets.

Indicators are developed to measure movement towards, or away from, a pre-defined target and are a mechanism for keeping track of progress towards an overall goal. There are some measures that can be used as both an indicator and a target. For example, Target 5 of the Millennium Development Goals is to reduce the under-five mortality rate by two thirds between, 1995 and 2015. The under-five mortality rate is also used as an indicator to monitor progress towards this overall target.

History of targets

Targets have been a feature of subnational, national and international health policy for over half a century and in that time have been through numerous iterations, however as the WHO states 'when it comes to implementation the track record of health targets is less clear and less perfect' (Kirch, 2008).

Targets for health policy have existed since the second half of the twentieth century and at that time were focused on ensuring the necessary supply of services to meet the newly realised demand for health care. The targets set were often phrased in terms of hospital beds or health professionals per head of population, their geographical spread and the number of individuals who did or did not have access to health services. In the late 1970s, the focus of health policies shifted from service expansion to reducing health care expenditure through improving the efficiency of health services delivery. Targets were now focused on reducing expenditure by controlling supply, for example through capped budgets for hospitals, through capitation fees for GPs, or by limiting the number of doctors in training and the number of hospital beds.

In the 1980s, WHO and some national governments were at the forefront of a campaign to place population health at the centre of health policy action. This change in focus was influenced by the growing availability of information on the risk factors for diseases and the evidence of effectiveness of treatments. Both of these could link policy action to the potential health benefits for the population. Both national and supranational policies started to translate policy priorities into health targets. For example, in 1982 the European region developed regional health targets to aid achievement of the WHO *Health for All* strategy. Many countries subsequently adapted these targets to their local situation.

The *Health of the Nation* strategy (HOTN) launched in England in 1992 signalled a shift in national health policy from health care to health. The strategy included 27 targets that were seen as a source of inspiration rather than a management tool. The targets quantitatively indicated what level of health in the populations should be attained and by when. They included infant mortality rates, prevalence of hypertension, deaths due to motor-vehicle accidents, and mortality rates due to coronary heart disease or lung cancer. Health targets were widely supported at this time as a helpful way of prioritising actions and focusing efforts, however, they were criticised for following a mainly disease based model. Targets were often based on arbitrary numbers and people argued that this resulted in some targets being set too low such as those for CHD and stroke.

In 1999 following a change of Government in the UK, and a review of HOTN, a new strategy, *Saving Lives: Our Healthier Nation* (OHN) was published. The new health policy had two key aims; to improve life expectancy and to narrow the gap in health between the worst off and best off in society. The strategy was also disease focused but in contrast to HOTN, OHN targets were focused on both improving health outcomes as well as ensuring that key policy objectives were being met.

Targets were also now increasingly used as a management tool integral to the governance of health services both to monitor progress in improving health and to manage the performance of services. To ensure that the policy objectives were achieved the government developed a performance management framework with performance indicators. Organisations were rewarded or sanctioned according to their performance against these targets and indicators. The rewards and sanctions included; budgetary allocation that was based on the measured performance (more money allocated to the better performing organisations); bonuses and renewed tenure for managers; reputational effects (shame or glory on the basis of league tables of performance).

OHN saw a shift in the emphasis of health targets from inputs and structures to processes, outputs and outcomes and there were considerable improvements in the reported public health performance of the NHS in England subsequent to its publication. However, there was widespread concern about the large number of indicators and the top down bias and centrally driven nature of these targets. There were numerous examples of organisations and services that engaged in undesirable practices in order to achieve their targets and opponents of this system strongly criticise targets for creating poor quality services (Fulop, 2000; Seddon, 2008).

In 2010 the newly elected coalition government published *Liberating the NHS*, its white paper for health and Healthy Lives, Healthy People, its public health white paper. Both white papers signalled an intention to replace top down process targets with evidence based and relevant outcome measures. An outcomes framework was constructed covering the three key areas of **public health**, the NHS and adult social care.

The value of targets

Targets help drive improvement in a number of ways:

* *Identify priorities and help define an agreed direction*: targets indicate which areas arc high

priorities for action and can be used to focus attention, efforts and resources on achieving the desired health outcome.

- *Provide accountability*: targets explicitly states what outcomes an organisation is working towards and demonstrate to the rest of the organisation, the public and other stakeholders what is regarded as important and that there is a commitment to deliver.
- *Motivate staff*: people are motivated in different ways and targets can be used as a tool to motivate people to find ways to improve outcomes. Targets can provide individuals with a clear understanding of why some things need to happen and their role in making them happen. Targets can provide staff with an overall goal and a sense of purpose especially if they reflect policy priorities. Targets can motivate staff if they are challenging but realistic and there is a sense of ownership. Rewards or sanctions associated with targets may also motivate staff.
- *Share learning and good practice*: targets provide an opportunity to focus on what has been achieved, to identify lessons learnt and share examples of good practice where possible. In this way targets that are not met can still lead to improvements and so should not be seen as a sign of failure.

Problems with targets

Target setting is an imperfect process, many targets are not set well and do not result in improvement. An understanding of the deficiencies and failures of targets can be highly instructive and aid the process of improvement. Common problems identified with setting targets include:

- *Perverse incentives*: A perverse incentive is an incentive that has an unintended and undesirable effect, which is against the interest of the policy makers. This occurs when the indicator does not accurately measure the health outcome and results in action that is focused on improving performance in respect of the indicator rather than action that achieves the intended health outcome. For example, a hospital that was having difficulty meeting a national target of giving access within 48 hours to patients wanting to attend a genito-urinary

medicine clinic decided to stop providing that service rather than fail a target.

Indicators should be reviewed to make them more reflective of the intended health outcome; this can be achieved with the use of a balanced suite of indicators and focusing on outcomes as far as possible.

- *Gaming*: The use of targets results in a distortion of practice, where people use targets to cheat the system rather than as a tool for improvement. This reduces the ability of policy makers to be confident that there have been genuine improvements when the reported performance meets the targets. For example a target that no one should wait more than four hours in accident and emergency departments was introduced. Acute trusts were penalised financially for not achieving this target and, in some instances, resorted to drafting extra staff into accident and emergency departments, operations being cancelled, and patients having to wait in ambulances until staff were confident of meeting the target (Bevan, 2006).

The introduction of uncertainty in the way that performance is assessed, for example varying the targets from time to time, can reduce the potential for gaming. Other suggestions for reducing gaming include focusing on outcomes as far as possible, better auditing of performance data or the introduction of an independent review of the reported improvements and the costs to other services.

- *Lack of attribution*: Targets are allocated to individuals/organisation that have little or no control over them and cannot be achieved by those who are made primarily responsible; this is particularly an issue with targets that are set in partnership with other organisations or people or require such partnership working to be achieved.

For example, it could be argued that it is contradictory to set local targets to reduce alcohol related harm whilst promoting other national policies that oppose changes in alcohol pricing and encourage alcohol consumption (Hadfield, 2009).

- *Conflicting targets*: Achievement of one target results in doing worse in another. This may occur because the performance indicators do not accurately reflect the whole picture and may require indicators that are more representative or the use of multiple indicators. In other instances this may arise because of real differences across policy areas. For example the installation of brighter street lights to reduce crime may conflict with the goal of reducing use of energy or promoting dark skies.

- *Wrong type of indicators*: The indicators do not provide an appropriate assessment of the outcome for which they have been set. For example four week quit rates for smoking cessation are used as an indicator of success; however, this is based on self reports and is not a reliable indicator of successful long term quitting (Ash, 2009).

  Outcome indicators are often preferred as they reflect what one is trying to achieve, however, input, process and output indicators may be required to provide a better understanding of what is going on and what action can be taken.

- *Unreliable data*: Data used to monitor performance are unavailable, inconsistent, incomplete or not timely. Targets should only be set if there is a robust mechanism for monitoring progress and indicators should be reviewed to ensure that they are consistent with what they are asked define.

  For example the 2008 Health Survey for England used two new methods to measure physical activity; all participants were questioned about their activity as done in previous years and a sub sample was also asked to wear pedometers for a week. The survey results highlighted enormous discrepancies between the two methods, emphasising the importance of using reliable methods to track trends over time (Cavill *et al.*, 2009).

- *Lack of ownership of targets*: Targets that are not agreed by partners risk a lack of ownership and are unlikely to attract sufficient support to achieve the intended improvements. For example clinicians may disengage with processes to improve performance and health outcomes if targets are externally set or set top down.

  Those responsible for the target need to be clearly identified and made aware of how they will be held accountable for the target.

- *Ambiguous indicators*: In some instances an indicator can be interpreted in different ways and it is generally considered inappropriate to set targets against these indicators. Indicators should be objective, and operationally precise. For example the percentage of individuals that eat healthily is ambiguous, instead the percentage of adults (18 or older) that eat five or more portions of fruit and vegetables in a day is

operationally precise and less open to interpretation.

- *Distorted activity*: Targets set for areas of health care are often limited to diseases or health problems that are easily measured and controlled and where quantitative and timely data is readily available. More complicated diseases that are more difficult to measure and not amenable to targets, such as many psychiatric conditions, are frequently ignored. It is clearly desirable that targets should measure aspects of public health and service delivery that are truly important rather than those that are easily measured.

  It is therefore necessary in some areas of practice to consider making use of a wider, and potentially unorthodox range of targets and indicators, or other methods such as qualitative or narrative reports.

- *Too many indicators*: A large number of targets and indicators may overwhelm those responsible for them and also become meaningless if they include everything. Therefore indicators should only be used if they provide useful information that can lead to action against the objectives and priorities identified. The application of an appropriate level of parsimony in the selection and imposition of targets is something that is rarely seen and often neglected entirely. Indeed, the desire to limit the number and range of indicators can generate opposition from vested interests who wish to see their own narrow subject area covered.

Characteristics of good targets

Targets should be set using the **SMART** criteria to ensure that they are properly constructed and successfully achieve their aim:

Specific – clearly indicate who or what is the focus of target and what is the intended outcome. The target should be clear, unambiguous and easy to understand by those who are required to use them.

Measurable – the change that is expected can be measured and the source of the measurement is identified. Targets should not be set when there is not a specific measure that can be used to gauge success.

Achievable – are challenging but realistic. A target should have aims that those achieving it feel can be realistically achieved with some effort: 'out of reach, not out of sight'.

Realistic – are achievable within existing conditions and with available resources, knowledge and time. Those responsible for meeting targets should have enough control over their work to be able to achieve their targets.

Time bound – clearly stated time period for the achievement the outcome. Open ended targets should be avoided as they do not encourage focussed efforts on improving performance.

Against the background of these characteristics of a good target it is important to consider the following factors when setting health targets in a specific context:

- *Local and national policies and priorities*: targets need to reflect both local and national priorities and a balance has to be struck where there are conflicting or inconsistent objectives. A criticism of target setting is that national policies are often not consistent or openly conflict with local strategies making it difficult to maintain momentum and enthusiasm for strategies at a local level
- *Consultation with key individuals and organisations:* the knowledge and experience of people responsible for the delivery of the target should be used to inform the targets to ensure that targets are appropriate, achievable and realistic and to encourage ownership of the target.
- *Purpose of the targets:* the type of target set must reflect the purpose of the target. For example, is the target intended to drive up performance, be a source of inspiration or used as a benchmark against which people and practice are assessed?
- *Control over target area*: targets should only be set when the intended outcome can be positively affected. It is inappropriate to set targets for an activity that cannot be directly influenced or controlled.
- *Level of the target*: targets need to be sufficiently challenging without being unrealistic. Targets should be set at an attainable level; targets that are set too low provide a disincentive for improvements while targets that are set too high risk demotivating those responsible for achieving them.
  The level a target is set at can be based on:
  ○ Benchmarking against similar organisations or services, the national average, a certain percentage of organisations or services (e.g. the top 25%), or against international levels of performance.
  ○ Trend analysis where targets are based on previous changes in performance over time.
- *Resources*: in some instances additional resources may be required to ensure targets are successfully met. Therefore, it is important that the necessary resources are identified and available otherwise there is a risk that the target becomes purely symbolic.
- *Time period*: the target needs to be achievable in the time period specified. Some diseases remain latent for a long time and have risk factors that have a long lag time. Therefore actions to reduce the prevalence of disease may take years to have an impact and will require a longer commitment to achieve an improvement in outcomes.
- *Evidence based*: the development of realistic targets requires an understanding of the epidemiology of disease and the estimated health benefits that would be achievable with the current interventions.
- *Indicators/measures*: indicators are used as proxy measures and so need to be a plausible measure of the outcome of interest. Indicators should be clearly defined from the outset and not be open to interpretation. Indicators are used to measure progress and therefore need to sensitive and responsive to changes in the outcome. The data should be already available or if not, could be easily collected. The data should be of good quality (complete, accurate and timely) and be comparable across individuals, organisations and services. The data collection systems must be robust and should be mapped to ensure that the data is consistent with the definition of the indicator.

Conclusion

Well-set targets have an important role to play in improving health outcomes and can be a powerful tool in managing performance. However, targets are just one method for improving outcomes and may not always be suitable. Setting targets is a complex and targets that are poorly set can be divisive and damaging to individual morale and service performance. Therefore before setting a target it is important to first consider if a target is necessary and appropriate; if a target is needed then it is essential that it is properly constructed and will result in genuine improvements in outcomes.

KEY LEARNING POINTS

- How target setting has developed from structural factors to public health related targets
- Their role in priority setting, motivating staff, providing accountability and sharing best practice
- The dangers of perverse incentives, gaming, distorting activities, lack of ownership, poor quality or too many indicators
- How SMART targets with widespread consultation and ownership, sufficient resources and control and a robust evidence base can lead to improvements in public health

 REFERENCES

Ash Briefing Document for HM Treasury Performance Management and Smoking Cessation Targets. November 2009. Available online http://www.ash.org.uk/files/documents/ASH_421.pdf

Bevan G, Hood C (2006) What's measured is what matters: targets and gaming in the English public health care system. *Public Administration* **84**(3): 517–38.

Cavill N, Rutter H and Ells L (2009) *Physical Activity Data in the 2008 Health Survey for England: Notes of a NOO/HSE Seminar 2009*. Oxford: National Obesity Observatory.

Fulop N, Hunter DJ (2000) The experience of setting health targets in England. *European Journal of Public Health*. **10** (4 supplement): 20–4.

Hadfield P, Lister S and Traynor P (2009) *Alcohol Insights: The Orientation and Integration of Local and National Alcohol Policy in England and Wales*. London: Alcohol Education Research Council.

Kirch W (2008) *Encyclopedia of Public Health*. New York: Spring Science and Business Media.

Seddon J (2008) *Systems Thinking in the Public Sector: The Failure of a Reform Regime and a Manifesto for a Better Way*. Axminster: Triarchy Press.

Wismar M, Ernest K, Srivastava D and Busse R (2006) Health targets and (good) governance. *EuroObserver* **8**(1): 1–5.

22

Global health

Sanjay Kinra, David L. Heymann and Shah Ebrahim
London School of Hygiene and Tropical Medicine

Learning objectives

In this chapter you will learn:

✓ What are the global burdens of disease and how they differ between low-middle income and high income countries?

✓ What are the wider determinants of health and the potential impact of demographic changes, migration and globalisation?

✓ What is the role for global initiatives to address these problems and

✓ What are the possible solutions to improve global health?

What is global health?

Global health can be defined as

> health problems, issues and concerns that transcend national boundaries, may be influenced by circumstances or experiences in other countries, and are best addressed by cooperative actions and solutions.
>
> (US Institute of Medicine, 2008)

Alternatively, and more comprehensively, global health is 'an area for study, research, and practice that places a priority on improving health and achieving equity in health for all people worldwide' (Koplan *et al.*, 2009).

Some examples are: avian flu; tobacco control; climate change to mention just a few.

Global health relies on people from a range of different disciplines, often outside of conventional health sciences, working together. Global health is exciting because it requires new thinking and there are no 'textbook' solutions. Most situations require different mixes of skills, there are different stakeholders, and different means of understanding and formulating problems – and sometimes solving them.

Global burden of death and disability

Reliable information on causes of death is essential to development of national and international policies for prevention and control of disease and injuries. However, data collection is often limited in many developing countries; medically certified information is available for less than a third of deaths worldwide.

The Global Burden of Disease (GBD) study, supported by the World Bank and the World Health Organisation (WHO), used various data sources and techniques to estimate the numbers of deaths

---

Epidemiology, Evidence-based Medicine and Public Health Lecture Notes, Sixth Edition. Yoav Ben-Shlomo, Sara T. Brookes and Matthew Hickman.

Table 22.1 Ten leading causes of death by income group.

	Low -and-middle-income countries			High-income countries		
	Cause	Deaths (millions)	% of total deaths	Cause	Deaths (millions)	% of total deaths
1	Ischaemic heart disease	5.70	11.8%	Ischaemic heart disease	1.36	17.3%
2	Cerebrovascular disease	4.61	9.5%	Cerebrovascular disease	0.78	9.9%
3	Lower respiratory infections	3.41	7.0%	Trachea, bronchus, lung cancers	0.46	5.8%
4	HIV/AIDS	2.55	5.3%	Lower respiratory infections	0.34	4.4%
5	Perinatal conditions	2.49	5.1%	Chronic obstructive pulmonary disease	0.30	3.8%
6	Chronic obstructive pulmonary disease	2.38	4.9%	Colon and rectum cancers	0.26	3.3%
7	Diarrhoeal diseases	1.78	3.7%	Alzheimer's disease and other dementias	0.21	2.6%
8	Tuberculosis	1.59	3.3%	Diabetes mellitus	0.20	2.6%
9	Malaria	1.21	2.5%	Breast cancer	0.16	2.0%
10	Road traffic accidents	1.07	2.2%	Stomach cancer	0.15	1.9%

Ten leading causes of death by income group, 2001
Source: Lopez *et al.* (2006), p. 1747.

and **disability adjusted life years (DALYs)**; numbers of years of life lost due to ill-health, disability or early death) attributable to specific causes.

Of the 56 million deaths worldwide in 2001, a third were from communicable, maternal, and perinatal conditions and nutritional deficiencies, while non-communicable diseases were the commonest causes of death worldwide (Table 22.1). Of these deaths, 10.6 million were children, 99% of whom lived in low- and middle-income countries.

Factors that influence research and public health action are:

(1) rankings of the numbers of deaths and DALYs;
(2) availability of technical solutions;
(3) cost of actions (and of not taking action);
(4) political will to take actions that may be unpopular.

Communicable diseases

Communicable diseases continue to take a heavy toll in developing countries: approximately half of all deaths in the least developed countries are estimated to result from communicable diseases, of which approximately 90% are attributed to: acute diarrhoeal and respiratory infections of children, AIDS, tuberculosis, malaria and measles.

These communicable diseases pose a great challenge because (a) lack of effective vaccines (except for measles), (b) those at risk or already infected are unable to access medicines and other goods such as bed-nets and condoms. The reasons for these include costs of health goods, as well as the lack of health systems capable of getting these goods to those at risk or in need.

The so-called neglected tropical diseases – such as leprosy, lymphatic filariasis, and onchocerciasis – continue to cause a great deal of human suffering and permanent disability, as well as being an economic burden on the individual (unable to join the workforce) and their families and society upon which they must often depend for economic support.

Economic consequences of these conditions are still not adequately appreciated by governments; tuberculosis alone causes an estimated annual loss of between US$ 1.4 and 2.8 billion in economic growth worldwide.

In addition to these endemic infections, there are often unpredictable infections such as rare outbreak-prone disease (Ebola, Marburg) to cholera, and seasonal or pandemic influenza. Not only do these diseases cause human suffering and death, often placing health workers at great risk, but they cause negative economic impact from control measures such as culling of livestock and animals from which many of these infections originate. Bovine Spongiform Encephalopathy (BSE), and the associated new human variant of Creutzfeld Jakob Disease (vCJD), cost the UK economy around £1.5bn during 1996/97; and the Food and Agricultural Organisation (FAO) estimates that H5N1 has cost South-East Asia's poultry farmers approximately $10 billion from 2003 to 2007 – strong reminders of the negative economic impact caused by emerging infectious diseases.

The power of vaccines in decreasing disease and death was clearly demonstrated by the eradication of smallpox, a major infectious cause of death.

In 1967 (the year that intensive efforts to eradicate smallpox began) there were an estimated 2.7 million smallpox deaths. In 1980 smallpox was certified eradicated.

Vaccines have had a major impact on polio, in the last phase of a global eradication programme, measles, tetanus, diphtheria and pertussis. Newer vaccines such as those for hepatitis B, haemophilus B (Hib), human papillomavirus (HPV) and rotavirus show great promise – once they have been successfully integrated into routine immunisation programmes in all countries – both in preventing acute illness, and chronic disease including hepatic and cervical cancers. Access to vaccines and other health goods has been facilitated by UNICEF and mechanisms for donor funding such as Global Alliance for Vaccines and Immunizations (GAVI) and the Global Fund on AIDS, TB, and Malaria. However, governments of many low income countries must also become more engaged in ensuring the systems that will deliver these goods to health facilities. Despite the almost universal provision of vaccines by UNICEF for many of the childhood vaccine preventable diseases, some countries have had routine vaccine coverage, as measured by 3 doses of DTP at age 12 years, at levels much below 50%. And peripheral health facilities in many countries have repeated rupture of stocks of vaccines, and also of medicines for AIDS, TB, malaria and other medicines on the WHO essential drugs list.

Maternal and child health

There are huge global differentials in maternal mortality: the risk of a woman dying as a result of pregnancy or childbirth during her lifetime is about one in six in the poorest parts of the world compared with about one in 30,000 in Northern Europe. Sub-Saharan Africa and south Asia have the highest burden of maternal mortality. Most maternal deaths happen around the time of delivery, most commonly due to haemorrhage. Other important causes include hypertensive diseases and infections, and in some parts of the world, unsafe abortion and puerperal infection carry a huge risk. Surprisingly, a large proportion of maternal death takes place in hospitals; these include women who come to the hospital in a moribund state too late to benefit from care, but also those who arrive with treatable complications but do not receive timely and effective interventions and those admitted for normal delivery that subsequently develop complications. A number of interventions are effective. A strategy of encouraging women to routinely deliver at health centres, with skilled midwives as the main providers of care, backed up by access to referral-level facilities, is among the most cost-effective options for low income settings. A broader perspective to health, reducing the economic and social vulnerability of pregnant women through education of girls, poverty reduction and women's empowerment is central to any strategy.

Although child mortality has been declining worldwide in recent times, yet 8.8 million children die every year before their fifth birthday. The most important causes of child death are pneumonia, diarrhoea and preterm birth complications (see Figure 22.1). Most of these deaths occur in Africa and south Asia, particularly, India, Nigeria, Democratic Republic of Congo, Pakistan and China. The majority of these deaths occur in the neonatal period, during which time preterm birth complications and birth asphyxia are particularly important. Interventions directed towards health education of families and communities to promote adoption of evidence-based home-care practices and improved care seeking, could avert majority of neonatal deaths in low income settings, but the coverage of these interventions remains poor.

Nutrition and health

WHO regards hunger and malnutrition as the gravest threats to global health. It is a challenge to human dignity, and also threatens the ability of nations to progress socioeconomically. Most deaths from hunger do not occur in high profile emergencies but in unnoticed circumstances. With economic development, the proportion of hungry people in the low-income countries has halved in the last four decades; despite this, maternal

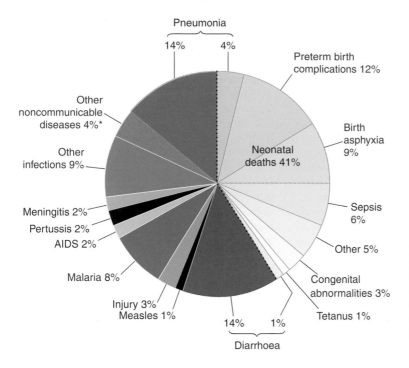

Figure 22.1 Global causes of child mortality in 2008. *Source*: Black RE; Cousens S, Johnson HL, *et al*. (2010) Global, regional, and national causes of child mortality in 2008: a systematic analysis. *The Lancet* **375**: 1969–87.

and child undernutrition remains highly prevalent in low income countries. Undernutrition is a largely preventable cause of over a third of child deaths. Vitamin A – which causes xeropthalmia – and zinc – which reduces immune function – are now among the most important micronutrient deficiencies, particularly as the burden of iodine and iron deficiencies have gone down, given the intervention programmes in many parts of the world. Suboptimal breast feeding, especially nonexclusive breast feeding in the first six months of life, is an important cause of child mortality, while maternal short stature and iron deficiency anaemia increase the risk of death of the mother at delivery. Apart from these short term consequences, damage suffered due to undernutrition in the early years of life may lead to irreversible damage, including shorter adult height, lower attained schooling, reduced adult income, and potentially greater risk of some chronic diseases due to these early life determinants.

Noncommunicable diseases

As countries move through economic development from a pre-industrial to an industrialised economy, transition occurs in the demographic and disease profile of the population. Deaths from acute infectious and deficiency diseases characteristic of underdevelopment decline, and deaths due to chronic noncommunicable diseases which result from modernisation and advanced levels of development rise – the 'epidemiological transition'. The rapid 'epidemiological transition' currently taking place in many low- and middle-income countries bears many similarities to the similar transition that took place in high income countries nearly a century ago, yet there are important differences.

The transition is happening at a much faster pace, and before the disappearance of the diseases of the old world (e.g. infections, malnutrition) leading to a double burden of disease. The speed of the transition is driven by:

(a) ageing population,
(b) greater urbanisation,
(c) migration and
(d) increasingly globalisation.

Each of these is accompanied by other challenges (see below). As a result of these forces, ischaemic heart disease and cerebrovascular disease are now the commonest causes of death in low- and high-income countries. Their risk factors (obesity, higher consumption of calorie and fat rich diets, salt intake, physical inactivity and tobacco use) are well established.

Most noncommunicable diseases require long-term treatment, and often expensive, treatments which people from low- and middle-income countries are least able to afford to pay, particularly as these countries usually lack free health care or health insurance coverage and health costs are borne by out-of-pocket expenses. The cost of treating chronic diseases and their risk factors is sizeable, ranging from 0.02 to 6.66% of the country's gross domestic product. These conditions generally affect those of working age which causes huge economic burden to developing country economies.

Most NCDs have a multifactorial aetiology and the risk factors for NCDs tend to cluster. NCDs also have pre-clinical phases where early detection may reduce clinical disease and many of the risk factors are amenable to both behaviour change of individuals and societal change. WHO recommend that both individually and population targeted interventions (see Chapter 16) are used together to gain maximum benefit. Population measures can have far reaching impact. In many western countries, the rates of cardiovascular disease have fallen dramatically and are probably explained by reductions in tobacco use, less saturated fat intake, and lower salt.

It is not always clear whether population-based interventions are effective. The *north Karelia project* in Finland, launched in 1972, used a multi-component approach (media activities, participation of health care and other workers and community organisations, environmental changes through collaborations with industry etc.). to reduce burden of cardiovascular disease Following first 25 years of project, it was able to show 68% reduction in cardiovascular mortality. However, death rates in the comparison county and across the whole country also fell by the same amount.

More promising was a population intervention on the island of Mauritius, when the Government banned the import of palm oil (a saturated oil), substituting this with Soya bean oil (a polyunsaturated oil). This was associated with a pronounced improvement in population lipid profile. It has also been estimated that a 10% increase in the price of tobacco in LMICs could reduce the number of smokers by 37.6 million (9.3 million deaths averted).

Injuries

Often injuries are overlooked in global health but are a major cause of avoidable death and disability. Road traffic injuries are among the most common causes of injury but the other causes of injuries (poisoning, falls, fires, drowning, self-inflicted, violence etc.) are about two to four times as common in developing countries as in the developed world. Exceptions are falls with are less common in developing countries, reflecting the younger age distribution and injuries due to wars which are about 300 times as common. Typically injuries are referred to as accidents which lead to the assumption that 'accidents will happen' and a fatalistic outlook.

Adequate surveillance systems are uncommon in developing countries and mitigate against strong advocacy for prevention, measurement of variation and evaluation of prevention programmes. Prevention is based on the conventional epidemiological understanding of host, vector and environment. For road traffic injury prevention the host factors relate to people's behaviour (e.g. drinking and driving), the vector relates to vehicles (e.g. cars with poor brakes) and the environment relates to issues of segregation of pedestrians from motorised vehicles, lighting, and signage, for example.

Trends are not encouraging: car ownership is rising globally but injury rates are not falling. In developing countries with adequate data increases in death rates from road injuries have increased by 40 to 200% between 1975 and 1998. Whereas in developed countries dramatic falls have occurred, reflecting the increased emphasis on road safety and implementation of effective strategies.

A World Health Organisation report in 2004 recommended global action on road traffic injuries that would be interdisciplinary, would focus on reasons for the inequalities between developing and developed countries, and would develop an evidence base on prevention of road traffic injuries of relevance to developing countries.

Population ageing and urbanisation

The proportion of older people has increased worldwide (resulting from declines in fertility and in infant mortality), and the change in most low

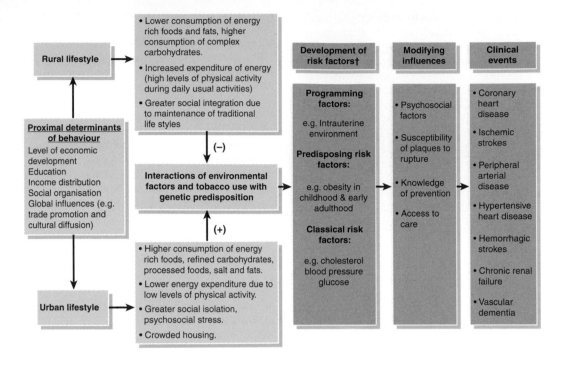

Figure 22.2 Conceptual approach to understanding how societal level influences lead to the development of cardiovascular diseases.
Source: Yusuf S, Reddy S, Ounpuu S, Anand S (2001) Global burden of cardiovascular diseases: Part I: general considerations, the epidemiologic transition, risk factors, and impact of urbanization. Review. *Circulation* **104**: 2746–53.

and middle income countries has been particularly dramatic due to concomitant economic and social developments.

Belgium took over 100 years to double the proportion of its 60+ population from 9% to 18%, China – which adopted a one-child per family policy – will take only 34 years to undergo the same transition.

Sub-Saharan Africa is the exception because of the continued mortality caused by HIV/AIDS. As many chronic diseases show an exponential increase with age, it is not surprising that the rise in chronic diseases have become one of the major global health challenges. A greater number of older people in the world raises the issue of who will support and care for their needs; few countries are facing up to this issue and introducing universal pensions for older people or other mechanisms for ensuring their rights.

Between 1990 and 2025, the urban population of the world is expected to double, and most of this is expected to happen in developing countries (~150,000 people per day) and this arises by expansion of urban areas as well as by migration from rural areas.

Urbanisation has important health effects through changes in the social and physical environment (see Figure 22.2).

Negative effects

(1) Adverse lifestyle changes: poor diets, less physical activity; alcohol and recreational drug use; and high risk sexual behaviour.
(2) Physical environment: over-crowding, traffic hazards, air pollution, greater risk of bacterial and vector-borne diseases through lack of potable water and good sanitation and risk of food poisoning.
(3) Social effects: marginalisation and isolation which can lead to depression.
(4) Ecological effects: ecological footprint (from greenhouse gases, waste), lack of recreational space and time wasted in attempting to move around.

Positive effects

(1) Socioeconomic: positive health benefits from improvements in socioeconomic circumstances.

(2) Access: better access to facilities such as education and health care.

Migration, globalisation and the environment

Migration has been a major force since our earliest history. However, what makes it more relevant today is its speed (possible to reach anywhere in the world within 1–2 days, while the incubation period of Ebola virus is 2–21 days) and scale (~1 billion international journeys each year worldwide and 150 million working as migrants). People migrate for a range of 'push' (e.g. natural disasters, civil unrest, poverty) and 'pull' factors (e.g. education and economic prospects). According to a model proposed by Marmot, the effects of migration on health can be understood as:

(a) selection of who migrates,
(b) process of migration itself,
(c) influences carried from the place of origin, and
(d) influences acquired from the place of migration.

Migration – whether international or internal – often entails movement to a more urban environment, which has attendant risks associated with urbanisation (see above). The process of migration itself, apart from stress and physical danger, also facilitates the transfer of the infectious agents that cause emerging and re-emerging infectious diseases. Infections can today spread around the globe and emerge in new geographic areas with amazing ease and speed. Some are transported by the flights of migratory birds. Others, such as disease-carrying mosquitoes, travel in the passenger cabin or luggage hold of jets, to cause tropical infections in temperate countries when they bite airport workers or those who live nearby.

Globalisation (*increasing interconnectedness of countries and openness of borders to ideas, people, commerce, and financial capital*) carries potential for harmful and beneficial effects on health of populations. The key determinants of chronic diseases (unhealthy diet, physical inactivity and tobacco use) are all strongly influenced by globalisation (see Box 22.1).

Box 22.1 Globalisation and health in developing countries

- Dietary changes
  - Westernised diets
  - Increased refined carbohydrates, saturated fats, low in fibre
- Food availability and pricing
  - trade agreements, corporate production, global distribution
  - reduced taxes on unhealthy food imports
- Food preferences and ways of consuming
  - pre-prepared and outside of home
  - multimedia and marketing of western lifestyles
  - carbonated chilled sweetened drinks
- Physical activity
  - promotion of car industry
  - urban design
- Tobacco
  - Aggressive marketing
  - Advertising, product placement
  - Political lobbying
  - Agricultural production

The environment

Climate change is a major global phenomenon that has its roots in excessive greenhouse gases (largely carbon dioxide) produced by over-reliance on burning of fossil fuels for energy requirements over the last century. The effect of greenhouse gases is to trap more heat in the lower atmosphere leading to global warming. The very existence of climate change has been questioned by some countries and some industries with vested interests in maintaining the current situation. Figure 22.3 shows some of the other pressures on the global environment that have impacts on human health.

Climate change is resulting in an increase in natural disasters – floods and hurricanes – that tend to affect developing countries much more the rest of the world, causing deaths, destruction and misery. Spikes of high temperatures also cause heat stroke and directly cause many deaths in rural areas of south Asia where there is no protection from high temperatures. Variable rainfall and failure of monsoons in the tropics is leading to water scarcity which in turn increases risks of diarrhoeal diseases, skin and eye infections. Lack of

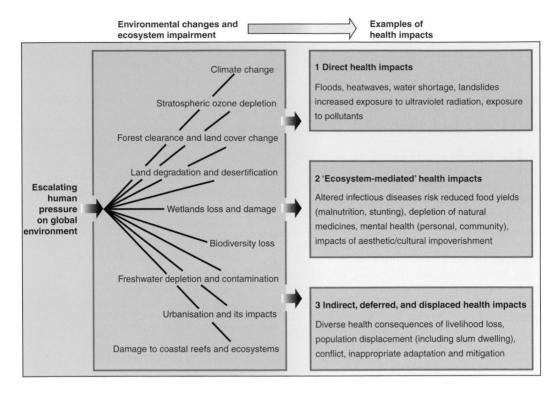

Figure 22.3 Impact of environmental change on health.
Source: WHO (2005) *Ecosystems and Human Well-being: Health Synthesis: a Report of the Millennium Ecosystem Assessment*. Core writing team. Carlos Corvalan, Simon I Iales, Anthony McMichael. Geneva: WHO.

water also leads to crop failures which may result in malnutrition and increases vulnerability of children to infectious diseases and malaria. Lowering greenhouse gas emissions globally is a major challenge. If individuals, organisations and countries lowered their emissions by reducing their reliance on motorised transport through wider use of bicycles and walking to cover short distances, overall health would improve as physical activity is a powerful means of improving many different health conditions, ranging from depression through osteoarthritis to cardiovascular diseases.

Wider determinants of health

Social inequalities in health

The Commission for Social Determinants of Health was set up in 2005 to examine what could

be done to reduce inequalities in health. The Commission's report *Closing the Gap in a Generation: Health Equity through Action on the Social Determinants of Health,* published in 2008, has highlighted comprehensively the invidious nature of most societies in which people live with massive gaps in life expectancy between those with and those without sufficient material resources.

Traditional thinking has been that economic growth would result in benefits for all through trickle down of wealth and pro-poor social programmes promoted by the World Bank and development programmes of major donor countries. The policies arising from this old thinking have not worked and have actually increased income and other social inequalities in most developing countries. The Commission noted that some countries – notably Cuba, China and the state of Kerala in India – have achieved great improvements in life expectancy without concomitant increases in wealth.

Tackling social determinants of health cannot be done by health services but requires a radical approach targeted at the root causes of these social causes. Much of what is required has to focus on implementing a charter of human rights to life, food, shelter, health care, and employment. The distribution of wealth is increasingly determined by global forces but within countries much can be done to ensure that policies are not regressive in their impacts on the poorest populations and that corruption is weeded out. The act of actually measuring the scale of the problem is also one of the levers for achieving action (see Box 22.2). In the UK, activist researchers published the life expectancy of every political constituency in the country and sent the information to each member of Parliament. Similar actions in developing countries may increase ideas of accountability among politicians but will require better health information systems.

Global solutions to global health challenges

There have been increasing global collaborations on health research and policy. These reflect the growth in the global health movement and the recognition of a need for new approaches in response to new problems such as HIV/AIDS. The funding difficulties that have beset World Health Organisation and other UN agencies over the last two decades have also triggered new funding streams and a greater impact of global philanthropic activities (e.g. Bill & Melinda Gates Foundation, Buffett Foundation).

Examples of global collaboration on research abound. One important effort is the Disease Control Priorities in Developing Countries project (http://www.dcp2.org/main/Home.html), which aimed to collate information on the cost-effectiveness of different interventions for use in developing countries. Attempting to make choices about which programmes to fund and where to spend available resources is not straight forward. Decision makers in developing countries now have a wide range of options to consider. The figure shows the cost-effectiveness of a range of interventions for diseases causing a high burden in sub-Saharan Africa. It is clear that traditional expanded programme on immunisation is strikingly cost-effective – less than US$10 per disability adjusted life year (DALY) averted compared with around US$1,000 per DALY averted from treating adults with a 'polypill' (a combination of blood pressure lowering and cholesterol lowering drugs) to reduce risk of stroke and hypertensive heart disease. (See Table 22.2.)

Another avenue for international collaboration is the through advocacy and agreements. The Tobacco Free Initiative was established in 1998 to provide global leadership and advocacy in tobacco control (see Chapter 16 for more about tobacco controls). One of its major activities was to support the WHOs Framework Convention on Tobacco Control (WHO FCTC); it became the world's first public health treaty when it came into force in 2005. It has been ratified by ~150 countries, and includes a host of measures to reduce the impact of tobacco through limits on production, distribution, advertisement and taxation.

The widely publicised concerns about the appearance in Asia of a new and highly contagious disease, SARS (Severe Acute Respiratory Syndrome) in 2002, and currently H5N1, an avian influenza virus that was first identified as the cause of human illness in 1997, may have been instrumental in revising the International Health Regulations (IHR), adopted by the World Health Assembly in 2005 to prevent the spread of disease across international borders. They provide the first comprehensive legal framework for global disease surveillance, notification, and response – designed to ensure international public health security. Under the IHR, any event that may constitute a potential public health emergency is assessed by the Member State in which it is occurring using a decision tree instrument, and if the particular criteria for a Public Health Emergency of International

Table 22.2 Cost-effectiveness ratio for various interventions.

Intervention	Cost-effectiveness ratio (US$ per DALY averted)				
	0	10	100	1,000	10,000
Polypill for stroke + heart disease					
Oral rehydration packages, diarrhoea					
MCH + neonatal care					
Maternal primary care					
HIV condom promotion + distribution					
Expanded immunisation programme					

Source: Laxminarayan R. *et al.* (2009) Intervention cost-effectiveness: overview. In DT Jamison, JG Breman, AR Measham, *et al.* (eds), *Disease Control Priorities in Developing Countries* (2nd edn), Oxford: Oxford University Press.

Concern (PHEIC) are met, an official notification must be provided to WHO.

Finally, perhaps the most important example of international cooperation is in the area of joint international goal setting which resulted in the **Millennium Development Goals** which have galvanised global action. These were established at a Millennium Summit in 2000 and are recognised by 123 United Nations member states and are supported by many international organisations concerned with health and development. The goals (see Box 22.3) and their associated targets are intended to focus resources on tractable global health problems.

The MDGs have operated globally and have provided a new forum for international organisations and country development programmes to work together towards a common purpose. Perhaps not surprisingly, not all countries have managed to meet the ambitious targets set for 2015.

Box 22.3 Millennium Development Goals

- Eradicate extreme poverty and hunger
- Achieve universal primary education
- Promote gender equality and empower women
- Reduce child mortality rate
- Improve maternal health
- Combat HIV/AIDS, malaria, and other diseases
- Ensure environmental sustainability
- Develop a global partnership for development

A global health system: reinventing primary health care

In every country there is some sort of health system and at the centre of it is *primary health care.* Primary health care is essential for the rational use of resources and for achieving many health outcome goals. Attempts have been made to develop primary health care globally.

The Alma Ata declaration of 1978 aimed to achieve universal access to primary health care under the logo of 'Health for All by the Year 2000'. It failed for multiple reasons, but during the 1980s indebtedness of developing countries was perceived as a major problem and the World Bank response was to introduce economic restructuring and stringent controls on spending. In primary health care, the introduction of user charges did not generate sustainable services and led to the decline of primary care in many of the poorest countries.

Learning the lessons of these earlier policies, The World Health Report 2008 titled, perhaps more realistically, 'Primary Care Now More Than Ever', called for four major reforms: (a) universal health care coverage and social health protection; (b) service delivery reform to make them more responsive to people's needs and expectations; (c) public policy reforms to integrate public health actions into primary care and cross-sectoral action for health; (d) and leadership reforms to develop inclusive and participatory negotiated leadership.

KEY LEARNING POINTS

- Global health is concerned with the ways in which health of populations is shaped – for better or worse – by factors operating across countries
- The balance between non-communicable and communicable diseases is changing in most developing countries but dual burdens are common
- Avoidable maternal and child mortality are largely confined to developing countries and require substantial and continued investment to achieve Millennium Development Goals
- New determinants of risk – urbanisation, migration, travel, population ageing, social inequalities – affect health globally
- Global health movements are rising to these new challenges through research on technical solutions, advocacy frameworks for control of risk factors, focusing on social determinants of health, and promoting primary health care

 REFERENCES

Commission for Social Determinants of Health (2008) *Closing the Gap in a Generation: Health Equity through Action on the Social Determinants of Health.*

 FURTHER READING

Beaglehole R, Epping-Jordan J, Ebrahim S, Chopra M, Patel V, Kidd M, Haines A (2008) Improving the management of chronic disease in low- and middle- income countries: a priority for primary health care. *Lancet* 372: 940–9.

Frenk J (2010) The global health system: strengthening national health systems as the next step for global progress. *PLoS Med* 2010, 7:e1000089.

Haines A, McMichael AJ, Smith KR *et al.* (2009) Public health benefits of strategies to reduce greenhouse-gas emissions: overview and implications for policy makers. *The Lancet* 374: 2104–14.

Heymann DL, Rodier GR (2001) WHO operational support team to the global outbreak alert and response network. Hot spots in a wired world: WHO surveillance of emerging and re-emerging infectious diseases. *Lancet Infect Dis* 1: 345–53.

Koplan J, Bond C, Merson M *et al.* (2009) Towards a common definition of global health. *Lancet* 373: 1993–95.

Lewin S, Lavis JN Oxman A *et al.* (2008) Supporting the delivery of cost-effective interventions in primary health-care systems in low-income and middle-income countries: an overview of systematic reviews. *Lancet* 372: 928–39.

Lopez A, Mathers C, Ezzati M (2006) Global and regional burden of disease and risk factors, 2001: systematic analysis of population health data. *Lancet* 27: 367: 1747–57.

Marmot M (2005) Social determinants of health. *Lancet* 365: 1099–1104.

McKee M (2008) Global research for health. *British Medical Journal* 337: 1249–50.

Self-assessment questions – Part 3: Public health

Q1 Public health interventions

Which of the following are public health interventions:
(a) A smoking cessation programme as part of antenatal care in order to prevent low birth weight
(b) Cognitive behavioural therapy in order to increase treatment compliance among patients with drug and alcohol or mental health problems
(c) An offer of screening to identify people with a genetic susceptibility to obesity
(d) Increasing paid maternity leave in order to lengthen the duration of breastfeeding
(e) Implementation of standards for folic acid fortification of breads and cereals

Q2 Screening

Screening programmes for abdominal aortic aneurysm (AAA) exist in the UK and elsewhere. For AAA screening;
(a) What is the eligible population?
(b) What is the 'sieve', i.e. the screening test or tests?
(c) Is there a 'sort' phase, i.e. the diagnostic test or tests, and if so what does this involve?
(d) What is the intervention that is offered?
(e) What is the purpose of the screening i.e. the adverse outcome that it aims to reduce the risk of?

Q3 Health protection and surveillance

With regards to health protection and surveillance which of the following statements are true/false?

(a) Only vaccine preventable diseases are notifiable
(b) A disease can be eradicated even if some people remain susceptible
(c) Public health surveillance is information for action
(d) The larger the R_0 the easier an infection may be to contain
(e) Treatment of cases can prevent future disease

Q4 Inequalities in health

The graph that follows shows the average of life expectancy for men in England and Wales from 1972–1996, by occupational social class. Interpret the data shown in this graph. What possible reasons could underlie these patterns? List possible points of intervention that medical professionals can play to address the inequalities shown.

Q5 Public health evaluation

The Ballabeina study sought to evaluate the effect on fitness and adiposity of a multicomponent, school-based intervention for primarily migrant children aged 4 to 6 years old in Switzerland. The intervention lasted for a year and was delivered to school classes containing children in the target age group. The intervention included in-school physical activity sessions for the children and lessons on healthy nutrition, media use and sleep. Workshops for teachers were held before the intervention was delivered to the children so that teachers understood its overall purpose and their role in its delivery. Teachers

Epidemiology, Evidence-based Medicine and Public Health Lecture Notes, Sixth Edition. Yoav Ben-Shlomo, Sara T. Brookes and Matthew Hickman.
© 2013 Y. Ben-Shlomo, S. T. Brookes and M. Hickman. Published 2013 by John Wiley & Sons, Ltd.

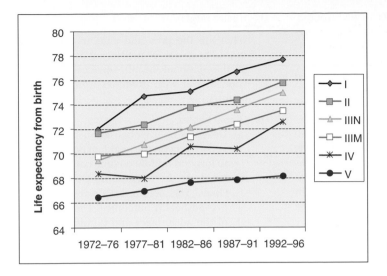

Average life expectancy for men in England and Wales, 1972–1996.

received lesson plans and were given advice on how to change the physical environment of the school to promote physical activity. Some additional pieces of play equipment such as climbing walls and balls were provided. Parents of the children were also invited to attend three information and discussion evenings which focussed on the importance of children being physically active, eating healthily, getting enough sleep and not watching too much TV. Classes with children in the target age group not receiving the intervention continued with the usual curriculum and their parents were invited to one information and discussion evening.

The study was undertaken in two different parts of Switzerland both area with high migrant populations but one in a French speaking and the other in a German speaking area. The study's authors noted that 'Randomisation of classes (1:1) was performed separately for the German (n=20) and French (n = 20) speaking areas. Classes were randomised with the use of opaque envelops. For practical reasons, and to minimise contamination, preschool classes affiliated to the same school building were randomised in the same group. The 40 classes were affiliated to 30 schools, but the schools had no role during the intervention as all activities were performed at the class level.' The study authors also reported that 'Teachers, parents,

and children were informed that the intervention was designed to promote children's health but were unaware of the main objectives of the study.'

The findings of the study were that children who were in classes that randomised to receive the intervention were more aerobically fit than those in classes randomised to the control arm, but there was no difference in BMI observed between intervention and control groups. You can read full details of the study and its findings in the report published in the *British Medical Journal* (Puder JJ, Marques-Vidal P, Schindler C *et al.* (2011) *BMJ* **343**: d6195 doi:10.1136/bmj.d6195).

(a) What kind of study design do you think the Ballabeina study use?

(b) Explain what the term contamination means and describe the steps taken in this study to prevent it? Given what you know about the study design how successful do you think such steps would have been in preventing contamination?

(c) The randomisation of classes was undertaken separately for German and French speaking areas. (i) What is the term used to describe this type of randomisation? (ii) Why do you think this might have been done?

(d) Why do you think teachers, parents and children were not fully informed about the main objectives of the study?

(e) Written, informed consent to participation was given by parents or legal representatives of each child in the study. Is this 'opt in' or 'opt out' consent?

(f) Opt out consent is more commonly used in population health improvement research. Why is this and how is opt out consent justified in this context?

(g) If health and education authorities had already to take the decision to gradually implement this intervention throughout Switzerland making a cluster randomised trial impossible how else might it still have been possible to evaluate the effect of the intervention?

Q6 Health targets

You have been asked to set local targets for the reduction of deaths from cervical cancer. Describe the factors you would need to take into consideration as part of this task and indicate any reservations you might have regarding the appropriateness of targets for this disease.

Q7 Health targets

What are the pros and cons of the use of targets as a tool for measuring performance in the national health services? Illustrate your answer with examples from a named country.

Q8 Global health

(a) Describe how globalisation has an adverse effect on the health of people living in low and middle income countries.

(b) What are the Millennium Development Goals? Has setting MDGs result in improved health outcomes? Discuss some of the advantages and disadvantages of setting MDGs.

Q9 Health improvement

(a) Define primary, secondary and tertiary prevention.

(b) Describe the relative strengths and weaknesses of high-risk and population approaches to disease prevention.

(c) Describe how medical practitioners can contribute to health improvement.

Glossary of terms

abnormal *see* **normal**

accuracy How close on average is the sample statistic to the population parameter that it estimates

adoption studies Comparing a trait or disease risk between an individual and their adopted relatives to determine the relative importance of the shared and nonshared environment since these individuals are genetically unrelated

aetiology The science of causality

allele The alternative form of a gene that can exist at a single locus

allocative efficiency Providing a mix of health services that optimises the health of a population from a fixed budget or set of resources.

ascertainment The process of determining what is happening in a population or study group, e.g. finding cases

audit An examination or review that establishes the extent to which a condition, process or performance conforms to pre-determined standards or criteria

bar chart A graph used to presenting discrete data. Each observation can fall into only one category. Frequencies of each group of observations are represented by the heights of the corresponding bars

baseline group The exposure group (often the unexposed group) with which other exposure groups are compared; also known as **reference** group

baseline comparisons In a RCT, it is conventional to compare characteristics of the participants across the treatment arms to check that randomisation has been effective in balancing both known (and unknown) confounders between groups. Any imbalance may either occur by chance or by failure of randomisation

basic reproduction number (R0) Average number of secondary cases produced by one primary case in a wholly susceptible population

bias Departure from the **true** value when one observes a prevalence in a cross-sectional study or an association between an exposure and an outcome in an analytical study

detection bias: refers to the biased assessment of outcome, where the outcome assessor or the participant is more or less likely to report a specific outcome in the treatment or control group depending on their beliefs or preferences

language bias: can occur in a systematic review or meta-analysis when the review is restricted to studies reported in specific languages. For example, investigators working in a non-English-speaking country may be more likely to publish positive findings in international, English-language journals, while sending less interesting negative or null findings to local-language journals

loss to follow-up bias: subjects are often lost over a follow-up period. If this loss is unrelated to both the exposure and outcome the results will not be biased. But this assumption may not be true. If loss to follow-up is associated with exposure and outcome then the results will be biased. This could operate in either directions so that the risk estimate may be greater or less than the true risk

measurement bias: a bias in how exposure and/or outcome is measured or classified that results in different quality (validity) of information collected between comparison groups

performance bias: relates to the unequal provision of care between the treatment and control group, apart from the treatment under evaluation. For example, if a health care professional knows that an individual is receiving a placebo or other control they may offer

Epidemiology, Evidence-based Medicine and Public Health Lecture Notes, Sixth Edition. Yoav Ben-Shlomo, Sara T. Brookes and Matthew Hickman.
© 2013 Y. Ben-Shlomo, S. T. Brookes and M. Hickman. Published 2013 by John Wiley & Sons, Ltd.

additional therapies. Alternatively, if the patient knows what they are receiving they may change other health behaviours

publication bias: refers to the nonpublication of study results because of the strength or direction of the findings. By excluding such studies in a meta-analysis, it is common for the summary results to over-estimate the treatment benefits

recall bias (reporting bias): where subjects have to recall past exposures (such as in a case-control study) there is likely to be an element of error. If this recall if differential across those with and without a specific outcome we have recall bias

referral bias: subjects ascertained from specialist centres are often atypical, (more severely ill) that subjects ascertained from the general population leading to nongeneralisable conclusions. This is important in prognostic studies

selection bias: a systematic difference in the likelihood of selecting subjects to take part in the study on the basis of their association between exposure and outcome status

spectrum bias: in an ideal diagnostic study, all consecutive patients, or a random sample (*spectrum*) of patients, with suspected disease should be enrolled and criteria for enrolment should be clearly stated. Studies that avoid inclusion of 'difficult to diagnose patients' or 'grey cases' but take clear cut clinical cases and healthy controls (see diagnostic case control study) may result in overoptimistic estimates of test accuracy

verification bias (also known as **work-up bias, (primary) selection bias** or **sequential ordering bias**): this occurs when not all of the study group receive confirmation of the diagnosis by a reference standard, or if some patients receive a different reference standard. If the results of the index test influence the decision on whether to perform the reference standard, or on which reference standard to use, this may result in biased estimates of accuracy

bimodal (multimodal) A probability distribution with two (or multiple) modes

blinding This is where subjects and/or the outcome assessors are unaware of treatment allocation in a trial until the study is completed

brief interventions These involve opportunistic advice, discussion, negotiation or encouragement provided by clinicians to support patient behaviour change

burden of disease/ global burden of disease Measure of the impact of a health problem on mortality and morbidity – in WHO burden of disease project burden is measured in **DALYs**

carrier state An individual may be infected and able to infect others without displaying any symptoms of disease

case control study An epidemiological study design where subjects are recruited on the basis of the presence or absence of disease (cases or controls) and exposure is measured retrospectively. In this way it is possible to estimate the risk of disease associated with exposure usually by calculating an odds ratio. A **diagnostic case-control** is a variation of this design where the exposure is an index test to calculate its diagnostic utility

case definition A set of diagnostic criteria used to classify individuals as having disease. Often but not always the same as what is used to normal clinical care

case fatality rate The proportion of cases of a specific condition that die after a specified time period, e.g. 1 year or 5 years

case series Collections of individual cases reports. May be helpful in recognising new diseases but cannot be used to test for the presence of a valid statistical association

causal Something that influences the probability of an outcome due to its direct effect on the disease process

censoring The truncation of follow-up time for subjects in a cohort study who are lost to follow-up so any future outcomes are unknown. This is used in survival analysis

central randomisation In an RCT selection bias can be avoided if proper randomisation is carried out, usually using a computer-generated sequence at a site remote from the trial location so that local recruiters cannot manipulate the randomisation process. Investigators' knowledge of treatment allocation can result in them either knowingly or unknowingly adjusting allocation based on prognostic factors which would mean that allocation is no longer random

central tendency The centre or middle value of a frequency distribution. Commonly known as the average. Mean, median and mode are examples of measures of central tendency

chance Variation which is due to random fluctuations

clinical epidemiology The use of epidemiological methods to study clinical problems such as the effectiveness of a treatment, how to best reach a diagnosis, or the prognosis of a disease

clinical equipoise A state of genuine uncertainty about the benefits or harm that may result from each of two or more regimens. This is an ethical pre-requisite for a randomised controlled trial. In practice, some evidence or 'hunch' is required that the new treatment may be better then the old

clinical iceberg The phenomenon that doctors are only aware of the relatively small proportion of disease that presents to them.

Cochrane collaboration An international venture to systematically appraise and synthesise the evidence for medical interventions (though it now also includes observational studies)

cohort study (from Latin *cohors* warriors, tenth part of a legion) An epidemiological study whereby a defined subset of the population can be identified and classified according to exposure status. The main feature of a cohort study is that it can determine the incidence rate of disease amongst exposed and unexposed individuals. Common synonyms include longitudinal or follow-up study
diagnostic cohort: a cohort of patients who present with symptoms of a target conditions; in this scenario exposure is the use of a diagnostic or index test (one or more) and follow-up is to determine the final diagnosis on the basis of a reference standard so that one can calculate the diagnostic utility of the index test
occupational cohort: the definition of the cohort is based primarily on a common occupational exposure, e.g. workers in the nuclear power industry; in this way the risk of disease can be compared with the general population or other occupational groups to determine the occupational risk
prospective cohort: healthy individuals are recruited, though some may already have the disease at baseline, and followed up for future disease occurrence, often for decades; exposure status is measured at baseline and repeat measures for change in exposure may be undertaken over the follow-up period
retrospective cohort: disease status for a defined subset of the population is ascertained at baseline

but this is linked to pre-existing historical data on exposure either from routine records or an earlier research project so that the cohort's experience of disease risk can be reconstructed

communicable disease An infectious disease that can be transmitted directly or indirectly from person to person

complex intervention A health care intervention that consists of several separate components, each of which is considered essential to the functioning of the intervention as a whole

concealment of allocation Concealment is where random allocation is hidden from investigators making it impossible for them to have any influence over allocation of patients

confidence interval An interval with given probability (e.g. 95%) that the true value of a parameter such as a mean, difference between proportions or risk ratio is contained within the interval

confounding A situation in which a measure of the effect of an exposure is distorted because of the association of exposure with other factor(s) (**confounders**) that influence the outcome under study

contamination Contamination occurs when individuals randomised to intervention or control receive the wrong intervention – usually with the control being exposed to the intervention. This can happen by accident or deliberately and can introduce bias. Using a cluster RCT design is one solution to concerns over 'contamination'.

contingency table A table showing the frequencies of observations for two categorical variables such that subcategories of one variable (exposure) are indicated in rows and subcategories of the other variable (outcome) are indicated in columns. The simplest form is the **2 × 2 table**, when both variables are binary (dichotomous). The notation for the cells of a 2 × 2 table used in this course is shown in the table below:

		Disease		
		Yes	**No**	**Total**
Exposure	**Yes**	d_1	h_1	$n_1 = d_1 + h_1$
	No	d_0	h_0	$n_0 = d_0 + h_0$
	Total	$d = d_1 + d_0$	$h = h_1 + h_0$	$n = d_1 + d_0$ $+ h_1 + h_0$

d = disease, h = healthy, 1 = exposed, 0 = unexposed

correlation co-efficient A measure of association that indicates the degree to which variables change together

cost-benefit analysis This analysis values the costs and benefits of healthcare in monetary terms; treatments with the highest benefit-cost ratio are the most efficient

cost consequences study A form of economic evaluation where there is more than one important health outcome and where outcomes are tabulated but not weighted or combined

cost-effectiveness acceptability curve (CEAC) A graph that presents the degree of certainty about the result of an economic evaluation. A steeper curve typically indicates a greater degree of certainty

cost-effectiveness analysis This analysis aims to determine the cost of one or more treatments to achieve the same degree of benefit e.g. reduce blood pressure by 10 mmHg

cost-effectiveness plane A graph showing the difference between two treatments in terms of effects (x-axis) against monetary cost (y-axis). Treatments in the North East quadrant have better outcomes but are more costly. Whether they are considered affordable or cost-effective will depend on the wealth of society

cost-utility analysis A form of economic evaluation that compares the efficiency of health care on a single common scale, cost per QALY gained

counterfactual A hypothetical situation where we run a thought experiment of what would have happened under different circumstances to see if this influences outcomes. Ideally we would observe someone who was treated or exposed and then using a time machine replay their life without treatment or exposure to see if this made a difference to their developing the outcome

Cox proportional hazard regression A multivariable regression method that is used in survival analysis that calculates the relative hazard of an event for exposure groups. It assumes that this hazard remains proportional over time

critical incidence analysis The investigation of an unplanned major serious event to try an understand what went wrong. For example the confidential enquiry into peri-operative mortality would be one such example

cross-product ratio This is equivalent to the **odds ratio** and is defined as $(d_1 \times h_0)/(h_1 \times d_0)$ in a 2×2 contingency table

cross-sectional study A study that examines the relationship between diseases (or other health-related characteristics) and other variables of interest in a particular population at one particular time. Cross-sectional studies may be used to estimate the prevalence of disease, but not the incidence of disease

crude association The estimated association between exposure and outcome, before possible confounding variables are taken into account

cumulative frequency plot This is a graph that illustrates the cumulative frequency of a variable. It is useful for identifying particularly common values

cumulative incidence *see* **risk**

demography The study of populations, especially with reference to size, density, mortality, fertility, growth, age distribution and the interaction of these with social and economic factors

denominator The lower portion of a fraction used to calculate a rate or a ratio; the population at risk; often person-years

descriptive studies A study concerned with and designed only to describe the existing distribution of variables. This is in contrast to an analytical study which examines a hypothesis

determinants of health Include the range of genetic, behavioural, personal, social, economic and environmental influences or factors on the health status of individuals or populations

difference in means The observed difference in a continuous outcome between two exposure (or treatment) groups

disability adjusted life years (DALYs) Years of life lost due to premature mortality and years of life lost due to time lived in states of less than full health

disease Literally dis-ease, the opposite of ease when something is wrong with bodily function.

The terms disease, illness and sickness are often used synonymously but are not. Disease is a physiological/psychological dysfunction, illness is a subjective state when a person feels unwell but may not have disease, sickness is a state of social dysfunction, a role an individual assumes when ill

disease progression bias If there is a delay between the application of an index test and reference standard, misclassification due to recovery or progression to a more advanced stage of disease may occur which will bias the results

dominant A relationship between two alleles at the same locus. When one allele (A) masks the expression of another allele (B), A is said to be dominant over B

dose-response effect The pattern of association between increasing exposure and disease risk, i.e. more exposure the bigger the effect

ecological fallacy The bias that may occur because an association observed between variables on an aggregate level does not necessarily represent the association that exists at an individual level

ecological study A study in which the unit of analysis are populations or groups of people, rather than individuals. An example is the association between median income and cancer mortality rates in administrative jurisdictions such as Primary Care Trusts or Regions

effective reproduction number (R) The actual average number of secondary cases produced by an infectious primary case

elimination Refers to a reduction to zero of the incidence of disease or infection in a defined geographical area

endemic Infection is one that occurs regularly in a given population and can be maintained in that population without external influence (i.e. R is around 1)

epidemic An epidemic occurs when the incidence of disease, in a given population and during a given period, substantially exceeds the expected incidence. If R is greater than 1 then the incidence of the disease is increasing in the population

epidemic curve Figure of number of cases by data of inset in order to characterise an outbreak. The epidemic curve provides a great deal of information and can show how the outbreak is spread through the population, at what point we are in the epidemic and its overall pattern

epidemiology The study of the **distribution** and **determinants** of health-related conditions or events in specified **populations** and the application of this study to the **control** of health problems
descriptive epidemiology: observations relating measures of disease occurrence with basic characteristics such as age, sex, geography, ethnicity, socioeconomic status and secular trends (Time, Place, Person). Often used to generate aetiological hypotheses
analytical epidemiology: identifying and measuring the effects of risk factors on disease. Analytical study designs include cross-sectional, case control, cohort studies and randomised controlled trials

equipoise A state of uncertainty in the evidence base as to whether a specific intervention is more or less effective than a comparator intervention or no intervention – a pre-condition for a clinical trial to be ethical

eradication The permanent reduction to zero of the worldwide incidence of infection

error factor (EF) A measure of precision for a ratio measure. For example the error factor for a risk ratio (RR) is $\exp(1.96 \times$ s.e. of log RR). It is used to calculate the 95% confidence interval; for example the 95% C.I. for the RR is RR/EF to $RR \times EF$

evidence-based medicine The conscientious, explicit and judicious use of current best evidence in making decisions about the care of individual patients

experimental study A study in which the investigator intentionally alters one or more factors under controlled conditions in order to study the effects of doing so; usually a randomised controlled trial

exposure variable A variable whose influence on the outcome variable we wish to assess. Exposure variables are also known as **risk factors**, **explanatory variables**, **independent variables** or *x*-variables. In the context of a randomised trial the exposure variable is the **treatment** being assessed

forest plots This displays the results of a systematic review and meta-analysis. Such plots display a square centred on the effect estimate from each individual study, a horizontal line showing the corresponding 95% confidence intervals. The area of the square is proportional to its weight in the meta-analysis, so that studies that contribute more weight are represented by larger squares. The result of the meta-analysis is displayed by a diamond at the bottom of the graph: the centre of the diamond corresponds to the summary effect estimate, while its width corresponds to the corresponding 95% confidence interval. A dashed vertical line corresponding to the summary effect estimate is included to allow visual assessment of the variability of the individual study effect estimates around the summary estimate

frequency distribution The complete summary of the frequencies of the values or categories of a measurement made on a group of persons. The distribution tells either how many or what proportion of the group was found to have each value (or each range of values) out of all the possible values that the quantitative measure can have

funnel plot A graphical method used in meta-analyses that enables one to examine for differences in effects by size of study. If there is evidence of asymmetry, so that smaller studies tend to show larger effects than larger studies, or there are fewer than expected smaller studies showing negative or adverse effects then this suggests reporting biases (negative small studies are not published) or that smaller studies are usually methodologically less rigorous and produce inflated estimates. It could also be that smaller studies provide a more intensive intervention and are therefore genuinely more effective

Gaussian distribution *see* **Normal distribution**

gene A segment of the genome that codes for a functional product such as a protein

generalisability The degree to which the findings of a study can be applied to another external population

genetic epidemiology The study of the role of genetic factors in determining health and disease in families and in populations, and the interplay of these genetic factors with the environment

genome-wide association studies (GWAS) A genetic association study that examines hundreds of thousands of genetic markers simultaneously across the genome, rather than just analyzing a few markers in a candidate region. It is a hypothesis free approach

genotype Usually refers to an individual's genetic make up at a single location in the genotype. For example, a person's genotype at the ABO blood locus might be A/A meaning that they have two copies of the gene that codes for the A blood group protein

geometric mean The back transformation (antilog) of the mean log value

global health Health problems, issues and concerns that transcend national boundaries, may be influenced by circumstances or experiences in other countries, and are best addressed by cooperative actions and solutions; and is an area for study, research, and practice that places a priority on improving health and achieving equity in health for all people worldwide

Haddon matrix Part of injury prevention and attempts to identify and describe risk and protective factors in terms of the person, environment, and agent, and whether the risks occur before, during or after the injury event

hazard ratio This is derived from Cox proportional hazard models and is used in survival analysis. The hazard ratio is similar though not identical to the relative risk so a hazard ratio greater than one indicates increased risk whilst less than one indicates a reduced risk

health care evaluation Evaluation of health care services to inform which services should be provided by identifying which interventions work and are affordable

Health Impact Assessment (HIA) HIA is defined by WHO as 'a combination of procedures, methods and tools by which a policy, programme or project may be judged as to its potential effects on the health of a population, and the distribution of those effects within the population'

health improvement This is about preventing disease and death, and improving quality of life and well-being. Interventions can be implemented at different stages of the natural history of disease (see Table 19.1) and at individual, community and population levels.

health inequalities Have been defined as 'differences in the prevalence or incidence of health problems between individual people of higher and lower socio-economic status' (Kunst and Mackenbach, 1995)

Health Inequality Impact Assessment (HIIA) A process that intends to assess the likely positive and negative health, equality and human rights impacts of a policy (including unintended impacts) and the population groups who will bear them

health inequities Variations in health (health inequalities) that are attributable to the external environment and conditions mainly outside the control of the individuals concerned, i.e. are unfair

health promotion The process of enabling people to increase control over, and to improve, their health

health protection Concerns prevention of communicable disease, protection against noncommunicable environmental hazards, and emergency planning and response

healthy screenee effect The people who come for screening tend to be healthier than those who do not, therefore outcome in screened individuals tends to be better than in the background population

herd immunity The protection conferred in the population (including nonimmunised or 'susceptible') by the portion of a host population which is immune to an infection

herd immunity threshold The proportion of the population that needs to be vaccinated to prevent sustained spread of the infection $(1 - 1/\mathbf{R0})$

heritability The proportion of variance in a trait due to genetic factors

heterozygote An individual having different alleles of a particular gene.

hierarchy of evidence This is a simple guide in helping assess evidence from different study designs. RCTs are viewed as the highest level of evidence followed by cohort, case control, cross-sectional studies, ecological studies and case series or anecdote. This should not be applied too rigorously as a well conducted cohort study may be superior to a badly designed RCT

histogram A graphic representation of the frequency distribution of a variable. The area of the bar represents the frequency of the variable

homozygotes An individual having identical alleles of a particular gene

hypothesis An idea expressed in such a way that it can be tested and refuted

I^2 statistic This quantifies the percentage of total variation across studies in a meta-analysis that is due to heterogeneity rather than chance. I^2 lies between 0% and 100%; a value of 0% indicates no observed heterogeneity, and larger values show increasing heterogeneity

immunity Following infection or vaccination individuals may become immune (resistant) to future infections. Some pathogens are strongly immunogenic (e.g. measles infection provokes long-lasting immunity that protects against future infection), others are weakly immunogenic (e.g. gonorrhoea) and therefore people may become infected again

imputation A statistical method to generate values for missing data which can be used to check whether excluding missing data may bias the results

incident rate The number of new cases of a disease, divided by the total population at risk by the time interval

incremental cost effectiveness ratio (ICER) This is the difference in cost between the intervention and the comparator $(C_i - C_c)$ divided by the difference in effectiveness $(E_i - E_c)$

incubation period Time between infection onset/occurrence and time when symptoms develop

index of multiple deprivation This can be used to characterise small geographical areas where individuals live

index test This is usually a new diagnostic test which is being evaluated against some form of reference standard to determine its diagnostic usefulness

infectious disease An illness resulting from the transmission of a pathogenic biological agent – including some viruses, bacteria, fungi, protozoa, parasites and prions – to a susceptible host

informed consent Consent given by the subject or responsible person for participation in a study. For informed consent to be ethically valid the investigator must disclose all risks and benefits, the participant must understand the condition and all the risks and benefits, the participant must be competent and consent must be given voluntarily

intention to treat analysis Intention to treat analysis (ITT) is where all participants are analysed according to their group allocation, regardless of whether they completed the trial. The alternative is 'on-treatment' analysis, which is limited to those who completed the trial according to protocol. On treatment analysis defeats the main purpose of random allocation and may invalidate the results

interaction (effect modification) When the direction and/or magnitude of an association between an exposure and outcome depends on the value of a third variable (the effect modifier)

interquartile range The interquartile range describes the spread of data around the median. It is the distance between the lower quartile value and the upper quartile value of a distribution

intervention study An investigation involving intentional change in some aspect of the status of subjects; introduces a therapeutic or preventive regime; designed to test a hypothesis; usually a randomised controlled trial

Joint Strategic Needs Assessment Describes a process that identifies current and future health and wellbeing needs in light of existing services and informs future service planning taking into account evidence of effectiveness. It is intended that Joint Strategic Needs Assessment identifies 'the big picture', in terms of the health and wellbeing needs and inequalities of a local population

Kaplan-Meier estimates A statistical method to estimate survival probabilities using life tables. This can be visually presented as a Kaplan-Meier

graph from which one can determine 5-year survival or the median survival time

latency period Time between initial pathology until clinical diagnosis or screen detection

latent period Time during which the person infected is not infectious (not able to transmit the disease to others)

lead time effect Survival time for people with screen-detected disease appears longer because you start the clock sooner

length time effect Screening is best at picking up long-lasting nonprogressive or slowly-progressive pathological conditions, and tends to miss the poor prognosis rapidly-progressing cases. Outcome is therefore automatically better in screen-detected cases compared with clinically detected cases even if screening makes no difference to outcome

life course (epidemiology) framework The study of long-term effects on chronic disease risk of physical and social exposures during gestation, childhood, adolescence, young adulthood and later adult life. It includes studies of the biological, behavioural and psychosocial pathways that operate across an individual's life course, as well as across generations, to influence the development of disease.

likelihood ratio Describes how much more likely a person with the target condition is to receive a particular test result than a person without the target condition. Thus positive LRs describe how much more likely a person with the condition is to receive a positive test than a person without the condition, and negative LRs how much more likely a person with the condition is to receive a negative test than a person without the condition

linkage analysis The co-segregation of genetic markers with a disease or trait of interest in pedigrees of related individuals

linkage disequilibrium Genetic markers that are in close physical proximity to each other on the genome will be correlated with each other. This is known as linkage disequilibrium

locus A location in the genome

logarithmic transformation Data are transformed by converting it to its natural log values, in order to give it a Normal distribution.

This facilitates some statistical analysis. Other transformations are possible but log transformation is the most common

logistic regression (see regression) Type of regression model used when the outcome is binary/dichotomous

Mantel-Haenszel A method for controlling for confounders. The association between exposure and outcome is estimated separately for each level or strata of the confounder. Information from the separate strata is then combined

mean The average of a set of observations, derived by adding their values and then dividing by the total number of observations

measurement error Measurement error is a form of misclassification bias either in the exposure or the outcome that can bias the measurement of the effect of exposoure on outcome.
If **differential** then the bias is systematic across groups of study subjects and may lead to an over or under-estimate of the intervention or treatment effect.
If **nondifferential** then all study subjects experience the same error rate which tends to make the groups more similar and therefore lead to a dilution of the intervention or treatment effect

median A measure of central tendency, which is useful if the data is skewed. It is the value that halves the distribution. It is the middle value when the values in a set are arranged in order. If there is an even number of values the median is defined as the mean of the two middle values

Mendelian randomisation Studies that use genetic variants in observational epidemiology to make causal inferences about modifiable (non-genetic) risk factors for disease and health related outcomes

meta-analysis A statistical analysis that aims to produce a single summary estimate by combining the estimates reported in the included studies. This is done by calculating a weighted average of the effect estimates from different studies
fixed effects: in fixed-effect meta-analyses, the weights are based on the *inverse variance* of the effect in each study. Because large studies estimate the effect, this approach gives more weight to the studies that provide most information

random effects: in a random-effects meta-analysis, the weights are modified to account for the variability in true effects between the studies. This modification makes the weights (a) smaller and (b) relatively more similar to each other

meta-regression analyses Trying to explain variability in study findings by using study characteristics as explanatory factors. For example unblended trials tend to show larger drug benefits than double blind studies

migration studies Studies of people who migrate from one country to another with different physical, social, environmental and cultural backgrounds. Comparisons are made between morbidity and mortality of the migrant group and the indigenous group

Millennium Development Goals Eradicate extreme poverty and hunger; Achieve universal primary education; Promote gender equality and empower women; Reduce child mortality rate; Improve maternal health; Combat HIV/AIDS, malaria, and other diseases; Ensure environmental sustainability; Develop a global partnership for development

mode The mode, another measure of central tendency, is the most frequently occurring value in a set. It is rarely used in epidemiological practice. When there is a single mode, the distribution is known as **unimodal.** If there is more than one peak the distribution is said to be **bimodal** (two peaks) or **multi-modal**

monogenic diseases (Mendelian diseases) These are predominantly the result of a single gene variant. In other words, if an individual has a copy of the risk allele (in the case of a dominant disease/phenotype), or the risk genotype (in the case of a recessive disease/phenotype) then they have a high probability of developing the disease

Moral hazard The theory that patients are likely to use more healthcare sometimes for trivial reasons, because they do not bear the full cost of healthcare

mortality rate The proportion of the population who die after a specific time period. The numerator is the number of deaths and the denominator is the population at risk – usually estimated from mid-year estimates if using routine census data

motivational interviewing A client-centred, directive method for enhancing intrinsic motivation to change by exploring and resolving ambivalence. The overall goals is to increase intrinsic motivation, so that the behaviour change arises from within the individual

multivariable models A form of regression analysis that adjusts for several variables at the same time often used to adjust for confounding

natural experiments Events, interventions or policies which are not under the control of researchers, but which are amenable to research which uses the variation in exposure that they generate to analyse their impact. The key features are that: the intervention is not undertaken for the purposes of research; and the variation in exposure and outcomes is analysed using methods that attempt to make causal inferences

needs assessment An objective way of prioritising health services. Measuring the 'need' for services in a population includes measuring the burden of illness in a population, the effectiveness of therapeutic or preventive services, their economic efficiency (e.g. cost-effectiveness), and the effect of services on equity (i.e. who gains and who loses)

net monetary benefit (NMB) This statistic quantifies the net benefits to health of an intervention after subtracting the costs of that intervention. Interventions with a positive NMB are cost effective

normal/abnormal This term has distinct meanings and conceptual difficulties may arise if this is not clear:

(a) within the usual range of variation; this is a statistical definition which defines, arbitrarily that values more or less than 2 standard deviations (bottom and top 2.5%) as abnormal;

(b) associated with pathological process; a blood measure may be abnormal as it is a measure of an abnormal metabolic pathway that results in disease;

(c) predictive of future disease. Individuals may be abnormal as they are at greater risk of developing future disease

Normal (Gaussian) distribution This is a continuous symmetrical frequency distribution where both tails extend to infinity, the arithmetic mean, mode and median are identical and its shape is determined by the mean and standard deviation

null hypothesis The hypothesis that there is no difference between two groups. Statistical methods look for evidence against the null hypothesis by calculating a **P value**

number needed to treat (NNT) The number of people with a specified condition, who need to be treated for a specified period of time according to a specified protocol, in order to prevent one beneficial (NNT to benefit) or adverse outcome (NNT to harm). It is the inverse of the risk difference

numerator The upper portion of a fraction used to calculate a rate or a ratio

observational study Nonexperimental study; Epidemiological study that does not involve any intervention, experimental or otherwise; nature is allowed to take its course, with changes in one characteristic being studied in relation to changes in other characteristics. Case control and cohort studies are observational studies because the investigator is observing without intervention other than to record, classify, count and statistically analyse

odds of disease The number of people with a disease divided by the number of people without the disease

odds ratio The ratio of odds of exposure amongst subjects with disease compared to the odds of exposure amongst a control group. It is equal to the **cross-product ratio**

$$\text{odds ratio (OR)} = \text{odds in exposed} \div \text{odds in non-exposed} = (d_1/h_1) \div (d_0/h_0) = (d_1 \times h_0) \div (d_0 \times h_1)$$

opportunity cost The true cost of using a scarce resource in one way is the lost opportunity to use it for another purpose which might bring more benefits

outbreak The occurrence of more cases of a specific infection than expected in a particular time and place and/or among a specific group of people

outcome variable A variable, often a measure of disease occurrence, whose occurrence we wish to investigate and which is therefore the focus of interest of our analysis. Outcome variables are also known as **response variables**, **dependent variables** or **y-variables**. In a case-control study the outcome variable is case-control status
clinical outcomes: outcomes defined by health professionals such as, survival, remission, admission to hospital, cholesterol levels
composite outcome: combines multiple end-points. An RCT may combine coronary deaths with nonfatal coronary events and surgical interventions such as by-pass grafting. This is often done to increase the power of a trial but may complicate the interpretation of the results
patient reported outcomes are reported by the patient or participants themselves. They provide a patient's perspective and usually **generic** or **disease-specific** questionnaires or a **symptom-specific** measure such as a pain score
surrogate outcome refers to a measure that whilst may not be of direct practical importance, is associated with an outcome that is important. For example, a trial of a treatment to prevent dementia may use MRI scans to look at differences in brain atrophy, a surrogate for Alzheimer's disease

P value The probability that the difference between groups would be as big as or bigger than that observed, if the null hypothesis of no difference is true. The smaller the P value, the stronger is the evidence against the null hypothesis of that there is no difference between the groups

pandemic A worldwide epidemic – one which occurs over a wide geographic area and also affects a high proportion of the population

per-protocol or on treatment analysis An analysis that only includes those patients who adhered to their allocated treatment in contrast to an intention to treat analysis. This may produce biased results as nonadherence to protocol is likely to be associated with prognostic risk factors

pharmacogenomics The branch of pharmacology which deals with the influence of genetic variation on drug response

phenotype An observable trait

PICO **P**atient, **I**ntervention, **C**omparator, **O**utcome

pie chart A circular diagram divided into segments, each representing a category or subset of data

placebo An inert medication or procedure, i.e. having no pharmacological effect. It is intended to give patients the perception that they are receiving treatment for their complaint. From the Latin *placebo* 'I shall be pleasing'

polygenic diseases Diseases or traits caused by the combined action of many genes of small effect plus environmental influences. Polygenic diseases are sometimes referred to as complex diseases or common diseases

polymorphisms A variation in DNA sequence between matching chromosomes or DNA regions; at least two or more alleles at one locus with frequencies greater than 1% must be present in the population

population attributable risk An absolute measure of risk calculated as the overall risk (ignoring exposure status) minus the risk among the unexposed only. It tells us how much of the overall population risk of a disease is due to a specific exposure

population-based epidemiology The use of epidemiological methods to study the causes of disease

population mean The true mean in the population from which a sample has been drawn. This is the value that we infer from the sample mean

power The ability of a study to demonstrate an association if one exists. The power of a study is determined by several factors, including the frequency of the condition under study, the magnitude of the effect, the study design and the sample size. It is the probability of observing evidence against the null hypothesis, if it is indeed false

precision The amount of variation in the sample statistic; the greater the variation the smaller the precision

predictive value These are summary measure of probability that the target condition is present or absent given a positive or negative index test result. The Positive Predictive Value is the (post-test) probability that a patient with a positive test result has the target condition, while the Negative Predictive Value (NPV) is the probability that a patient with a negative test result does not have the target condition

pre-test probability The pre-test probability of the target condition can be defined either at the population or the patient level. At the population level it corresponds to the prevalence of the target condition. The pre-test probability of the target condition at an individual patient level can be estimated based on their clinical history, results of physical examination, and clinical knowledge and experience. It is the clinician's prior prediction of whether the patient has the target condition

prevalence The total number of individuals, who have an attribute or disease at a particular time or during a particular period, divided by the total population at risk

prevention Prevention of disease or the consequences of disease has three levels: **primary** prevention: prevent occurrence of the disease in people who are disease free and susceptible to the disease (e.g. vaccination or strategies that can prevent onset of smoking or HIV transmission); **secondary** prevention: prevent or cure the disease by diagnosing and treating the disease (e.g. diagnosis and treatment of Chlamydia or H pylori which causes peptic ulcers); **tertiary** prevention: prevent consequences or adverse prognosis of disease (e.g. annual diabetic checkups)

prevention paradox Whereby an intervention delivered at the population level confers relatively little advantage to the majority of low-risk persons, but achieves benefit at the population level

primary prevention The prevention of the occurrence of disease in the population

prognosis Prognosis begins at diagnosis. It concerns 'the expected course of a disease' or natural history – derived from the Greek 'knowledge beforehand' or 'foretelling'. Patients can have mild, moderate or severe prognoses depending on how rapidly their disease progresses

prognostic risk factor These are risk factors that influence disease progression and may be used to target treatment especially if it is costly or has serious side effects

proportion The number of occurrences of an event divided by the total number of observations

public health The science and art of preventing disease, prolonging life, and promoting health through organised efforts of society

Public Health Intervention Ladder As defined by the Nuffield School on Bioethics classifies interventions according to the degree of social control on individual choice

public health surveillance aka information for action Refers to the ongoing, systematic collection, analysis and interpretation of data essential to the planning, implementation, and evaluation of public health practice, closely integrated with the timely dissemination of these data to those responsible for prevention and control

qualitative methods A nonnumeric method that involves collecting textual data from interviews of individuals or groups and using this to generate themes that may explain health-related behaviours or attitudinal factors. These methods are often used in developing complex outcomes measures such as quality of life which are then operationalised into quantitative scales

quality adjusted life year (QALY) QALYs provide a summary measure of morbidity and mortality. Life expectancy is weighted by a factor indicating health related quality of life. The weights are anchored at 1 (perfect health) and 0 (a health state considered to be as bad as death)

quality of life A summary measure based on a quantitative scale that attempts to capture the impact of illness on both physical, psychological and social aspects of well-being

quantitative methods Methods that involve collecting numerical data from individuals or groups to explore the prevalence of disease or associations between an exposure and outcome

R *See* **effective reproduction number**

R0 *See* **basic reproduction number**

random allocation, randomisation Allocation of individuals, in randomised controlled trials, to the intervention group or the control group, by chance alone

randomised controlled trial A study in which individuals or groups are randomly allocated to two or more groups. Often, one of these groups will be the treatment group while the other will be a placebo group that receives no treatment other than standard care

cluster randomised trial: the unit of randomisation is a group (e.g. hospital, general practice, school, factory etc. rather than an individual). This is usually done for either ethical, pragmatic reasons or because the intervention by definition has to be given to a group, e.g. media campaign

crossover trial: this is an individual level trial where subjects got either treatment A or B in a random order and then crossover so that the act as their own control. This method is more efficient in terms of recruiting fewer subjects but is only suitable for stable chronic conditions and there may be problems with a carryover effect

parallel arm: this is where treatments are allocated at random and run in parallel to each other

range The lowest to highest values in a sample of data

rate A measure of the frequency of occurrence of a phenomenon. The components of a rate are; the number of cases (numerator), the number at risk (denominator), a specified period of time. Unlike a risk, the denominator is usually comprised of precise 'person years at risk'

recessive A relationship between two alleles at the same locus. When one allele (A) masks the expression of another allele (B), B is said to be recessive to A

reference group *see* **baseline** group

reference range This range measures how much variation there is between the individual observations in a sample. It tells us the likely values for an individual in the population

reference standard The reference standard is the method used to determine the presence or absence of the target condition. Estimates of diagnostic accuracy are based on the assumption that the reference standard is 100% sensitive and specific

regression Finds the best mathematical model to describe y, the outcome, with respect to x, the exposure. The most common form is linear regression. In this case the regression co-efficient is an estimate of the change in outcome (y) for a unit change in exposure (x) according to the equation is $y = a + bx$, where a is the intercept and b is the slope. The regression line is a diagrammatic presentation of a regression equation

relative risk The ratio of risk in an exposed to an unexposed group

research governance This can be defined as the broad range of regulations, principles and standards of good practice that exist to achieve, and continuously improve, research quality across all aspects of healthcare in the UK and worldwide. This usually involved independent review by a research ethics committee

residual confounding An association between an exposure and outcome which is noncausal but reflects confounding due to variables that have not been measured or measured inadequately and so cannot be incorporated into an analysis or do so imperfectly

reverse causality This term is applied to an exposure - outcome association which is thought to be due to the outcome actually causing the exposure rather than the other way round

risk The probability that an event will occur; number of new cases of a disease(numerator) / number of people initially disease free and at risk over a specified time (denominator)

risk difference (attributable risk) The difference in risk between exposed subjects and nonexposed subjects

$$\text{risk difference} = \text{risk in exposed}$$
$$- \text{risk in nonexposed} = (d_1/n_1) - (d_0/n_0)$$

risk factor A factor or characteristics that might alter the risk of disease

risk ratio (sometimes also referred to as the **relative risk** and often abbreviated to **RR**) The risk ratio is the risk of developing disease associated with an exposure divided by the risk of developing the disease in the absence of exposure

$$\text{risk ratio (RR)} = \text{risk in exposed} \div \text{risk}$$
$$\text{in nonexposed} = (d_1/n_1) \div (d_0/n_0)$$

Relative risk (Genetic Epidemiology): The relative risk is the risk that a relative of an affected proband will be affected with disease divided by the risk of disease in the general population. For example, a sibling relative risk of 3, means that the sibling of an affected proband is 3 times more likely to suffer from the disease than an unrelated individual randomly drawn from the population.

sample A selected subset of a population
selected sample: usually a random sample of individuals that have been selected from the target population
study sample: the subgroup of subjects from the selected sample that actually agree to take part and contribute data to the study

sample mean *see* **mean**

sample size calculation The mathematical process of deciding before the study begins, how many subjects should be studied. In order to calculate the required sample size, the investigator needs to specify four things:
(1) the expected level of outcome in the control (placebo) group;
(2) the smallest difference they wish to detect (% difference);
(3) the strength of the evidence (p value) they wish to find, usually 5%;
(4) the probability of detecting a difference at a specified p value, if the true difference is the size they expect. This is called the power of the study and is often set at 90%

sampling The process of selecting a number of subjects from all the subjects in a particular population

sampling distribution The distribution that would be observed if we derived a sample statistic, such as a mean or a difference between proportions, from repeated samples from the same population

sampling error That part of the difference between the observed value of a sample statistic (such as a mean or a difference between proportions) and the true value in the population, caused by random variation

scatter plot This is a graphical display of the association between two numerical values

screening The process of identifying early or asymptomatic disease or risk factors for disease in

populations in order to intervene and alter the natural history

secondary prevention Interventions including early diagnosis, use of referral services, and rapid initiation of treatment to stop or slow disease progression

sensitivity Sensitivity is a measure of a diagnostic test's usefulness. It is the proportion of those with the target condition who have a positive index test result (better sensitivity lower percentage with false negative rate)

sensitivity analysis Additional analyses which are undertaken to assess the robustness of the main findings by checking assumptions, including different population or looking at missing data using imputation

service evaluation This can be considered even one stage earlier than audit as its primary purpose is simply to measure what and how services are actually delivered without reference to any specific quality standard as in audit

single nucleotide polymorphism (SNP) A single base mutation in the genome that varies across a population of individuals

skewed An asymmetrical frequency distribution

SMART Criteria to measure targets: **S**pecific; **M**easurable; **A**chievable; **R**ealistic; **T**ime bound

SNP *see* **single nucleotide polymorphism**

social class or socioeconomic status or socioeconomic position (SEP) Refers to the social and economic factors that influence what positions individuals or groups hold within the structure of a society

specificity specificity is a measure of a diagnostic test's usefulness. Specificity refers to the proportion of those without the target condition who have a negative index test result (better specificity lower percentage with false positive result)

standardisation This is a method for controlling for confounders and is used to control for differences in the age (or gender) structure between two populations

standard deviation A measure of how widely dispersed are the individual observations in a distribution. The standard deviation is the square root of the **variance**

standard error The standard deviation of the sampling distribution of a sample statistic such as a mean or a difference between proportions

statistics The science of collecting, summarising, presenting, interpreting data, **estimating** the magnitude/strength of relationships and testing **hypotheses**

Statistical Process Control charts This is a graphical method to plot health care performance either between centres or across time and potentially identify units or time periods that are outliers by either performing worse or better than expected. This can be used either as feedback to units or as the basis of a more detailed enquiry

stratum-specific estimates Risk ratios or odds ratios estimated in different strata defined by the levels of a confounding variable. These are then combined into a summary estimate of the risk ratio or odds ratio controlled for the effect of the confounding variable

stepped wedge design Whereby all clusters receive the intervention but some receive it immediately whilst others receive after a delay so there is a period of time when they act as the control arm, i.e. the time when the cluster receives the intervention is randomised

study sample The sample of subjects who actually participate in the study and provide data, i.e. this does not include nonresponders

Supplier induced demand The theory that financial gain might lead doctors to encourage under-informed patients to use more healthcare than is necessary

survival analysis A set of statistical techniques that are used to analyse time to event data such as death or incident disease. These can be used to identify aetiological or prognostic risk factors

survival rate The proportion of cases of a specific condition that are alive after a specified time period, e.g. 1 year or 5 years

statutory notifications Key source of surveillance information in the UK. Clinicians have a legal requirement under public health legislation to notify, on suspicion, each case of a notifiable disease. The current list of notifiable infectious diseases in the UK is given below

systematic review A structured approach to the collection, appraisal and synthesis of quantitative data which may or may not also include a summary measure as part of a meta-analysis

T distribution This is a symmetrical, bell-shaped distribution with slightly wider tails than the Normal distribution. It is used when deriving confidence intervals for small sample sizes and produces slightly wider intervals than the Normal distribution

target population The collection of individuals about whom we wish to draw inferences or be able to generalise too

technical efficiency Providing care that optimises the health of a patient group from a fixed budget or set of resources.

test performance *see* **sensitivity, specificity, positive predictive value and likelihood ratios**

threshold effect A pattern of association between exposure and disease in which only subjects whose exposure is above a certain level are at increased risk

time series A method of analysis that examines data points over time and takes account of an internal structure, pattern of relatedness, between the data points (such as autocorrelation, or trend or seasonal variation) and can be used to investigate whether there is evidence that patterns of disease changed after an intervention or exposure

treatment effect The effectiveness of a treatment compared to the control (for example usual care).

trend test A statistical method that tests whether there is a linear increase or decrease in risk associated with an increase in exposure. This is usually used to examine the association of an ordered categorical exposure variable with a binary outcome

type I error Wrongly rejecting the null hypothesis thereby declaring there is an association when in fact there is not (false positive)

unimodal A probability distribution with a single mode

utilities The value of a particular health state used in health economic analyses

vaccines An inoculation of live, attenuated, modified, killed or simulated parts of bacteria or viruses which stimulate the immune system to produce antigen-specific antibodies against the bacteria or virus

variability The extent to which the values of a variable in a distribution are spread out from the centre

variable A quantity that varies. An attribute, phenomenon, or event that can have different values
numerical variable: variables given a numerical value
continuous: a variable with a numerical value, which has a potentially infinite number of possible values along a continuum, within a specified range
discrete: a variable with a numerical value, which cannot take on any intermediate values e.g number of children, number of deaths
categorical variable: a variable, which refers to categories. It is given a 'value label', which is usually a number
dichotomous or **binary**: a variable where only two categories are possible
ordered categorical: a variable where values are ranked according to an ordered classification
unordered categorical: a categorical variable where categories have no order to them

Wilson and Junger criteria A set of criteria for appraising the viability, effectiveness and appropriateness of a screening programme

 REFERENCE

Kunst AE, Mackenbach JP (1995) *Measuring Socioeconomic Inequalities in Health.* Copenhagen: World Health Organization.
Porta M. (2008) A dictionary of epidemiology. Oxford University Press, UK.

Self-assessment answers – Part 1: Epidemiology

Q1

(c) An increase in the mean
The mean is particularly sensitive to extreme values (outliers).

Q2

(c), (d) and (e)
Incidence relates to how fast new cases are occurring so we need to know how many new cases there have been in a specific period of time. Since only children in private schools were measured, this estimate of the prevalence may be biased and so should not be assumed representative of all 11-year-olds in Bristol. The researchers should have randomly selected the study sample from all schools in Bristol. Although cross-sectional studies are used primarily for measuring prevalence, they can also be used to test for aetiological associations. Prevalence is calculated as the number of cases (numerator) divided by the population at risk (denominator).

Q3

(b) The sample size increases
Anything which decreases the standard error (i.e. a decrease in the standard deviation, or an increase in the sample size) will reduce the width of the 95% CI. Similarly if we take a lower level of confidence then this will reduce the confidence coefficient multiplier, e.g. from 1.96 (95%) to 1.64 (90%).

Q4

(b) and (e)
The P stands for Probability. The probability of an event varies between 0 (never occurs) and 1 (always occurs). The P value is defined as the probability of getting a difference at least as big as the one in our study, if the null hypothesis is true. P values thus measure the strength of the evidence against a null hypothesis about the population. The smaller the P value, the stronger the evidence against the null hypothesis.

Q5

(c) Hypertension
Sickle cell anaemia is caused by a mutation in the haemoglobin beta globin gene, Huntington's chorea by an expanded trinuclotide repeat (CAG)n in the gene encoding huntingtin, and cystic fibrosis by a mutation in the cystic fibrosis transmembrane conductance regulator gene. All of these conditions are transmitted according to simple Mendelian inheritance patterns. In contrast, hypertension is caused by many different genetic and environmental factors of small effect. Its inheritance is complex and does not follow simple Mendelian inheritance patterns.

Q6

(d) Technology is not yet sufficiently advanced to assay genetic polymorphisms
Answers (a) through (c) are all reasons for why genetic testing of complex diseases is likely to be limited. However, the technology for assaying genetic polymorphisms has been available for many years, and so this is not a limitation.

Q7

(a) Classical twin design
The classical twin design enables investigators to partition a trait's variance into genetic and nongenetic sources of variation and hence estimate the trait's heritability. Adoption studies are useful for estimating the relative contribution of shared and unique environmental influences on a trait of interest. Whilst migration studies can provide

Epidemiology, Evidence-based Medicine and Public Health Lecture Notes, Sixth Edition. Yoav Ben-Shlomo, Sara T. Brookes and Matthew Hickman.
© 2013 Y. Ben-Shlomo, S. T. Brookes and M. Hickman. Published 2013 by John Wiley & Sons, Ltd.

evidence for a genetic component underlying a trait, related individuals are required (e.g. as in the classical twin design) in order to estimate heritability accurately. Genome-wide association studies allow the identification of specific mutations associated with a trait/disease but do not provide overall estimates of heritability.

Q8

The standard deviation is a measure of how widely dispersed individual observations in a distribution are. The standard error is the standard deviation of the sampling distribution of a sample statistic such as a mean or a difference between proportions.

Q9

The reference range tells you the likely values for an individual, while the confidence interval gives you likely values for the mean of a group of individuals.

Q10

(a) This is a case-control study, since participants were chosen on the basis of the outcome, and exposure was assessed retrospectively. This is the most appropriate study design, as an RCT would not be ethical or feasible (we could not withhold seasonal flu vaccine from those who are eligible). A case-control is better than a cohort study in this instance as at the time of the study the outcome was still relatively rare / case-control so this is more efficient.

Q10

(b) The null hypothesis is that there is no association between seasonal flu vaccination and influenza A/H1N1.

Q10

(c) Measurement bias relates to random or systematic error in the measurement or classification of either or both the exposure and outcome measures. Measurement bias can be differential or nondifferential. Recall bias is measurement error in the exposure, which is differential between cases and controls. It is possible that this occurred in the current study. Data on vaccination was obtained by interview with the patient or with next of kin, rather than from medical records. Those who have/do not have A/H1N1 may be more/less likely to recall prior vaccination.

If there was recall bias, it could result in the over-estimation or under-estimation of results.

Q10

(d) Selection bias is a systematic difference in the likelihood of selecting subjects to take part in the study on the basis of their association between exposure and outcome status. In case-control studies, cases and controls should be selected irrespective of their exposure status. Since in this study, controls were chosen from among patients presenting to a respiratory disease hospital, it is likely that their vaccination status was different to that of the general population, since the seasonal flu vaccine is recommended for people with conditions conferring a higher risk of influenza-related complications. It is therefore likely that exposure was over-represented in the control group and the odds ratio was underestimated.

Q10

(e) There is a relative reduction of 73% in the odds of having received a seasonal flu vaccine amongst A/H1N1 patients compared to controls. The CI shows that we can be 95% confident that the odds are reduced by between 34% and 89%. Although this is a relatively wide CI, indicating low precision, even the lower limit of the CI is consistent with an important reduction in risk. The P value shows that there is strong evidence against the null hypothesis, and therefore that it appears that the seasonal flu vaccine is associated with a reduction in influenza A/H1N1 risk.

Q11

(a) The exposure is the presence of a family history of asthma which is recorded as yes/no so is a dichotomous/binary variable. The outcome is presence or absence of an adverse perioperative event. This is also a dichotomous/binary variable.

Q11

(b) This is a cohort study, since individuals are measured on their exposure at baseline, and subsequently followed up during/after the operation when outcome data are collected. This is the most appropriate design as an RCT is not feasible since we cannot randomise to receiving a history of asthma.

A cohort avoids reverse causality and so is preferable to a case-control or cross-sectional study.

Q11

(c) Individuals with a positive family history of asthma were 2.93 times more likely to experience an adverse event than individuals without a positive family history of asthma. The CI shows that we can be 95% confident that individuals with a positive family history of asthma are between 2.21 and 3.89 times (or 121 and 289 %) more likely to have an adverse event as compared to those without a positive family history of asthma, hence we can rule out no effect or a protective effect of a positive family history of asthma. The P value is very small, showing that there is strong evidence against the null hypothesis of no association between family history of asthma and risk of adverse perioperative events.

Q11

(d) The authors carried out an adjusted analysis because they were concerned about confounding. For example children who have parents that smoke are more at risk of asthma and also more likely to experience adverse perioperative events. Adjusting for sex, age or parental history of smoking in the analysis reduced the association between family history of asthma and perioperative events from 2.93 to 1.86.

Q12

(a) Individuals from least deprived areas have on average 0.02mm thinner carotid intima-media. The 95% CI shows that we can be sure that the least deprived group has between 0.03 mm and 0.01 mm reduced thickness compared to the more deprived group ruling out increased thickness in the least deprived group. The low P value provides strong evidence against the null hypothesis of no association between atherosclerosis and socio-economic deprivation.

Q12

(b) Chance –The observed association is unlikely to be due to chance as the P value provides strong evidence against the null hypothesis. Selection bias is unlikely here as it was a random sample taken from the electoral roll. Measurement error is a possibility with ultrasound measurement. Recall bias and follow-up bias are not relevant in this study design. Reverse causality – possibly an issue if poor health causes unemployment and consequently living in more deprived area. Confounding – residual confounding likely to exist.

Self-assessment answers – Part 2: Evidence-based medicine

Q1

(a) The null hypothesis is that the intervention schedule does not reduce or increase the rate of serious medical errors compared to the traditional schedule.

(b) The rate (or risk) ratio is 0.74 suggesting a 26% relative reduction in the rate (or risk) of errors with the intervention schedule compared to the traditional schedule. We can be 95% confident that the true effect lies between a relative reduction of 5% and 43% so ruling out any detrimental effect of the intervention. The P value is small and provides some evidence against the null hypothesis. Whilst there is some evidence that the intervention schedule reduces the rate of serious medical errors, the confidence interval is wide and the true reduction could be small.

(c) The intervention schedule is most effective at reducing the number of diagnostic errors. The rate ratio suggests an 82% relative reduction, the CI is more precise than for other errors and excludes any detrimental effect of the intervention and suggests at least a 41% reduction. The P value is small providing strong evidence against the null hypothesis.

(d) So that randomisation is not corrupted or biased in any way (to avoid selection bias), as, if known, the characteristics of the PRHO may influence which arm they get allocated to. This design feature is known as 'concealment of allocation'. If this had not been done, better PRHOs may have been allocated to the intervention arm and hence the reduction in serious errors might not be due to the intervention but the different clinical abilities of the PRHOs.

(e) In this study blinding refers to when either the subject or the outcome assessor or both are unaware of treatment allocation. In this study the physician observers knew which schedule the PRHO was working hence they were not blinded and clearly the doctors themselves knew whether they were doing the traditional or intervention schedule. Lack of blinding may produce measurement (detection) bias – observers may record things differently if they know what schedule the PRHO is on. For example, if the observers believed that the intervention schedule should be better, they may have under-recorded errors in the intervention and/or over-recorded errors in the traditional schedule. In addition, lack of blinding may lead to performance bias if physicians offer more help to certain PRHOs.

(f) Randomised trials are also prone to follow-up bias. During the year of the trial some interns may have dropped out or withdrawn from the study. However, we are told that all the interns who consented did actually undertake the study and were observed (with the exception of one that dropped out), so this was not a problem.

(g) Could be a chance finding, there is just over a 1 in 100 probability of observing this result, or more extreme, if the null hypothesis is true – P=0.016. Confounding

Epidemiology, Evidence-based Medicine and Public Health Lecture Notes, Sixth Edition. Yoav Ben-Shlomo, Sara T. Brookes and Matthew Hickman.
© 2013 Y. Ben-Shlomo, S. T. Brookes and M. Hickman. Published 2013 by John Wiley & Sons, Ltd.

is unlikely to be an explanation as it is a randomised trial and the patients' and interns' characteristics in each schedule are similar. Reverse causality is not possible here.

(h) Preventable adverse events may be a more important outcome. If reducing errors has no impact on the rate of preventable adverse events then the implementation of the intervention schedule may not be justified. There may be other detrimental effects of the intervention which have not been measured e.g. patient satisfaction with care, relationship with doctor, training experiences etc.

(i) The rate (or risk) ratio suggests a 21% reduction in preventable adverse events with the intervention schedule. However, the P value is large and provides no (or *very* weak) evidence against the null hypothesis and the confidence interval is wide and imprecise – there may be a relative reduction as large as 61% or an increase of up to 54% with the intervention schedule. This imprecision is due to small numbers of events.

(j) The study was done in two units in one academic hospital in the US. The findings may not be generalisable to nonacademic hospitals or other units where the traditional schedule may not be the same. There may also be differences between the US and the UK. Would not suggest implementation until a similar trial had been performed in a range of units in the UK.

Q2

(a) Both patients and researchers can be blinded – by making the tablets identical neither the patient or researcher will know which treatment they have been allocated and hence the outcome measure, though subjective, should not be biased.

(b) Researchers – It is impossible to blind the participants to whether they have received group or individual sessions but the researcher assessing the recording can be kept blinded. It is possible that the participant may try to speak better if they have received more one-to-one care out of loyalty to the therapist so even though the outcome assessor is blinded there may be some bias introduced

(c) Possibly neither – In this case whilst it is not possible to identify the medications, because beta-blockers slow down one's heart rate (usually to at least 60 beats per minute) it is very likely that the nurse will guess who is on the beta-blocker which may effect how she takes the blood pressure. Similarly any patient who measures their own pulse and who knows this drug effect, may also work out which drug they are on and may alter other aspects of their lifestyle, e.g. salt in diet. In this case though the study should be double blind and we are using an objective outcome measure, the side effects of the drug make it hard to maintain this.

(d) Patients and researchers – Clearly the surgeon who will undertake the operative procedure will know which prosthesis has been used. The patient, unless told, will not know as the scar will look identical and hence their report of quality of life should not be biased. Similarly, as long as the assessor is not the surgeon and does not access the medical records, they can also be kept blinded to the intervention.

(e) Patients and researchers – It is possible to use sham acupuncture so that patients either receive real acupuncture needles that are placed in specific points and pierce the skin versus false needles that are placed randomly and provide the experience of pressure but do not actually go through the skin. As long as the participants are unaware of what 'real' acupuncture feels like, they will probably be unaware of the difference (one can check this by asking them and if they are blinded then they will be correct on average only 50% of the time). In this case if the sham procedure is convincing then the outcome is blinded to the treatment allocation and is not biased.

Q3

(a) i. Resource use from the NHS/health service provider perspective could include: hospital outpatient consultations; hospital inpatient stays; general practitioner (GP) consultation at the GPSI service; nurse consultation at the GPSI service; GP consultation at the GP surgery; GP consultation at home; practice nurse consultation at the GP surgery; district nurse home visit; tests, e.g. biochemistry, haematology, histopathology, immunology, microbiology, mycology, patch test, radiology, skin prick test, virology; investigations and treatments, e.g. excision biopsy, punch biopsy, curettage and cautery; and prescribed medication.

ii. In addition to the above mentioned resource use from the NHS/health service provider perspective, resource use from a societal perspective could include: use of personal social services e.g. home care worker (home help); food at home service (meals on wheels); over the counter medication; consultations with private health care practitioners e.g. private doctor, homeopath, acupuncturist, herbalist, reflexologist, aromatherapist, faith healer; travel costs of patient and companion; child care costs; absenteeism from work (both paid and unpaid).

(b) The use of self-completed questionnaires to measure patient costs and time off work may be affected by nonresponse and recall bias.

(c) The **PICO** for the **cost-effectiveness analysis** is:

Patient Group: Patients who were referred to a hospital outpatient dermatology clinic and were deemed suitable to be managed by a general practitioner with special interests

Intervention: The General Practitioner with Special Interest Service

Comparator: Usual Care i.e. Hospital Outpatient Care

Outcome: Incremental cost per increase in the dermatology life quality index score

(d) A **cost-consequence analysis** could be used for the second type of evaluation, whereby all the costs (to the health service and wider society) are tabulated alongside all the outcomes (e.g. quality of life, access, satisfaction etc.) of the intervention. The decision-maker is left to judge whether any additional costs of GPSI are justified by an improved range of outcomes.

(e) In order for the evaluation to aid the creation of an allocatively efficient health care system then either the **QALY** could be used as an outcome measure in a **cost utility analysis**. Alternatively, a monetary value could be placed on the outcomes of the intervention using techniques such as willingness to pay in a **cost-benefit analysis**.

(f) This means that GPSI service is more costly and more effective in terms of an improvement in the dermatology life quality index score compared with usual outpatient care. In this journal article, the **incremental cost-effectiveness ratio** for general practitioner with special interest care over outpatient care was £540 per one point gain in the dermatology life quality index. The decision-maker must judge whether the additional costs of GPSI are justified by the improvement in quality of life.

(g) **Confidence intervals** or a **cost-effectiveness acceptability curve** are typically used to represent uncertainty in a cost-effectiveness analysis.

(h) The **sensitivity analysis** was conducted because of the longer waiting period for the initial hospital outpatient consultation compared with a GPSI consultation. This meant that there was a possibility that not all the resources in the hospital outpatient arm needed for the treatment and resolution of the dermatological condition would occur within the time horizon of the trial.

Q4

(a) i. *50%*
ii. *86%*
iii. *2%*
iv. *11%*
v. *Ruling in*

(b) i. F: if important not to miss new cases then needs high sensitivity
ii. F: depends on sensitivity and specificity and whether more cost-effective to introduce better more costly test
iii. T: high positive predictive value means that high proportion of subjects with positive test results are correctly diagnosed
iv. F: ideally, a trial randomizing new test against current practice with a

relevant health outcome would be the best design

v. T: therefore no false positives or false negative tests

Q5

(a) T: asking about health consequences of a diagnosis of glue ear

(b) T: asking about survival after diagnosis of lung cancer

(c) F: asking about aetiology/causes of a diagnosis

(d) T: asking about risk of consequences of a diagnosis of hepatitis C

(e) F: asking about transmission risk to others

Q6

(a) F: it is a forest plot

(b) T: the outcome is total mortality, the horizontal axis shows whether treatment reduces mortality Odds Ratio of <1 or increases mortality OR>1 compared to control

(c) T the pooled effect is less than 1 (OR 0.76 95% CI 0.59 to 0.98) favouring treatment over control, i.e. that reduces the outcome (mortality).

(d) F: the length of the bars relates to confidence interval of individual effect which is related to power or size of trial. Longer bars are less precise and hence have less power to detect an effect.

(e) F: The size of the square is proportional to the weight given to each study in the meta-analysis (study weight as a percentage has also been presented). This is not the same as the precision, shown by the 95% confidence interval, but is related to it i.e. studies with greater weight will have more precise estimates as the weight in a fixed effect model is the inverse of the variance (square of the standard error).

Self-assessment answers – Part 3: Public health

Q1

(a) T: This is a population-based approach to help women who smoke give up and hence increase the birth weight of their child. As smoking as fairly common, if the intervention is effective, this should shift the birth weight distribution of all infants to the right so that the mean birthweight (adjusted for gestation) should increase.

(b) F: This is a clinical intervention amongst a client group with drug, alcohol or mental health problems.

(c) F: This test will simply identify an increased risk on average for individuals rather than diagnosing a disorder.

(d) T: This intervention would apply to all mothers who have had a baby and by providing financial support may encourage women to stay at home longer and continue to breast feed their child.

(e) T: This would increase the total population intake of folic acid and hence reduce the risk of any adverse effects of deficiency.

Q2

(a) Men at age 65, and self-referral for older unscreened men

(b) Abdominal ultrasound

(c) In AAA screening the result of the ultrasound is diagnostic, and participants with aneurysm of 5.5 cm and above are referred to an accredited surgeon. The surgeon may choose to carry out a CT scan if there is a need to assess the shape and extent of the aneurysm

(d) Elective (i.e. planned rather than emergency) surgical repair of abdominal aortic aneurysm

(e) Reduced risk of death from ruptured aortic aneurysm

Q3

(a) F: Several notifiable diseases do not yet have an effective vaccine e.g. Leprosy, Food poisoning, Legionnaires' Disease

(b) T: As a result of herd immunity

(c) T: As coined by Communicable Disease Centre, US

(d) F: The larger the Ro the more infectious (the more secondary infections per index case) so the harder the infection is to contain

(e) T: Successful treatment averts future secondary infections that may occur if an infection is left untreated, and so can reduce incidence

Q4

A good answer would include most of the following points.

Data interpretation:

- The social gradient is apparent at all time periods and the magnitude of health inequalities has increased over time.
- Life expectancy improved in all occupational groups.
- The rate of improvement in life expectancy was fastest in group I and slowest in group V.
- The absolute inequality in life expectancy between groups I and V widened from five to 10 years over the 20-year time period.

Possible reasons for inequalities in life expectancy are socio-economic differences in:

- smoking rates
- access to affordable healthy food
- opportunities for physical activity
- working conditions and exposures
- demographic composition of the groups, e.g. higher rates of ethnic minority men in group V

Epidemiology, Evidence-based Medicine and Public Health Lecture Notes, Sixth Edition. Yoav Ben-Shlomo, Sara T. Brookes and Matthew Hickman. © 2013 Y. Ben-Shlomo, S. T. Brookes and M. Hickman. Published 2013 by John Wiley & Sons, Ltd.

- cumulative effects of parental deprivation (which is more likely in men with manual occupations)
- access to prompt medical care (although NHS is free at the point of service, opportunity costs across socioeconomic groups differ, e.g. if you are paid wages by the hour, the personal cost of going to the doctor is higher than if you received a salary)

The role of doctors in tackling health inequalities:

- ensuring a system of equal access to all (access in the broadest sense)
- directly targeting health behaviours
- targeting the determinants of health behaviours
- political advocacy
- health inequality impact assessment

Q5

(a) Cluster randomised controlled trial with class as the unit of randomisation.

(b) Contamination means that those randomised to the control arm have been exposed to parts of the intervention: in effect the intervention has leaked into the control arm. In this study classes were randomly allocated to the intervention or control arm but with the added stipulation that classes who shared the same school building had to be in the same arm of the trial. Given that the intervention involved targeting children, teachers, parents and the school environment, ensuring that classes sharing the same building were in the same trial arm should have prevented most contamination as far as the environment was concerned, but the children may have passed on some of what they learnt to friends and siblings in other classes in different school buildings, as might teachers. Parents may also have had other children in classes the control arm and so those children may have been exposed to parts of the intervention via their parents.

(c) (i) Stratified randomisation. (ii) Stratifying in this way would have ensured balance in the trial arm between classes from the different language and cultural traditions and having these two traditions represented in a balanced way would enhance the generalisability (external validity) of the trial findings.

(d) Giving detailed information about the purpose of an RCT in which the intervention is designed to produce behaviour change, always runs a risk of a 'Hawthorn effect' whereby people change their behaviour by virtue of being in a trial, and knowing all about the intervention being tested. This is most likely to happen in the control arm where participants, having been told that the purpose of this trial was to test the effectiveness of the intervention in improving fitness and reducing BMI, and knowing that they would not be receiving the intervention, may have been encouraged to seek additional physical activity outside of school and change their families diet, patterns of sedentary behaviour and sleep routines. Were this to happen then it would reduce the chances of observing a difference in outcomes between the intervention and control arms.

(e) Opt in consent.

(f) Opt out consent is more commonly used because the interventions being tested are usually noninvasive and directed at populations rather than in closely defined groups of patients as is the case in clinical research. In these circumstances there are concerns that obtaining individual, written consent may introduce bias by limiting recruitment to certain types within the population (e.g. the more educated, those in good health) and therefore potentially seriously compromising the validity of the research. It is argued that in public health research where there is a low risk of harm, individual consent should be waived where (a) the benefits to society are potentially high, (b) the risk to individuals low, and (c) the effort and cost of obtaining individual consent may be prohibitive.

(g) As the programme was to be gradually implemented across the country a stepped wedge design could be used.

Q6

Key points in approximate order of importance

A well-structured, systematic approach to the question, and demonstration of a thorough understanding of all the characteristics of good targets, context within which targets are set and the potential pitfalls of using targets.

Key factors
- Targets — Structure, process and/or outcome; SMART.
- Identify national and local standards — NHS Cancer Plan, relevant NICE guidance etc.
- Information requirements: local and national data sources to help describe the epidemiology of disease and to monitor progress against the target for e.g. mortality statistics (outcome), hospital activity (mainly structure and process), Cancer Registry data (outcome).
- Assessment of evidence base to determine what would be a realistic reduction given current available treatment.
- Availability of resources e.g. monetary and human resources, to ensure that the target is successfully met.

Reservations about appropriateness
- Comparisons (with national or other local data) may be difficult – e.g. variation in case definition(s), problems with age-standardisation
- Small numbers – aggregate data over several years – but this makes monitoring more difficult
- Demotivation of unrealistic targets
- Deflect resources away from areas with more priority
- Targets can lead to 'gaming'

Q7

Key Points
Pros
- Targets can identify priorities and provide an agreed direction for action, e.g. reduction in the prevalence of disease correlates with target attainment, e.g. Hib immunisation programme, or reduction in mortality with a population screening coverage, e.g. breast or cervical screening.
- Motivates staff by providing a common agenda with shared objectives for professional and managerial endeavours: possibility of team cohesion, individual/team/ organisational rewards and sanctions.
- Provide a means of accountability for Governments and are a prominent part of national strategies e.g. Health of the Nation, NHS Plan, National Service Frameworks.

- Can be used to share learning and practice and can lead to improvements even when target not met.

Cons
- Focus clinicians and organisations on the 'measurable' and the masking of clinical priorities, e.g. waiting lists and the prioritisation of those waiting longest over those with urgent clinical need.
- Conversely aspects of care which are important but difficult to measure may not appear as targets, e.g. in UK sexual health is an example.
- A target may oversimplify and mask complexity making valid comparisons difficult, e.g. debate over use of postoperative mortality statistics that ignore case mix monitoring targets can be costly, e.g. new GP contract, hospital targets require staff, computerised systems, data entry costs etc.
- Targets may create undesirable effects or be subject to gaming by those responsible for delivering the target.

Q8
(a) Outline answer
- Urbanisation: less physical activity/over-crowding → CVD, diabetes; road injuries
- Migration: internal →lone men - risky sexual behaviour, alcohol
- Trade policies: dumping of palm oil → cholesterol increases; tobacco markets moving to LMICs
- Connectivity: pandemics of infectious diseases
- Global ecosystem: direct health impacts → climate change: flooding, drought, heatwaves
- Indirect health impacts→ loss of work, social drift, conflict; eco-system mediated→ food scarcity, infections increase (e.g. malaria)
(b) Outline answer
- MDGs were established in 2000 at a United Nations Millennium Summit. They comprise: Eradicate extreme poverty and hunger; Achieve universal primary education; Promote gender equality and empower women; Reduce child mortality rate; Improve maternal health; Combat HIV/AIDS, malaria,

and other diseases; Ensure environmental sustainability; Develop a global partnership for development.

- The MDGs have operated globally and have provided a new forum for international organisations and country development programmes to work together towards a common purpose.
- Indicators of progress: infant mortality, maternal mortality; money going into programmes; countries setting up monitoring systems; greater focus on MCH, education and poverty alleviation in international agencies and aid programmes.
- Improved health outcomes: The MDGs have had variable success with some countries improving maternal and child health. Setting the goals does not equate to changing the political system.
- Advantages: focus; attracts funds, encourages transparency, promotes greater equity, works around political differences, brings new thinking.
- Disadvantages: problems not subject of MDGs are neglected (e.g. NCDs, ageing), monitoring is difficult and health systems not equipped to do it, failing to meet goals is discouraging.

Q9

(a)
- Primary prevention aims to reduce the incidence of disease by controlling the risk factors for morbidity and mortality, e.g. immunisation.
- Secondary prevention aims to reduce the prevalence of disease by shortening its duration through early identification and prompt intervention, e.g. cancer screening.
- Tertiary prevention aims to reduce the progress and severity of established disease, e.g. stroke rehabilitation.

(b) The high risk approach targets intervention at those at significant individual risk of disease and is most successful when the largest burden of disease is borne in specific segments of the population, for example tuberculosis in migrant, homeless, and substance-dependent groups in the UK.
- Strengths – strong patient and clinical motivation and a high benefit to risk ratio on an individual level.
- Weaknesses – resources required to identify and contact members of high risk groups.

The population approach intervenes across the whole of society and is most effective when risk is spread widely, for example in high blood pressure or excess sodium intake.
- Strengths – reduces incidence in both high risk and low risk segments of the population and is highly efficient as it does not require targeting.
- Weaknesses – the prevention paradox: most individuals will not directly benefit from intervention.

(c) At an individual level, by encouraging and enabling healthy living and self-care behaviours for patients, staff and themselves

Brief interventions for smoking cessation and alcohol misuse, for example, and clinical skills such as motivational interviewing to support patient behavioural change are important parts of best clinical practice.

At a service level, by leading the development of quality healthcare that promotes the health of staff and patients.

At a community level, by advocating for interventions that address the determinants of health.

Index

614.4 BEN(B)   30/5/13

Epidemiology, Evidence-based Medicine and Public Health

Lecture Notes

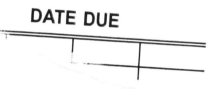
£23.99.

This new edition is also available as an e-book.
For more details, please see
www.wiley.com/buy/9781444334784
or scan this QR code: